Stent-Grafts

Current Clinical Practice

Stent-Grafts

Current Clinical Practice

Edited by

Bart L. Dolmatch, M.D.
Section Head
Vascular and Interventional Radiology
The Cleveland Clinic Foundation
Cleveland, Ohio

Ulrich Blum, M.D.
Professor
Department of Radiology
University Hospital Zurich
Zurich, Switzerland

2000

Thieme

New York • Stuttgart

Thieme New York
333 Seventh Avenue
New York, NY 10001

Stent-Grafts
Bart L. Dolmatch, M.D.
Ulrich Blum, M.D.

Executive Editor: Jane Pennington, Ph.D.
Editorial Director: Avé McCracken
Editorial Assistant: Todd Warnock
Director, Production & Manufacturing: Anne Vinnicombe
Senior Production Editor: Eric L. Gladstone
Marketing Director: Phyllis Gold
Sales Manager: Ross Lumpkin
Chief Financial Officer: Seth S. Fishman
President: Brian D. Scanlan
Compositor: Compset
Printer: Maple-Vail

Library of Congress Cataloging-in-Publication Data

Stent-grafts / [edited by] Bart L. Dolmatch, Ulrich Blum.
    p.;cm.
    Includes index.
    ISBN 0-86577-893-0 (TNY)–ISBN
    1. Stents (Surgery) 2. Blood vessel prosthesis. I. Dolmatch, Bart L. II. Blum, Ulrich,
M.D.
    [DNLM: 1. Vascular Diseases–surgery. 2. Blood Vessel Prosthesis Implantation. 3.
Blood Vessel Prosthesis. 4. Stents. WG 170 S826 2000]
RD598.55. S74 2000
617.4'13059–dc21

                                                        99-044547

Important note: Medical knowledge is ever-changing. As new research and clinical experience broaden our knowledge, changes in treatment and drug therapy may be required. The authors and editors of the material herein have consulted sources believed to be reliable in their efforts to provide information that is complete and in accord with the standards accepted at the time of publication. However, in view of the possibility of human error by the authors, editors, or publisher of the work herein, or changes in medical knowledge, neither the authors, editors, publisher, nor any other party who has been involved in the preparation of this work, warrants that the information contained herein is in every respect accurate or complete, and they are not responsible for any errors or omissions or for the results obtained from use of such information. Readers are encouraged to confirm the information contained herein with other sources. For example, readers are advised to check the product information sheet included in the package of each drug they plan to administer to be certain that the information contained in this publication is accurate and that changes have not been made in the recommended dose or in the contraindications for administration. This recommendation is of particular importance in connection with new or infrequently used drugs.

Some of the product names, patents, and registered designs referred to in this book are in fact registered trademarks or proprietary names even though specific reference to this fact is not always made in the text. Therefore, the appearance of a name without designation as proprietary is not to be construed as a representation by the publisher that it is in the public domain.

Printed in the United States of America
5 4 3 2
TNY ISBN 0–86577–893–0
GTV ISBN 3–13–124061-X

For Kimberly Elaine Dolmatch, who has shown an ever-expanding capacity to endure the many endeavors which take me late into the night.

BD

Contents

Foreword

When asked to write the foreword for a new text, I usually take a quick look at the chapter titles, take into account the authors, and proceed to write my comments. However, for *Stent-Grafts: Current Clinical Practice*, I found the text so interesting and well written that I literally read the whole book before proceeding to write this Foreword.

A great proportion of this book is dedicated to stent-grafts. From a historical perspective, it is interesting to note that endograft development is not the result of blending stent or graft technologies. In 1975 the first prototype for a stent was called a "cage"[1] and the metal component of the original cage was designed to replace surgical suture. Subsequent concepts led to the use of tubular graft materials self-supported with stents, and the contemporary "stent-graft" concept was born. The use of stent-grafts today is just beginning to revolutionize the treatment of a number of disorders such as aortic aneurysms and peripheral atherosclerotic occlusive disease.

Because there are few places to look for a comprehensive discussion of stent-grafts, this book is a welcome addition to the field of endovascular therapies. Furthermore, it consistently provides a scholarly approach towards clinical problem solving. It is designed to provide an overview of the clinical challenges, a discussion of currently accepted therapies, and the role of stent-grafts in clinical care. For these reasons, I believe that this book will be a real asset for both beginners and accomplished interventionalists alike.

Juan Carlos Parodi, M.D.

1. Parodi JC. Endoluminal treatment of arterial diseases using a stent-graft combination: Reflections 200 years after the initial concept. J Endovasc Surg 1997; 4(1):3–4.

Preface

Change is inherent to any new emerging technologies, such as endoluminal grafting techniques. Since Dotter and colleagues first proposed the use of endoprostheses in the late 1960s, Balko and colleagues performed the repair of artificially induced aneurysms with polyurethane prostheses in animals in 1986, and Parodi and colleagues treated abdominal aortic aneurysms successfully by inserting an endovascular graft retrogradely through an open femoral artery into the abdominal aorta in 1991, endografting has become a technique of increasing interest for vascular surgeons, interventional radiologists, and cardiologists.

Stent-Grafts: Current Clinical Practice provides a state-of-the-art overview of endovascular treatment focusing on the latest technology, grafting techniques, clinical applications, and results available to-date, as well as indications. For this purpose, we brought together a well-balanced composition of experienced authors of various disciplines involved in this exciting new operative field.

The development of stents and stent-grafts is rapidly changing and improving. Although there is need for long-term proof of safety and efficacy of endoluminal techniques before their widespread use may be recommended, we are deeply convinced that the future holds promise, because such techniques offer potential economical advantages and—even more important—improved patient care.

Bart L. Dolmatch, M.D.
Ulrich Blum, M.D.

Acknowledgments

We would like to thank Antoinette Schumacher and Reba Gaddis for their administrative assistance in putting this book together. Their hard work typing, retyping, and re-retyping and their assistance to correspond with domestic and international authors has been greatly appreciated. We would also like to thank S. Wildermuth, M.D., for creating the cover figures.

Contributors

Robert T. Andrews, M.D.
Dotter Interventional Institute
Oregon Health Sciences University
Portland, Oregon

James F. Benenati, M.D.
Medical Director, Peripheral Vascular Laboratory
Interventional Radiologist
The Miami Cardiac and Vascular Institute
Baptist Hospital
Miami, Florida

Bernard M. Beyssen, M.D.
Cardiovascular Radiology Department
Broussais Hospital
University Paris VI
Paris, France

Ulrich Blum, M.D.
Professor
Department of Radiology
University Hospital Zurich
Zurich, Switzerland

Lucas H. Brennecke, D.V.M., D.A.C.V.P.
Vice President
Pathology Associates, Inc.
Fredrick, Maryland

Abbas Chamsuddin, M.D.
Fellow, Division of Cardiovascular/
 Interventional Radiology
University of Minnesota
Minneapolis, Minnesota
Assistant Professor of Radiology
Division of Cardiovascular/
 Interventional Radiology

University of Tennessee
Memphis, Tennessee

Andrew H. Cragg, M.D.
Suburban Radiologic Consultants
Fairview University Medical Center
Minneapolis, Minnesota

Michael D. Dake, M.D.
Associate Professor of Radiology and Medicine
Chief, Cardiovascular Interventional Radiology
Stanford University Medical Center
Stanford, California

Asok Dasgupta, M.B.B.S., M.R.C.P.
Staff Physician
Department of Pulmonary and Critical
 Care Medicine
Kelsey-Seybold Clinic
St. Luke's Episcopal Hospital
Houston, Texas

Mark M. Davidian, M.D.
Fellow
The Miami Cardiac and Vascular Institute
Baptist Hospital
Miami, Florida

Michael DeGroot, M.D.
Resident
Interventional Radiology
Stanford University Medical Center
Stanford, California

Bart L. Dolmatch, M.D.
Section Head
Vascular and Interventional Radiology

The Cleveland Clinic Foundation
Cleveland, Ohio

Yong Hua Dong, M.D.
Principal Research Scientist
Vascular and Interventional Radiology
The Cleveland Clinic Foundation
Cleveland, Ohio

Jean-Claude Gaux, M.D.
Cardiovascular Radiology Department
Broussais Hospital
University Paris VI
Paris, France

Frederick S. Keller, M.D.
Dotter Interventional Institute
Oregon Health Sciences University
Portland, Oregon

Robert Leonardo, M.D.
Clinical Instructor
Department of Radiology
New York Medical College
Valhalla, New York

Michael L. Marin, M.D.
Department of Surgery
Mount Sinai Medical Center
New York, New York

Claudie S. McArthur, M.D.
Department of Surgery
Mount Sinai Medical Center
New York, New York

Atul C. Mehta, M.B.B.S.
Professor of Medicine
Department of Pulmonary and Critical Care Medicine
The Cleveland Clinic Foundation
Cleveland, Ohio

Julio C. Palmaz, M.D.
Professor of Radiology
Section of Cardiovascular and Interventional Radiology
Department of Radiology
University of Texas Health Science Center at San Antonio
San Antonio, Texas

Juan Carlos Parodi, M.D.
Vice Director
Post-Graduate Training Program in Cardiovascular Surgery
University of Buenos Aires
Buenos Aires, Argentina
Professor of Surgery
Wayne State University

Harper Hospital
School of Medicine
Detroit, Michigan

Alex Powell, M.D.
Interventional Radiologist
The Miami Cardiac and Vascular Institute
Baptist Hospital
Miami, Florida

Alain C. Raynaud, M.D.
Cardiovascular Radiology Department
Broussais Hospital
University Paris VI
Paris, France

Mahmood K. Razavi, M.D.
Assistant Professor
Vascular and Interventional Radiology
Stanford University Medical Center
Stanford, California

Josef Rosch, M.D.
Dotter Interventional Institute
Oregon Health Sciences University
Portland, Oregon

Michael S. Rosenberg, M.D.
Assistant Professor
Department of Radiology
Cardiovascular Interventional Section
Fairview University Medical Center
Minneapolis, Minnesota

Grigory N. Rozenblit, M.D.
Associate Professor of Clinical Radiology
Departments of Radiology and Surgery
New York Medical College
Valhalla, New York

John H. Rundback, M.D.
Assistant Professor of Radiology and Surgery
Department of Vascular and Interventional Radiology
New York Medical College
Valhalla, New York

Marc R. Sapoval, M.D., Ph.D.
Professor of Medicine
Cardiovascular Radiology Department
Broussais Hospital
University Paris VI
Paris, France

Richard R. Saxon, M.D.
North County Radiology Medical Group
Diagnostic Imaging and Interventional Radiology

Tri-City Medical Center
Oceanside, California

Peter K. Schoenwald, M.D.
Staff Anesthesiologist
Head, Section of Vascular Anesthesia
Department of General Anesthesiology
The Cleveland Clinic Foundation
Cleveland, Ohio

Robert S. Schwartz, M.D.
Professor of Medicine
Division of Cardiovascular and Internal Medicine
Mayo Foundation
Rochester, Minnesota

Charles P. Semba, M.D.
Associate Professor of Radiology
Department of Cardiovascular-Interventional Radiology
Stanford University Medical Center
Stanford, California

Juraj Sprung, M.D., Ph.D.
Staff Anesthesiologist

Department of General Anesthesiology
The Cleveland Clinic Foundation
Cleveland, Ohio

Daniel Y. Sze, M.D.
Assistant Professor
Vascular and Interventional Radiology
Stanford University Medical Center
Stanford, California

Luc Turmel-Rodrigues, M.D.
Cardiovascular Radiology Department
Broussais Hospital
University Paris VI
Paris, France

Patrick L. Wyffels, M.D., F.A.C.S.
Saint Francis Medical Center
Peoria, Illinois

Gregory Zuccaro, Jr., M.D.
Department of Gastroenterology
The Cleveland Clinic Foundation
Cleveland, Ohio

1

Peripheral Vascular Stents

JOHN H. RUNDBACK, ROBERT LEONARDO, AND GRIGORY N. ROZENBLIT

> Once a pathway has been created across the occluded segment, repeated dilatation or the temporary use of a Silastic endovascular (or, in some cases, paravascular) splint could maintain an adequate false lumen until the natural processes of fibrosis and reintimalization had taken place.
>
> Dotter CT and Judkins MP, *Circulation*[1]

Since this first visionary description,[1] and early reports by Dotter of endoluminal coil spring stent implantation in canine[2] and human[3] arteries, there has been a remarkable evolution in the development and clinical utilization of intravascular prostheses. Stents have revolutionized endovascular practice not only by reducing angioplasty failures and expanding treatment thresholds, but also by allowing intervention[4,5] in new vascular territories such as carotid arteries. Considerable information regarding the biology of stent healing has spurred new approaches and device modifications to help maintain vessel patency. Perhaps most importantly, the widespread clinical acceptance and efficacy of stents as well as industry support have paved the way for a new evolution of vascular endoprostheses: stent-grafts.

■ The Rationale for Stenting

Percutaneous transluminal angioplasty (PTA) has become an established treatment option for patients with vascular obstructions. However, PTA has several limitations. It is less successful in eccentric and calcified vessels,[6] presumably due to an inability to cause either plaque fracture or local intimal-medial dehiscence.

While focal lesions usually respond well, PTA of long segment obstructions has higher rates of thromboembolic complications and restenosis.[7] Hemodynamic failures after PTA are not uncommon, and often occur owing to flow limiting dissection or elastic recoil. Even when technically optimal results are achieved, PTA continues to be plagued by early and late restenosis caused by fibrocellular proliferation at the site of balloon-induced vessel injury.[8]

The rationale for endoprostheses is the theoretical advantage of providing an internal scaffold to the vessel wall, thus eliminating or preventing post-PTA luminal compromise due to elastic recoil, dissection, or geometric remodeling.[9,10] In addition, the smoother luminal surface and increased internal vessel diameter after stenting may result in a more normal pattern of laminar flow and thus incite less of a cellular response and correspondingly lower rates of restenosis than seen after PTA alone.[11,12]

■ Stent Characteristics

The ideal vascular stent should have certain features.[13] It must be easily delivered via a small profile introducer, yet have an adequate expansion ratio to accommodate large target vessel diameters. The stent should be radiopaque to assure adequate visualization, and the implanted stent length and position should be easily recognizable prior to final deployment. Longitudinal flexibility is critical to accommodate tortuous and flexible anatomic sites. There must be sufficient radial strength to prevent elastic recoil and to oppose dissection flaps and calcified plaques. Secure anchoring after placement is critical to prevent migration. In the long-term, the stent must be biocompatible, maintain its structural integrity, be nonthrombogenic, and promote the development of a mature and functional endothelialized neointima to limit restenosis. Finally, technical and clinical results of stent use must outperform PTA alone.

Although numerous vascular stents are commercially available or investigational worldwide, none fulfill all of the criteria of the ideal device. Due to the rapid introduction of new stents, any attempt to describe all of the devices under development would be futile. However, all existing stents can be broadly characterized into two major categories: balloon-expandable and self-expandable. The mechanical characteristics of devices that have undergone a reasonable degree of clinical testing are listed in Table 1–1.

Balloon-Expandable Stents

The most widely used balloon-expandable stent and first to receive Food and Drug Administration (FDA) approval in the United States is the Palmaz stent (Cordis Corp., Johnson and Johnson Interventional Systems, Warren, NJ). It consists of a slotted, seamless, stainless steel tube measuring up to 78 mm in length, 3.1 mm in constrained diameter, and expandable to diameters ranging from 8 to 12 mm. The stent is either premounted or can be hand crimped on a balloon. The stent is delivered on the balloon and is deployed by the balloon inflation. The Palmaz stent has several advantages. Excellent radial strength prevents elastic recoil, especially in calcified vessels.[14] There is only minimal foreshortening, allowing for accurate placement. The major disadvantage of the Palmaz stent is its relative longitudinal inflexibility, thereby limiting placement through tortuous pathways. Finally, the stent cannot be used in vessels subject to extrinsic compression, which may cause permanent stent deformation.[15–17]

The Strecker stent (Boston Scientific Vascular, Watertown, MA) is premounted on an angioplasty balloon, and silicon retaining sleeves at each of the stent retract during balloon expansion. It is made of woven tantalum wire, is extremely radiopaque, and has increased flexibility when compared to the Palmaz stent. Another recently introduced balloon-expandable prosthesis is the Perflex stent (Cordis Corp., Johnson & Johnson Interventional Systems, Warren, NJ). This is composed of stainless steel in a sinusoidal wave configuration with soldered articulations. Although there is only minimal clinical experience, early data suggest that this stent provides excellent hoop strength and improved longitudinal flexibility when compared with the Palmaz stent. There is no FDA approval for vascular applications of the Strecker and Perflex stents and their use is restricted to off-label use in the United States.

Self-Expandable Stents

Self-expandable stents are made of either steel alloys or nitinol and are resistant to radial deformity. The Wallstent (Boston Scientific Vascular, Watertown, MA) is a woven steel mesh that is mounted on a 7-French (Fr) delivery system. This stent has FDA approval for iliac use. Approved stents are available in a wide assortment of lengths (24 to 69 mm) and range from 6 to 10 mm in nonconstrained width. Larger-diameter biliary stents are available for off-label use. Placement is accomplished by retraction of a thin outer sleeve that covers the stent, with resulting deployment occurring from the distal end toward the catheter hub. The stent can be reconstrained and repositioned after release of up to 80% of its length; positioning can also be facilitated by withdrawal of the delivery system after partial stent deployment. The Wallstent has the advantage of being relatively easy to use and having a large expansion ratio. Crossing points of the wire braid are nonsoldered, resulting in excellent longitudinal flexibility. Postinsertion balloon dilatation is often performed to achieve maximal expansion and assure complete apposi-

TABLE 1–1. Relative Characteristics of Vascular Stents

Stent	Expansion Ration	Longitudinal Flexibility	Hoop Strength	Foreshortening
Balloon-expandable				
Palmaz	++	−	++++	+
Strecker	++	+	++++	+
Perflex	++	++	++++	+
Self-expandable				
Wallstent	+++	+++	++	+++
Z-stent	+++	+	+++	++
Nitinol	++++	+++	+++	+

An increasing number of "+" signs denotes a more favorable presence of the stent characteristic.

tion with the vessel wall. The major disadvantage of the Wallstent is unpredictable foreshortening following deployment, particularly at the trailing end, which makes exact placement of the Wallstent somewhat more difficult than with balloon-expandable endoprostheses. Another disadvantage of the Wallstent is the possible obstruction of stent-spanned side branches.[18–20]

The Gianturco Z-stent (Cook, Inc., Bloomington, IN) is not yet approved for vascular use. This stent is composed of stainless steel wire bent into a zigzag pattern connected at the ends to form a cylinder. Barbs are available to provide anchoring to the vascular wall. The Gianturco stent has a maximum diameter of 35 mm and is therefore well suited for larger vessels. The stent is spring loaded into a delivery sheath and deployed by retraction of the sheath while the stent is held in place by a pusher catheter. The Gianturco stent has less longitudinal flexibility than the Wallstent, although there is higher hoop strength and only mild foreshortening upon insertion.

The Memotherm (Bard, Covington, GA) and Symphony (Boston Scientific Vascular, Watertown, MA) stents consist of cross-hatched nickel-titanium alloy strands with thermal memory properties. These have limited longitudinal flexibility, although somewhat better in Memotherm. More recently introduced, the S.M.A.R.T. stent (Cordis, Inc.) provides improved longitudinal flexibility. In comparison to steel endoprostheses, nitinol stents have better hoop strength but cannot exceed the nominal diameter even when "overdilated." These stents do not foreshorten with deployment, although exact positioning can be difficult due to poor radiopacity and "jumping" of the delivery system resulting from friction between the outer catheter and the vessel wall. Stents are available in various lengths with expanded diameters up to 10 mm. None of these devices has yet received FDA approval.

■ Biological Response to Vascular Stents

The healing response to vascular stent placement is complex but essentially uniform with all devices.[21] Similar to PTA, medial injury results in smooth muscle cell (SMC) proliferation, SMC migration, intimal proliferation with production of an extracellular matrix (neointima), and reendothelialization.[22,23] These processes are mediated by the SMC release of basic fibroblast growth factor and transforming growth factor beta, as well as by the in situ production of platelet-derived growth factor, insulin growth factor-I, and thrombin. SMC proliferation is responsible for neointimal thickening, which if abundant may cause restenosis.[24] Platelet and fibrin deposition on the stent material and adjacent denuded luminal surface serves as a critical determinant of subsequent reendothelialization, with endothelial ingrowth occurring from intact endothelium at the stent margin as well as from residual nondenuded patches within the stent or through the graft lining.[25] The early development of a mature confluent endothelial monolayer inhibits excessive intimal SMC proliferation that may result in restenosis.[26,27]

The gross and histopathological findings after arterial stent placement have been well described.[24,28–33] In a landmark study by Schatz,[29] in which balloon-expandable stents were implanted in the coronary arteries of dogs, thrombus and fibrin covering of the luminal surface was noted 1 week after placement. At 3 and 8 weeks poststenting, SMC infiltration and progressive neointimal thickening was noted (Fig. 1–1). Thinning of the media was noted to begin immediately after stent placement, with continued medial atrophy seen for up to 32 weeks. More recently, Yee et al[33] provided an excellent overview of the healing process in 20 stented porcine iliac arteries.

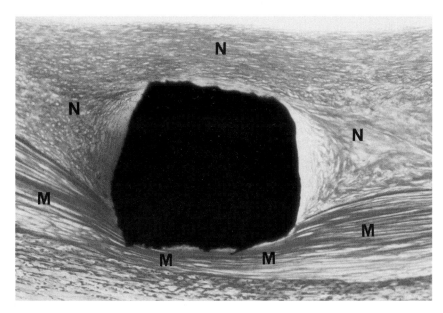

FIGURE 1–1. Neointimal formation in a canine iliac artery after stenting. Masson's trichrome stain, 10×. Tissue adjacent to and atop the stent is neointima (N). The media (M) has been compressed by the stent. (Courtesy of Dr. Bart Dolmatch.)

Swine were sacrificed at 1 week, 5 weeks, and 12 weeks, and stents were explanted for gross and microscopic evaluation. At 1 week, a patchy neointima was noted, with endothelial lining of stent struts but not the luminal surface. Examination at 5 weeks demonstrated a thin translucent neointima and luminal endothelial mono-layer (Fig. 1–2); the endothelial cells surrounding the stent tines was largely replaced by SMC. By 12 weeks, there was coverage of the stents by a thickened, more homogeneous neointima. While Yee et al observed no significant leukocyte infiltration, others have found an inflammatory reaction to be a potent mediator of neointimal hyperplasia.[34]

Although the significance of these findings is uncertain, several conclusions can be drawn. Early endothelialization is the primary determinant of improved early and late patency. While stents reduce the impact of elastic recoil and spasm on lumen loss, neointimal SMC proliferation is not substantially inhibited. An inflammatory (foreign body) reaction to the stent may contribute to restenosis. Finally, biological modifiers of the SMC response to vessel injury should further enhance the efficacy of endovascular stents.

■ Peripheral Vascular of Stent Implantation—Technical Considerations

Many of the principles underlying vascular stent insertion are similar to those guiding PTA.[8] The target lesion is imaged in the usual fashion and crossed using standard catheter-guidewire technique. Prior to stenting, a vascular sheath is inserted at the access site to allow nontraumatic insertion of the stent and delivery system. Procedures are generally performed over a stiff exchange wire to ease lesion crossing and prevent buckling of the delivery catheter. Pharmacological adjuncts including heparin and nitroglycerin are used to prevent procedure-related thrombosis and spasm. Postprocedural anticoagulation is not routinely utilized, but may be valuable in cases where marked luminal irregularity or stagnant flow is seen after intervention.[35] While poststenting anticoagulation has been shown in experimental studies to reduce acute thrombosis[36] and potentially limit intimal hyperplasia,[30] these findings have not been corroborated in clinical trials.[37,38] Aspirin is frequently prescribed beginning the day of the procedure and continued for at least several months, although it has not been clearly shown in either angioplasty[39] or stent[40] series to reduce the incidence of restenosis.

Stent implantation is also associated with a set of considerations not normally encountered with conventional PTA alone. Unlike PTA, stenting across a potential anas-

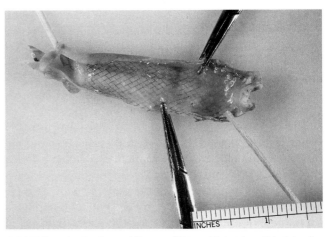

FIGURE 1–2. Explanted iliac wallstent. There is a thin translucent neointima covering the stent surface. The neointima is thickest at the stent margins.

tomotic site may interfere with subsequent surgical revascularization. Should surgery be necessary to salvage a stent failure, vascular control will require cross-clamping of the vessel above the stent margins, necessitating more extensive surgical dissection. Hence, an attempt should be made to use the shortest possible stent to match the lesion being treated.

Positioning the stent in the lesion is much more critical than with PTA alone. It is essential that the target vessel be imaged in the proper projection so that the lesion is seen exactly in profile, especially for ostial stenoses of the visceral vessels. The major technical failure is malpositioning of the stent, a problem that is especially difficult to avoid with the Wallstent.[41,42] The goal is to place the stent so that it covers the lesion and extends 1 to 2 mm past it on both sides; for ostial lesions within vessels arising from the aorta, the proximal end should extend 1 to 2 mm into the aorta to ensure that the ostium is covered. When inserting a Wallstent, many operators begin deployment with the leading end of the stent positioned 1 to 2 cm beyond the target site. After partial deployment, the stent and delivery catheter can then be pulled back into a more optimal position. Consideration must be made of further stent shortening that will occur with postdeployment balloon dilatation. Nitinol stents can also be difficult to accurately position due to a tendency of the delivery system to "jump forward" during retraction of the outer sheath. This tendency can be avoided by maintaining gentle traction on the delivery catheter to assure that the trailing (hub end) marker does not move during stent deployment.

It is important to select the proper stent to match target site anatomy. To assure adequate fixation of a self-expandable device, most clinicians use a stent with a non-constrained diameter 10 to 15% greater than the target vessel width. Tortuous or tapered vessels require the use of a prosthesis with greater longitudinal flexibility (i.e., Wallstent), as do crossover procedures performed from a contralateral access site. Since multiple overlapping stents are associated with an increased occurrence of restenosis,[43,44] an attempt should be made to use a single stent of sufficient length to fully cover the lesion.

Self-expandable stents usually continue to open toward their nominal diameter during the first several days after implantation (Fig. 1–3). Nonetheless, most operators advocate immediate postinsertion balloon dilatation to assure that all stent struts fully appose the vessel wall. Recent studies using intravascular ultrasound (IVUS) have shown that incomplete stent expansion appears to be a predictor of restenosis,[45] and IVUS appears to be superior to angiography in identifying incompletely expanded stents.[46–49] IVUS is also more accurate than angiography for determining true pretreatment target vessel diameter so that stent and balloon sizing is optimized.[50] An advantage for IVUS in evaluating in-stent restenosis has not been clearly established.[51,52]

■ Site-Specific Results of Peripheral Vascular Stenting

Aorta

Since 1980, PTA has been used with success for the management of focal aortic stenoses.[53] Stents have been described as a primary treatment option or following unsuccessful or suboptimal angioplasty[54–56] (Fig. 1–3). Sheeran and colleagues[57] treated 10 cases of mid-abdominal aortic stenosis with Palmaz stents. Seven of these 10 lesions were treated primarily by stenting and three were stented after suboptimal angioplasty. Technical success was 100%, with clinical success seen in eight of nine patients studied for a

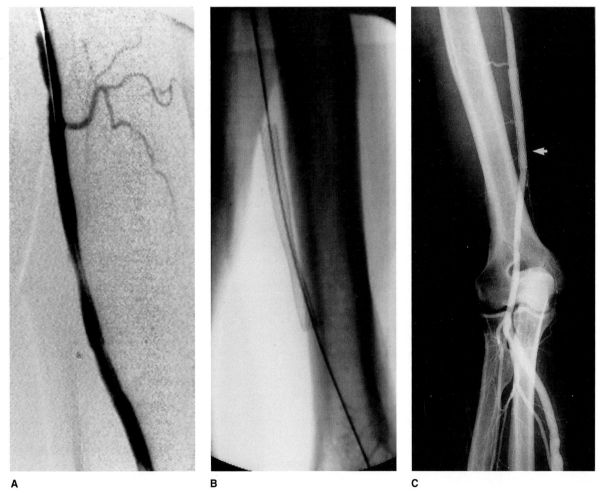

A   B   C

FIGURE 1–3. (A). Brachial artery Wallstent after percutaneous transluminal angioplasty (PTA) dissection in a patient with a forearm dialysis graft. There is persistent narrowing of the distal third of the stent. (B). The stent is incompletely expanded near the distal end. (C). Angiogram obtained 2 weeks later during graft revision shows that the stent is now fully expanded (arrow).

mean 1.6 years. Martinez et al[58] placed Palmaz stents in 24 patients with aortic stenoses ($n = 18$) or occlusions after unsatisfactory PTA, with a 5-year cumulative life-table primary patency of 100%. Likewise, Long and colleagues[59] managed seven patients with a combination of Wallstents and Palmaz stents, and found maintained stent patency in all cases at 2-year follow-up. However, despite this experience, stents have not clearly improved upon the results achievable with aortic PTA alone. In a comparison of aortic PTA with stent placement, Westcott and Bonn[60] found no differences in the percent stenosis reduction, decrease in transstenotic gradient, or initial clinical outcome. They concluded that aortic stent placement should be reserved for failed or suboptimal PTA results.

Iliac Arteries

PTA provides excellent initial results and durable benefit for focal iliac artery lesions, with reported 5-year patency rates up to 84%.[61] However, both technical and clinical results are lower when treating long-segment or nonconcentric lesions.[8] PTA is also hampered by a 40% incidence of technical failure due to elastic recoil or flow-limiting dissection.

Rousseau et al[62] first reported experimental iliac artery stenting in 1987, and Palmaz et al[63] described the technique of balloon-expandable iliac artery stent placement in humans in 1988. Since that early experience, both balloon-expandable and self-expanding stents have become widely utilized for the treatment of iliac disease (Fig. 1–4). Stent placement can be performed with high rates of technical success and limited complications. Initial technical success is achieved in 91 to 97% of stenotic lesions[18,64] and 71 to 98% of occlusions,[65,66] although treatment of occlusions is associated with lower rates of recanalization in most reports.[65,67,68] All stent types perform more or less equally. In a review of 18 series comprising 1,948 patients, Murphy[69] found major complications (defined as those requiring additional therapy or a change in treatment plan) in 6%. The most common events were distal embolization, arterial rupture, and puncture-site complications, many of which were amenable to further percutaneous treatment. Combined procedure-related and 30-day mortality occurred in 1.8% of cases. Stenting of occlusions has higher complication rates, particularly due to distal thromboembolism.[68,70] Early stent thrombosis is observed in approximately 5%[18,43,71] and is associated with the use of multiple stents[43] and the treatment of external iliac artery lesions, long-segment stenoses, occlusions, and extremities with poor femoral runoff.[71]

The overall experience with iliac stenting has resulted in very favorable rates of clinical success. In an analysis of 10 contemporary reports encompassing the treat-

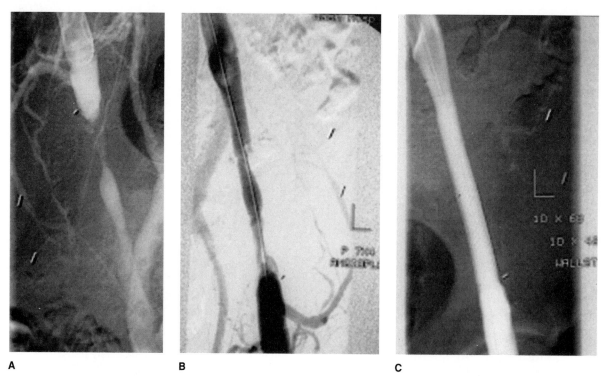

A   **B**   **C**

FIGURE 1–4. (**A**). Arteriogram shows a high-grade stenosis of the external iliac artery. (**B**). After PTA a flow-limiting dissection is evident. (**C**). There is wide patency after insertion of two overlapping Wallstents.

TABLE 1–2. Results of Iliac Artery Stents

First Author (Year)	Ref.	No. of Patients/ Limbs	Stent	Major Complications	Primary Patency First Year	Primary Patency Subsequently	Secondary Patency
Palmaz (1992)	32	486/567	Palmaz	10%	91%	84% 2 yr 69% 43 mo	
Cikrit (1995)	72	34/38	Palmaz	18%	87%	74% 3 yr 63% 5 yr	86% 5 yr
Henry (1995)	43	184/230	Palmaz	1%	94%	86% 4 yr	94% 4 yr
Martin (1995)	44	140/163	Wall	4%	81%	71% 2 yr	86% 2 yr
Long (1995)	73	61/64	Strecker	8%	84%	69% 2 yr	81% 2 yr
Sapoval (1996)	18	95/101	Wall	9%	80%	61% 4 yr	86% 4 yr
Strecker (1996)	71	289/289	Strecker	17%		85% 3 yr 70% 5 yr	
Vorwerk (1996)	55	109/118	Wall	3%	95%	82% 4 yr	91% 4 yr
Murphy (1996)	64	66/94	Wall	7%	78%	53% 3 yr	82% 2 yr
Sullivan (1997)	14	288/424	Palmaz/Wall	14%	84%	76% 2 yr	
Totals		**1,752/2,088**		**10%**	**87%**	**79% 2 yr 77% 3 yr 72% 4–5 yr**	**87% 2–5 yr**

ment of 2,088 limbs (Table 1–2)[14,18,32,43,44,55,64,71–73] primary patency rates at 1 year, 2 years, 3 years, and 4 to 5 years were 87%, 79%, 77%, and 72%, respectively. Although clinical deterioration due to in-stent restenosis or occlusion can be expected to occur in nearly one-fourth of patients at late follow-up, treatment with repeated PTA or other angiography techniques allows excellent long-term secondary patency in the majority of patients.[74,75] However, higher rates of restenosis are seen after redilatation than after the initial treatment.[74,76]

Although it is clear that selective iliac stenting is valuable as rescue technique after failed PTA, the role of primary stenting remains controversial. In a meta-analysis comparing iliac PTA and stent placement, Bosch and Hunink[77] concluded that stenting was superior to PTA alone owing to a reduced risk of long-term failure. However, much of their angioplasty data is derived from historical series prior to the widespread use of stents, and the impact of hemodynamically suboptimal PTA results on long-term outcomes is not clear. Other information suggests that long-term patency rates following primary stenting of focal iliac disease are equivalent to the results of angioplasty alone.[43,55] In the FDA-mandated U.S. multicenter iliac Wallstent trial, 2-year primary patency rates were 71%[44]—less than the calculated 81% 2-year patency following iliac PTA in a pooled series of 2,697 treated limbs reported by Becker et al[8]! More recently, the Dutch iliac stent trial[78,79] prospectively randomized 279 patients with intermittent claudication to either primary stent placement ($n = 143$) or primary angioplasty with selective stenting for a residual post-PTA gradient ≥ 10 mm Hg. Using this criterion, selective stenting was performed in 43% of the angioplasty group. No differences were observed in complications or initial hemodynamic success. Two-year clinical success was 78% in the primary stent group compared with 77% in the selective

stent group. Of note, a strategy of PTA with selective stenting was more cost-effective than primary stenting or PTA alone.[80]

Despite increased technical difficulty,[64,71,81] primary stenting can perhaps be advocated for complex long-segment stenoses and occlusions. For these lesions, primary stenting appears to provide higher clinical success and lower complication rates than angioplasty alone. Murphy et al[64] found a 78% cumulative 1-year patency rate after stenting of occlusions and long stenoses, which compares favorably with the 23% 6-month patency reported by Murray et al[6] for PTA of similar lesions. Overall, primary 1-year and 4-year clinical patency rates following primary stenting of iliac occlusions average approximately 83% and 75%, respectively.[43,44,64,71,82–85] (Table 1–3). Restenoses are generally easier to treat than the initial occlusion, and 4-year secondary patency rates as high as 88% have been noted.

Femoropopliteal Arteries

Similar to the experience with iliac stents, there is considerable variation in reported outcomes following the placement of stents in the femoropopliteal distribution (Table 1–4).[20,38,43,44,86–91] The preponderance of data suggests that stent use in the femoral and popliteal area should be limited to angioplasty failures and patients who present an unacceptably high risk for surgical revascularization (Fig. 1–5). A cumulative 2-year patency of 76% has been reported using stents as a "bailout" following unsatisfactory PTA in patients with focal femoral disease.[89,90,92] However, for long-segment or occlusive lesions, femoral stents have not proven equally beneficial either as a primary treatment or salvage therapy.[43,91,93] Zollikofer et al[93] treated 13 patients with 15 femoral lesions, 12 of which were long occlusions. At a mean follow-up of 20 months,

TABLE 1–3. Stents for Iliac Occlusions

First Author (Year)	Ref.	No. of Lesions	Stent	Primary Patency Short-Term	Primary Patency Long-Term	Secondary Patency
Henry (1995)	43	17	Palmaz		76% 4 yr	88% 4 yr
Vorwerk (1995)	82	127	Wallstent	87% 1 yr	78% 4 yr	88% 4 yr
Martin (1995)	44	15	Wallstent	84% 9 mo		
Strecker (1996)	71	66	Strecker	78% 1 yr	59% 4 yr	
Murphy (1996)	64	39	Wallstent	67% 1 yr		
Dyet (1997)	83	72	Mostly Wallstent (75/87)		85% 1 yr	83% 4 yr
Reyes (1997)	84	61	Wallstent	73% 2 yr		88% 2 yr
Raza (1998)	85	22	Memotherm	95% 1 yr		

9/11 (82%) patients developed stent stenosis or occlusion. In a series of 58 limbs with a mean lesion length of 13.5 cm, Gray et al[91] demonstrated a primary patency rate of only 22% at 1 year, although poor distal runoff may have contributed to the low patency rates in this study. Martin and colleagues[44] excluded patients with poor distal runoff. In their series of 154 lesions, a 61% and 49% primary patency rate was noted at 1 and 2 years, respectively, with a 2-year secondary patency rate of 72%. When patients were further stratified by lesion type and length, patency was seen in 53% of occlusions versus 66% of stenoses, and in 59% of lesions 10 cm or longer compared with 83% in those shorter than 10 cm. Henry et al[43] also noted poor results when treating occlusions, with a 4-year patency rate of only 39%.

Several other factors appear to contribute to stent failure. Stents placed distally in the superficial femoral artery (SFA) or within the popliteal artery have higher rates of clinical failure than proximal stent placement.[43] This phenomenon is probably due to lower flow rates and reduced lumen area as the vessel size decreases. In fact, Sapoval et al[88] found worse patency to be associated with stents less than 5 mm in diameter, with a similar trend noted by Gray et al[91] for stents postdilated to <6

mm. The impact of long-term anticoagulation to stent thrombosis remains less certain. Rousseau et al[92] noted a 100% cumulative 1-year benefit in nine patients treated for 2 months with oral acenocoumarol, compared with only 70% in patients not receiving the drug. This experience prompted most early investigators to routinely prescribe oral anticoagulation after femoral stenting. However, more recent studies by White et al[38] and Bergeron et al[89] used either aspirin alone or combined with ticlopidine, and these studies reported 1- to 2-year patency rates equivalent to those described in patients treated with long-term anticoagulation.

Renal Arteries

Renal artery stenting was first described by Palmaz et al[94] more than a decade ago. Since that time, stenting has become widely embraced as an efficacious adjunct to maintain arterial patency after ineffective or complicated PTA. Furthermore, stenting of ostial lesions may have a higher initial success rate and improved intermediate-term patency rates compared with PTA alone (Fig. 1–6). Consequently, stent placement is being increasingly used as a primary treatment of ostial lesions.

TABLE 1–4. Results of Femoral Stents

First Author (Year)	Ref.	n	Stent	Primary Patency	Secondary Patency
Rousseau (1989)	20	36	Wall		76% 1–2 yr
Gunther (1989)	86	45	Wall	84% 6 mo	
Do-dai (1992)	87	26	Wall		69% 1 yr
Sapoval (1992)	88	21	Wall	49% 1 yr	67% 1 yr
					56% 18 mo
Henry (1995)	43	126	Palmaz	81% 1 yr, 65% 4 yr (SFA)	95% 4 yr (SFA)
				50% 1 yr, 50% 4 yr (POP)	69% 4 yr (POP)
White (1995)	38	32	Wall	75% 18 mo	89% 18 mo
Bergeron (1995)	89	39	Palmaz	77% 2 yr	89% 2 yr
Martin (1995)	44	90	Wall	61% 1 yr, 49% 2 yr	72% 2 yr
Chatelard (1996)	90	35	Palmaz	80% 1 yr, 70% 2 yr	83% 2 yr
Gray (1998)	91	55	Palmaz and Wall	22% 1 yr	46% 1 yr
Totals		**505**		**63% 1 yr**	**78% 2 yr**
				60% 2 yr	

POP, popliteal artery; SFA, superficial femoral artery.

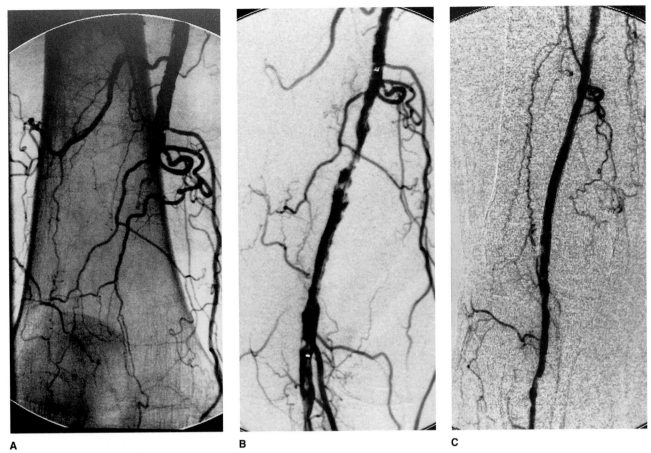

FIGURE 1–5. **(A)**. Angiography demonstrates occlusion of the popliteal artery. There is reconstitution of the vessel just above the knee joint. **(B)**. After thrombolysis and angioplasty a persistent irregular stenosis is noted. **(C)**. Patency is restored using a single stent. The stenoses of the tibioperoneal trunk was subsequently dilated.

Multiple reports of renal artery stent placement have now being published, and the results are summarized in Table 1–5.[37,42,95–110] A cumulative evaluation of nearly 1,000 stented arteries shows a 7% major complication rate and 58% hypertension benefit at roughly 1-year follow-up. Although a neointimal lining of the stent is routinely observed, restenosis of at least 50% of the arterial diameter occurs in 0 to 50% of treated sites at 6 to 30 months. Greater operator experience, maximal stent expansion, and complete stent covering of the lesion correlate with improved patency rates. Differences in reported patency rates are due to variable reporting standards and different imaging methods used for follow-up. In a recent series, Blum et al[106] reported on 74 Palmaz stents placed for ostial disease in 68 patients.[106] The mean clinical follow-up was 27 months (range 3–84 months). Hypertension was cured or improved in 78%, and there was an 11% angiographic restenosis rate. This study is probably an accurate reflection of contemporary results from experienced operators.

The use of arterial stents in patients with ischemic nephropathy has not been well described, and has only recently been the focus of some scrutiny. Henry et al[101] found no improvement in renal function following arterial stenting in 59 hypertensive patients despite high stent patency rates; however, only a small proportion of these patients were actually treated for renal insufficiency, and patients with stabilized serum creatinine levels were not considered to benefit from the procedure. In contrast, in a recent review of primary Palmaz-Schatz stent placement for atherosclerotic renal artery stenosis (RAS), Dorros et al[99] noted stabilized or improved serum creatinine levels in 55% of their patients at 6 months. Patients with higher initial creatinine levels ($\geq$2.0 mg/dL) were more likely to stabilize than to improve renal function. In an interesting study of Palmaz stent placement performed in 21 patients with a solitary kidney, Shannon et al[110] found a 71% renal function benefit at a mean of 15 months. In our own early experience,[100] improvement in renal function was seen in 7/11 patients at 6-month follow-up, with a statistically significant mean decrease in creatinine from 2.24 mg/dL at baseline to 1.91 mg/dL. Recently, we have reported our results with renal artery stent placement in 45 patients with ischemic nephropathy.[108] Stent placement was technically successful in

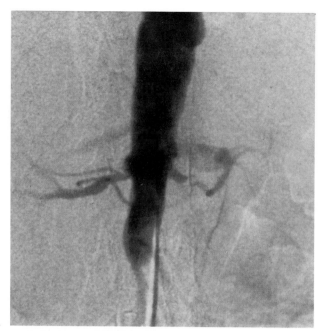

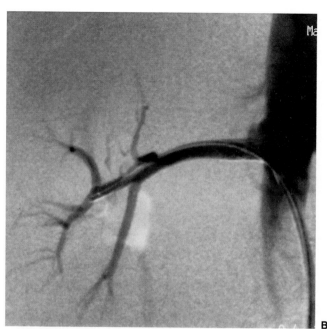

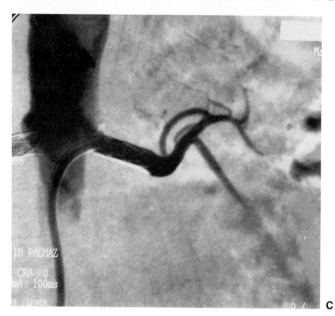

FIGURE 1–6. (A). A flush abdominal aortogram shows severe bilateral renal artery stenosis (RAS). On the right side, the stenosis extends to the aortic wall and was considered ostial. **(B)**. Primary Palmaz stent placement was done for the right RAS. The stent extends approximately 1 to 2 mm into the aorta. **(C)**. Stenting after unsuccessful PTA was performed for the left RAS.

51/54 (94%) of renal arteries, and angiographic follow-up of 28 stents at mean interval of 12.5 months showed a primary patency of 75%. Using life-table analysis, stabilization or improvement in renal function was observed in 72% at 1 year and 62% at 2 years. Benefit was noted in 84% of patients whose initial serum creatinine was 1.5 to 2.0 mg/dL versus only 38% for patients with creatinine >3.0 mg/dL. Stent patency appeared to correlate with clinical benefit. Ninety-three percent of patients with patent stents at angiographic follow-up maintained clinical benefit within the first year of treatment. Hence, rigorous surveillance of stent patency and early reintervention for stenotic stents may be critical to sustained clinical benefit.

Mesenteric Arteries

Chronic occlusive mesenteric ischemia is a rare clinical condition, and it is generally accepted that at least two of the major splanchnic arteries must be occluded before symptoms develop. Early descriptions of mesenteric PTA[111] as well as later studies[112–114] have demonstrated high technical success and symptomatic relief in 75 to 83% of cases. Early technical failures may occur secondary to extrinsic compression.[113] In addition, symptomatic restenosis is noted in approximately one-fourth of patients.

Several case reports have described the use of mesenteric stents for aortic dissection affecting the visceral vessels,[115–117] mesenteric stenoses seen in association with arteritis,[118,119] and in patients with atherosclerotic occlusive disease.[120,121] In these instances, stents appear to provide a viable treatment alternative for lesions refractory to PTA. While initial results are promising, follow-up data are necessary to determine long-term outcomes.

Subclavian Arteries

Subclavian artery stenting has been used to treat a variety of conditions including iatrogenic arterial dissection,[122] coronary-subclavian steal syndrome,[123] and

TABLE 1–5. Results of Renal Stents

First Author (Year)	Ref.	Stent	No. of Patients/RAS	Major Complications	Follow-Up	Hypertension Benefit	Azotemic Benefit[d]	Restenosis
Rees (1991)	37	Palmaz	28/28	17%	5 mo	64%	71%	39% 7 mo
Wilms (1991)	42	Wallstent	11/12	18%	6.7 mo		28%	28% 6 mo
Kuhn (1991)	95	Strecker	8/12	13%	10.6 mo	71%		17% 7 mo
Hennequin (1994)	96	Wallstent	19/19	5%	32 mo	100%	67%	21% 29 mo
MacLeod (1995)	97[a]	Palmaz	29/32	14%	10.6 mo	44%	24% improved	17% 7 mo
Van de Ven (1995)	98	Palmaz	29/28	8%	9 mo	67%		13% 6 mo
Dorros (1995)	99[b]	Palmaz	76/92	3%	6 mo	52%	55%	25% 6 mo
Rundback (1996)	100[c]	Palmaz	20/24	5%	6 mo	77%	86%	19% 6 mo
Henry (1996)	101	Palmaz	59/64	3%	14 mo	75%		2% 6 mo
Iannone (1996)	102	Palmaz (primary)	63/83	22%	10 mo	39%	82%	14% 11 mo
Boisclair (1997)	103	Palmaz	33/35	21%	13 mo	67%	76%	
Taylor (1997)	104[a]	Palmaz	29/32	3%	9.5 mo	50%	62%	16% 7 mo
White (1997)	105	Palmaz	100/133	1%	6 mo	76%	20% improved	19% 9 mo
Blum (1997)	106	Palmaz	68/74	0%	27 mo	62%		11% 27 mo
Fiala (1998)	107	Palmaz (primary)	21/25	14%	13 mo	53%		50% 13 mo
Rundback (1998)	108[c]	Palmaz	45/54	9%	12 mo		72%	25% 12 mo
Dorros (1998)	109[b]	Palmaz	163/202	2%	4 yr	49%		
Shannon (1998)	110	Palmaz (solitary)	21/21	19%	15 mo		72%	0% 9 mo
Totals			**815/966**	**7%**	**~1 YR**	**58%**	**69%**	**0–50%**

[a,b,c]Represents overlapping patient groups.
[d]Stabilization within ±20% of pretreatment levels or improvement of serum creatine levels.
RAS, renal artery stenosis.

subclavian occlusion.[124,125] Although the results of both PTA[126] and atherectomy[127] have been promising, stenting is useful for lesions failing PTA.[128] Sueoka[128] described his experience with stenting in seven patients with critical eccentric or ostial lesions failing angioplasty. Technical success was 100%, and symptoms resolved in all patients with no significant restenosis occurring over 2 years. Stents may also be considered a primary treatment for patients with markedly irregular stenoses or lesions proximal to an internal mammary artery bypass graft or patent vertebral artery. In such cases, initial stent placement may help to "tack down" any friable atheroma and prevent embolization.

Carotid Arteries

The North American Symptomatic Carotid Endarterectomy Trial (NASCET)[129] and Asymptomatic Carotid Atherosclerosis Study (ACAS)[130] have established carotid endarterectomy (CAE) to reduce the risk of stroke for selected patients with carotid artery stenosis exceeding 60 to 70%. The perioperative stroke and death rates for these two trials were 5.8% and 2.3%, respectively, with an additional 7.6% incidence of cranial nerve injury reported in NASCET. Recurrent stenosis is seen in up to 8% of patients after CAE, and usually occurs within the first 2 years.[131]

In recent years, there has been much interest in nonsurgical approaches (PTA and stent placement) for treatment of carotid artery disease. For these techniques to become feasible, a complication rate comparable to CAE must be achieved. Whether or not this is the case remains to be seen. A major limitation of carotid stent placement is cerebral embolization and ensuing strokes.[132] In a recent comparison of carotid angioplasty with stenting versus endarterectomy, Jordan and colleagues[133] found the total stroke and death rate to be 9.7% in the stented group compared to 0.9% for patients undergoing CAE. Further, stented patients had cardiopulmonary events requiring additional monitoring in 32.8% of cases. Naylor and colleagues[134] initiated a trial to prospectively compare CAE and angioplasty with stenting. The study had to be stopped when five of the seven patients treated percutaneously had cerebral events, three of which were disabling at 30 days.

In contrast, other authors have reported more favorable results with carotid stenting. Vitek et al[135] performed stent assisted carotid angioplasty on 392 arteries in 345 patients with a technical success of 98% and overall restenosis in 5%. The 30-day stroke and major stroke rate was 3.4%, with minor strokes in an additional 6.1% of patients. Technical and clinical outcomes were noted to improve with greater procedural experience. Wholey et al[136] surveyed 24 centers and recently presented the cumulative experience with extracranial carotid stent placement in 2,048 patients. Technical success was achieved in 98.6%, and there was a 5% overall rate of restenosis at 6 months. Perioperative mortality was 1.4%, and the total stroke rate was 4.4%, with only 1.3% described as causing a major permanent neurological deficit. These results compare very favorably with that described for carotid endarterectomy.

Patient selection affects the risk of procedure-related stroke. Mathur and colleagues[137] studied the effect of multiple variables on periprocedural stroke. In this series, advanced age was the single most important factor, with a stroke rate of 5.6% in patients younger than 80 years of age compared with 19.2% for patients 80 years of age and older. Increasing lesion severity also contributed to higher stroke incidence, especially with long or multiple lesions or stenoses greater than 90%. However, these lesions are also associated with increased stroke risk during CAE.[138] Using an ex vivo model of human atherosclerotic carotid plaque, Ohki et al[139] noted a greater embolic potential when dilating and stenting echolucent plaques or stenoses exceeding 90%, and suggested that these

criteria may also be useful for screening patients prior to percutaneous therapy.

There are certain clinical scenarios in which carotid stenting is less controversial. Stent placement may allow restored patency following spontaneous or iatrogenic carotid dissection.[140] We have also performed retrograde common carotid artery (CCA) stenting in three patients undergoing endarterectomy for carotid bifurcation disease and coexistent high-grade CCA stenosis refractory to angioplasty alone (Fig. 1–7). Finally, stenting may have a role in treating patients who are poor surgical candidates. Criado and colleagues[4] described the use of carotid stents in 33 patients with conditions thought to increase the risk of carotid endarterectomy, including distal internal carotid artery lesions, post-CAE restenosis, and a "hostile neck" due to previous radical neck surgery or radiotherapy. Technical success was 100%, with all patients remaining asymptomatic at 8 months. There was only a single case of restenosis. Yadav and colleagues[5] have also proposed using stents for restenosis following CAE. They treated 25 lesions in 22 patients. One minor stroke occurred, and at 6-month follow-up no restenosis greater than 50% was identified.

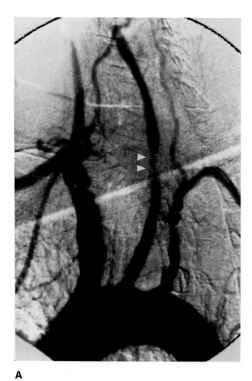

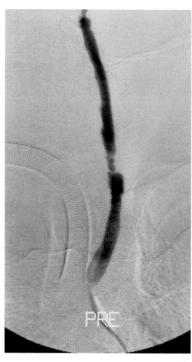

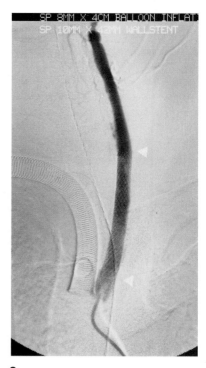

A

B

C

FIGURE 1–7. (A). Thoracic arch aortogram demonstrates severe atherosclerotic disease of the great vessels. A short stenosis is noted in the proximal left common carotid artery (arrowheads). There patient also had a focal stenosis of the left carotid bifurcation and complete occlusion of the right internal carotid artery. **(B)**. Selective left carotid arteriography reveals the severity of the stenosis. **(C)**. After retrograde stenting (arrowheads) at the time of carotid endarterectomy (CAE), the common carotid artery is patent.

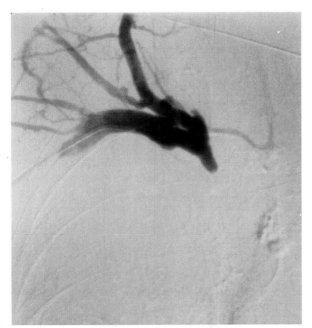

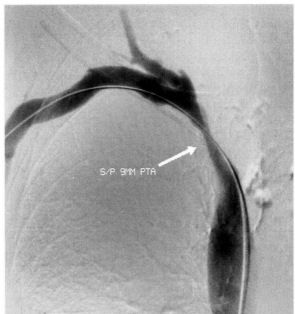

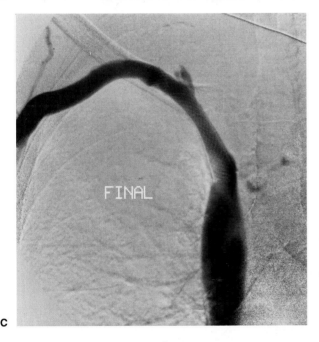

FIGURE 1–8. (A). Right subclavian arteriogram performed through a upper arm dialysis graft. There is complete occlusion of the subclavian-innominate venous junction at the site of previous catheter placement. The patient had arm swelling. **(B).** A residual stenosis is noted after 9-mm PTA. **(C).** There is restored patency of the innominate vein after insertion of a Wallstent. The patient had complete resolution of arm swelling in 24 hours.

Dialysis-Related Venous Stenosis

Over the past 20 years, PTA has become established as a mainstay of treatment for hemodialysis accesses failing owing to underlying central or peripheral venous stenoses,[141] with the recently published National Kidney Foundation (NKF) Dialysis Outcomes Quality Initiative (DOQI) document supporting this approach.[142–146] However, when PTA is insufficient due to elastic recoil or dissection, endovascular stenting allows preserved immediate graft function and acceptable early patency rates in the majority of patients.

Stents have proven particularly valuable for the treatment of central venous stenoses (Fig. 1–8). These lesions tend to be both fibrous and elastic and respond poorly to PTA, with reported 6-month patency rates of approximately 20%.[147] DOQI guideline number 20 suggests PTA as the initial treatment of choice for central stenoses and supports the use of stents for restenoses developing within 3 months of balloon dilatation. Stenting allows salvage of failed balloon angioplasty in almost all cases, with reported primary and secondary 6-month patency rates of 46% and 76%, respectively.[148] Rigorous clinical and hemodynamic surveillance and multiple reinterventions are necessary to assure acceptable long-term patency.[149] Self-expanding Wallstents (Boston Scientific Vascular) are the most commonly utilized endoprosthesis for refractory or recurrent central venous stenoses, although the use of nitinol stents is currently being investigated. Because of the inaccessible location of central venous lesions, surgical repair is discouraged.

Unlike central stenoses, stent placement for peripheral venous stenoses has not clearly been shown to improve access patency rates.[150] However, stents may still be utilized as a rescue technique for PTA complicated by the development of a flow-limiting dissection (Fig. 1–8). In this setting, percutaneous stenting may successfully preserve initial graft function, thereby avoiding the need for urgent surgical revision or the placement of a temporary hemodialysis catheter. Furthermore, stents allow a treatment option in patients having recurrent graft dysfunction despite repeated angioplasty. Turmel-Rodrigues et al[151] placed stents in 49 dialysis grafts for post-PTA elastic recoil ($n = 13$), and early ($n = 33$) or late ($n = 3$) restenosis. Primary patency was 47% at 6 months and 20% at 12 months. With repeated interventions it was possible to maintain access function in 88% of patients at 1 year. In patients treated for early restenosis after prior PTA, the interval between subsequent reinterventions was doubled after stent placement.

A newly recognized role for dialysis access stenting is in the management of post-PTA vein ruptures, a complication that occurs in 0.7 to 4.5% of cases. When observation (for limited extravasation) or prolonged balloon angioplasty at the site of vessel injury fails, recent reports have described Wallstent placement as an effective treatment for limiting further extravasation.[152,153] Presumably, the stent creates a "path of least resistance" toward the central veins, and may seal the site of vein rupture by apposing intact intima against the vessel defect.

Effort Thrombosis

Effort thrombosis, also known as primary axillosubclavian vein thrombosis or Paget-Schrötter syndrome, usually affects the dominant extremity in young patients with a history of unusual upper extremity activity or positioning.[154] Stents are best utilized as part of a multimodal approach[155–157] following thrombolysis, PTA, and surgical decompression of the thoracic inlet. This last component is critical to prevent stent deformation or breakage.[158]

Superior Vena Cava Syndrome

Until recently, the treatment of patients with malignant obstruction of the superior vena cava (SVC) was confined to radiotherapy and chemotherapy. These methods, however, result in either slow or incomplete resolution of symptoms.[159] Stents have been described to provide rapid symptomatic relief from this condition,[160–165] with immediate resolution of facial edema and resolution of peripheral edema over 1 to 7 days[166] (Fig. 1–9). Even in patients with complete obstruction of the SVC, a success rate of 85% has been reported.[167]

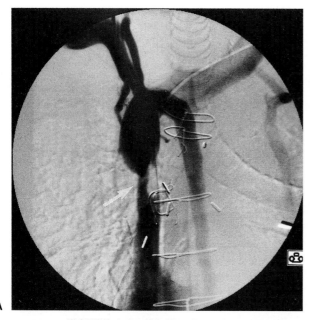
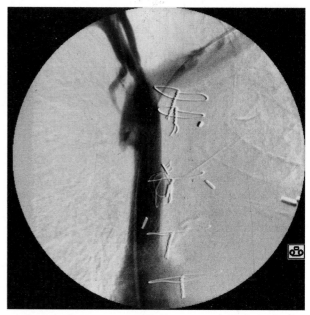

A   **B**

FIGURE 1–9. (A). Focal severe narrowing of the superior vena cava (SVC) in a patient with bronchogenic carcinoma (arrow). Retrograde filling of the azygous vein is evident. **(B).** The SVC stenosis is resolved using a stent. The azygous vein is no longer visualized.

Stents have also been used to treat benign causes of SVC syndrome, including trauma, intravenous catheter placement, fibrosing mediastinitis, and radiation therapy.[168–170] Although the long-term stent patency in patients with longer life expectancies remains uncertain, revision and repeat angioplasty of the restenosis should be expected to provide durable results.

Deep Venous Thrombosis–Related Iliac Vein Stenosis

Unrecognized chronic occlusion of the pelvic veins is a common cause of recurrent symptoms following venous thrombolysis or thrombectomy.[171] While most of these lesions are resistant to balloon dilation alone, metallic stents are able to provide adequate patency of the pelvic venous system in the majority of cases.[172–175] In fact, Nazarian et al[175] reported 81% 1-year and 75% 4-year assisted patencies in a series of 56 patients with percutaneously implanted pelvic venous stents.[175]

■ Limitations of Vascular Stents

Although stents have clearly expanded the limits of vascular intervention, there are several important limita-
tions. Stenting has greater technical complexity and higher complication rates when compared to PTA alone, increased procedural and material costs, and the uncertain biological effects of a long-term vascular implant. The latticework of bare stents is unable to seal aneurysms, arteriovenous malformations, or vessel ruptures (Fig. 1–10). The two most important shortcomings of current stent techniques are a relatively high poststent restenosis rate and an ineffectiveness in improving upon the results of PTA for many lesions.

While stents provide a scaffold to prevent elastic recoil and smooth luminal irregularities, they do not limit the process of restenosis (Fig. 1– 11). In fact, the greater initial luminal gain is largely offset by a more abundant fibrocellular response than noted following angioplasty alone. The process of restenosis is initiated immediately after stent placement as a result of vessel wall trauma, interactions at the stent-tissue interface,[176] and the inherent thrombogenicity of a metallic surface. Fibrocellular proliferation is invariable with all metal alloys[177] despite attempts at altering the metallic surface charge,[29] changing surface area,[178] varying radial force,[179] or applying a hydrophilic[180] or antithrombotic coating.[181] The open mesh between stent struts provides no physical barrier to this tissue ingrowth and encroachment on the treated vessel lumen. Although

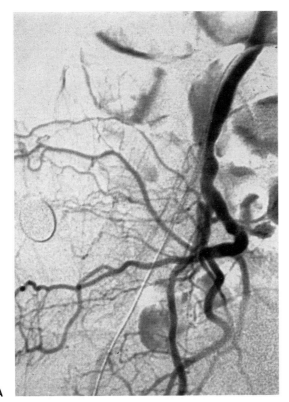
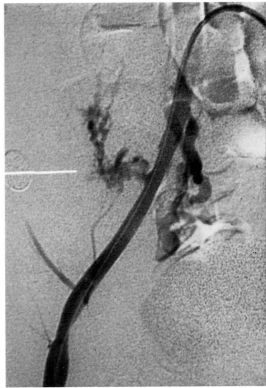

A   **B**

FIGURE 1–10. (**A**). An external iliac occlusion has been traversed with a guidewire. (**B**). Extravasation of contrast is seen after primary stenting and balloon dilatation. The vessel was surgically repaired.

geometric factors (e.g., implanted stent diameter) determine the relative hemodynamic significance of intimal hyperplasia in a given vessel, long-term patency is ultimately determined by the aggressiveness of the fibrocellular host response to stent implantation.

Despite initial enthusiasm, stents have also failed to provide a durable treatment option and thereby expand the role of percutaneous therapy for many lesions. This is particularly the case in smaller arteries, long-segment occlusions, or veins. Stenting of the superficial femoral artery has 2-year patency rates of 49 to 77%, not considerably different from the 67% pooled rate reported by Becker et al[8] for femoral PTA alone. In distal femoral and popliteal arteries, the patency after stent placement

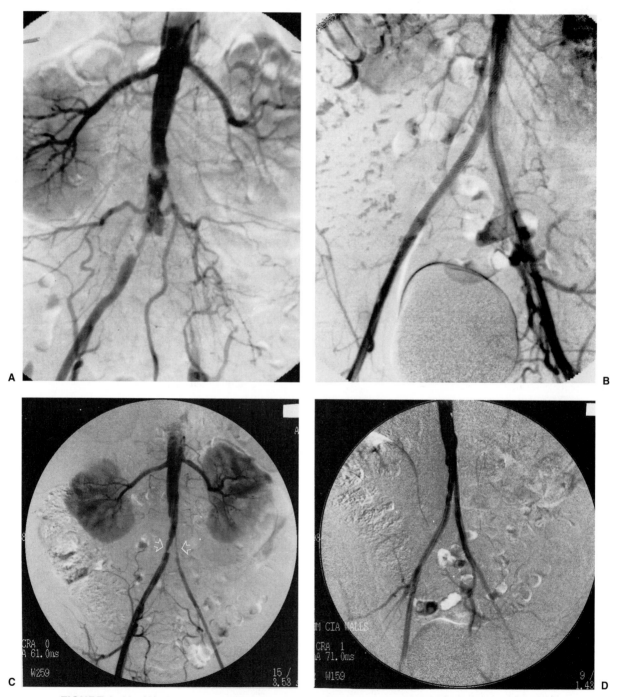

FIGURE 1–11. (**A**). Aortic and right common iliac artery (CIA) stenoses and occlusion of the left CIA. (**B**). After bilateral "kissing" stent placement, the aorta and iliac arteries are patent. (**C**). Six-month follow-up angiogram performed for recurrent symptoms shows bilateral instent stenosis of the CIA's (open arrows). (**D**). There is an improved appearance of both CIAs following repeat bilateral PTA.

is even lower,[43] and possibly worse than the results of PTA alone. As previously noted, stenting of long-segment femoral lesions has unacceptably poor results.[91] Stents in the peripheral veins also have not improved upon the results of PTA,[150] with 1-year unassisted patency of 12 to 25% for stents versus 11 to 40% for PTA alone.[148,150]

■ Future Stent Developments

The vexing problem of in-stent restenosis has yet to be solved. Stent-grafts, in which synthetic material covers the interstices of the stent, is one possible solution to prevent neointimal ingrowth, and is the topic of considerable review in this book. Stents may also be used as a vector for localized radiation or drug delivery.[27,182] Early experience with low-dose intravascular beta-particle radiation delivered via cyclotron modified or 32p-implanted Palmaz stents shows reduced neointimal hyperplasia.[183,184] Gene transfer techniques using vascular endothelial growth factor have produced marked reductions in cellular hyperplasia by promoting early stent endothelialization.[27] Perhaps in the future some combination of these and other techniques will produce long-term satisfactory results for all lesion types, and truly extend the limits of endovascular intervention.

REFERENCES

1. Dotter CT, Judkins MP. Transluminal treatment of arteriosclerotic obstruction. Circulation 1964;30:654–670.
2. Dotter CT. Transluminally placed coil-spring endarterial tube grafts, long term patency in canine popliteal artery. Invest Radiol 1969;4:329–332.
3. Dotter CT, Buschmann RW, McKinney MK, Rosch J. Transluminal expandable nitinol coil stent grafting: preliminary report. Radiology 1983;147:259–260.
4. Criado FJ, Wellons E, Clark NS. Evolving indications for and early results of carotid artery stenting. Am J Surg 1997;174:111–114.
5. Yadav JS, Roubin GS, King P, et al. Angioplasty and stenting for restenosis after carotid endarterectomy: initial experience. Stroke 1996;27:2075–2079.
6. Murray RR, Hewes RC, White RI Jr, et al. Long-segment femoropopliteal stenoses: is angioplasty a boon or a bust? Radiology 1987;162(2):473–476.
7. Capek P, McLean GK, Berkowitz HD. Femoropopliteal angioplasty. Factors influencing long-term success. Circulation 1991;83(suppl 2):I70–80.
8. Becker GJ, Katzen BT, Dake MD. Noncoronary angioplasty. Radiology 1989;170:921–940.
9. Becker GJ, Palmaz JC, Rees CR, et al. Angioplasty-induced dissections in human iliac arteries: management with Palmaz balloon-expandable intraluminal stents. Radiology 1990;176:31–38.
10. Hoffmann R, Mintz GS, Dussaillant GR, et al. Patterns and mechanism of in-stent restenosis. A serial intravascular ultrasound study. Circulation 1996;94:1247–1254.
11. Adams PC, Badimon JJ, Badimon L, Chesebro JH, Fuster V. Role of platelets in atherogenesis: relevance to coronary arterial restenosis after angioplasty. Cardiovasc Clin 1987;18(1):49–71.
12. Liu MW, Roubin GS, King SB 3d. Restenosis after coronary angioplasty. Potential biologic determinants and role of intimal hyperplasia. Circulation 1989;79(6):1374–1387.
13. Becker GJ. Intravascular stents. General principles and status of lower-extremity arterial applications. Circulation 1991;83(suppl I):I-122–I-136.
14. Sullivan TM, Childs MB, Bacharach JM. Percutaneous transluminal angioplasty and primary stenting of the iliac arteries in 288 patients. J Vasc Surg 1997;25:829–838.
15. Johnson SP, Fujitani RM, Leyendecker JR, Joseph FB. Stent deformation and intimal hyperplasia complicating treatment of a post-carotid endarterectomy intimal flap with a Palmaz stent. J Vasc Surg 1997;25(4):764–768.
16. Berry JL, Newman VS, Ferrario CM, Routh WD, Dean RH. A method to evaluate the elastic behavior of vascular stents. J Vasc Intervent Radiol 1996;7(3):381–385.
17. Rosenfield K, Schainfeld R, Pieczek A, Haley L, Isner JM. Restenosis of endovascular stents from stent compression. J Am Coll Cardiol 1997;29(2):328–338.
18. Sapoval M, Chatellier G, Long AL, et al. Self-expandable stents for the treatment of iliac artery obstructive lesions: long-term success and prognostic factors. Am J Roentgenol 1996; 116:1173–1179.
19. Long A, Page P, Raynaud AC, et al. Percutaneous iliac artery stent: angiographic long-term follow-up. Radiology 1991;180:771–778.
20. Rossseau H, Raillat C, Joffre FG, et al. Treatment of femoropopliteal stenosis by means of self-expandable endoprostheses: midterm results. Radiology 1989;172:961–964.
21. Schurmann K, Vorwerk D, Kulisch A, et al. Neointimal hyperplasia in low-profile nitinol stents, Palmaz stents, and Wallstents: a comparative experimental study. Cardiovasc Intervent Radiol 1996;19(4):248–254.
22. Castaneda-Zuniga WR, Formanek A, Tadavarthy M, et al. The mechanism of balloon angioplasty. Radiology 1980;135:565–571.
23. Consigny PM, Cragg AH, Waller BF. Pathophysiology of vascular intervention. In: Strandness DE, Van Breda A, eds. Vascular Disease: Surgical and Interventional Therapy. New York: Churchill-Livingstone, 1994.
24. Kearney M, Pieczek A, Haley L, et al. Histopathology of in-stent restenosis in patients with peripheral artery disease. Circulation 1997;31(2):1998–2002.
25. Palmaz JC, Tio FO, Schatz RA, Alvarado R, Rees C, Garcia O. Early endothelialisation of balloon-expandable stents: experimental observations. J Intervent Radiol 1988;3:119–124.
26. Liu MW, Roubin GS, King SB 3d. Restenosis after coronary angioplasty. Potential biologic determinants and role of intimal hyperplasia. Circulation 1989;79(6):1374–1387.
27. VanBelle E, Tio FO, Couffinhal T, Maillard L, Passeri J, Isner JM. Stent endothelialization. Time course, impact of local catheter delivery, feasibility of recombinant protein administration, and response to cytokine expedition. Circulation 1997;95(2):438–448.
28. Schatz RA, Palmaz JC, Tio FO, Garcia F, Garcia O, Reuter SR. Balloon-expandable intracoronary stents in the adult dog. Circulation 1987;76:450–457.
29. Schatz RA. A view of vascular stents. Circulation 1989;79(2):445–457.
30. Robinson KA, Roubin G, King S, Siegel R, Rodgers G, Apkarian RP. Correlated microscopic observations of arterial responses to intravascular stenting. Scanning Microsc 1989;3(2):665–678.
31. Rousseau H, Puel J, Joffre F, et al. Self-expanding endovascular prosthesis: an experimental study. Radiology 1987;164:709–714.
32. Palmaz JC. Intravascular stenting: from basic research to clinical application. Cardiovasc Intervent Radiol 1992;15:279–284.
33. Yee DC, Williams SK, Salzmann DL, et al. Stent versus endovascular graft healing characteristics in the porcine iliac artery. J Vasc Intervent Radiol 1998;9:609–617.
34. Kornowski R, Hong MK, Tio FO, Bramwell O, Wu H, Leon MB. In-stent restenosis: contributions of inflammatory responses and

arterial injury to neointimal hyperplasia. J Am Coll Cardiol 1998;31(2):224–230.

35. Bucx JJ, de Scheerder I, Beatt K, et al. The importance of adequate anticoagulation to prevent early thrombosis after stenting of stenosed venous bypass grafts. Am Heart J 1991;121:1389– 396.

36. van der Giessen WJ, Serruys PW, van Woerkens LJ, et al. Arterial stenting with self-expandable and balloon-expandable endoprostheses. Int J Card Imaging 1990;5:163–171.

37. Rees CR, Palmaz JC, Becker GJ, et al. Palmaz stent in atherosclerotic stenoses involving the ostia of the renal arteries: preliminary report of a multicenter study. Radiology 1991;181:507–514.

38. White GH, Liew SC, Waughn RC, et al. Early outcome and intermediate follow-up of vascular stents in the femoral and popliteal arteries without long-term anticoagulation. J Vasc Surg 1995;21: 270–279.

39. Schwartz L, Bourassa MG, Lesperance J, et al. Failure of antiplatelet agents to reduce restenosis after PTCA in a double blind placebo controlled trial. J Am Coll Cardiol 1988;11: 236A–241A.

40. Rodgers GP, Minor ST, Robinson K, et al. The coronary artery response to implantation of a balloon-expandable flexible stent in the aspirin and non-aspirin treated swine model. Am Heart J 1991;122:640–647.

41. Joffre F, Rousseau H, Bernadet AL, et al. Midterm results of renal artery stenting. Cardiovasc Intervent Radiol 1992;15:313–318.

42. Wilms GE, Peene P, Baert AL, et al. Renal artery stent placement with the use of the Wallstent endoprosthesis. Radiology 1991;179:457–462.

43. Henry M, Amor M, Ethevenot G, et al. Palmaz stent placement in iliac and femoropopliteal arteries: primary and secondary patency in 310 patients with 2–4 year follow-up. Radiology 1995;197:167–174.

44. Martin EC, Katzen BT, Benenati JF, et al. Multicenter trial of the Wallstent in the iliac and femoral arteries. J Vasc Intervent Radiol 1995;6:843–849.

45. Arko F, Mettauer M, McCollough R, et al. Use of intravascular ultrasound improves long-term clinical outcome in the endovascular management of atherosclerotic aortoiliac occlusive disease. J Vasc Surg 1998;27:614–623.

46. Arko F, Mettauer M, McCollough R, et al. Use of intravascular ultrasound in the endovascular management of atherosclerotic aortoiliac disease. Am J Surg 1996;27:546–549.

47. Werner GS, Diedrich J, Schunemann S, et al. Additional luminal area gain by intravascular ultrasound guidance after coronary stent implantation. Int J Card Imaging 1997;13:311–321.

48. Schiele F, Meneveau N, Vuillemenot A, et al. Impact of intravascular ultrasound guidance in stent deployment on 6-month restenosis rate: a multicenter randomized study comparing two strategies—with and without intravascular ultrasound guidance. RESIST study group. Restenosis after IVUS guided stenting. J Am Coll Cardiol 1998;32:320–328.

49. van Sambeck MR, Qureshi A, van Lankeren W, van der Lugt A, Honkoop J, Gussenhoven EJ. Discrepancy between stent deployment and balloon size used assessed by intravascular ultrasound. Eur J Vasc Endovasc Surg 1998;15:57–61.

50. Korogi Y, Hirai T, Takahashi M. Intravascular ultrasound imaging of peripheral arteries as an adjunct to balloon angioplasty and atherectomy. Cardiovasc Intervent Radiol 1996;93:1–9.

51. Schurmann K, Vorwerk D, Uppenkamp R, Klosterhalfen B, Bucker A, Gunther GW. Determination of stent stenosis: an in vivo experimental comparison of intravascular ultrasound and angiography with histology. Cardiovasc Intervent Radiol 1998;21:189–198.

52. Schwarzenberg H, Muller-Hulsbeck S, Gluer CC, Wesner F, Heller M. Restenosis of peripheral stents and stent grafts as revealed by intravascular sonography: in vivo comparison with angiography. AJR 1998;170:1181–1185.

53. Morag B, Garniek A, Bass A, et al. Percutaneous transluminal aortic angioplasty: early and late results. Cardiovasc Intervent Radiol 1993;16:37–42.

54. Wolf YG, Schatz RA, Knowles HJ, et al. Initial experience with the Palmaz stent for aortoiliac stenoses. Ann Vasc Surg 1993;7: 254–261.

55. Vorwerk D, Gunther RW, Schurmann K, Wendt G. Aortic and iliac stenoses: follow-up results of stent placement after insufficient balloon angioplasty in 118 cases. Radiology 1996;198:45–48.

56. Vorwerk D, Gunther RW, Bohndorf K, Keulers P. Stent placement for failed angioplasty of aortic stenoses: report of two cases. Cardiovasc Intervent Radiol 1991;14:316–319.

57. Sheeran SR, Hallisey MJ, Ferguson D. Percutaneous transluminal stent placement in the abdominal aorta. J Vasc Intervent Radiol 1997;8:55–60.

58. Martinez R, Rodriguez-Lopez J, Diethrich EB. Stenting for abdominal aortic occlusive disease: long-term results. Tex Heart Inst J 1997;31:15–22.

59. Long AL, Gaux JC, Raynaud JM, et al. Infrarenal aortic stents: initial clinical experience and angiographic follow-up. Cardiovasc Intervent Radiol 1993;16:203–208.

60. Westcott MA, Bonn J. Comparison of conventional angioplasty with the Palmaz stent in the treatment of abdominal aortic stenoses from the STAR registry. SCVIR transluminal angioplasty and revascularization. J Vasc Intervent Radiol 1998;9:225–231.

61. In der Maur GA, de Boo T, Boeve J, Kerdel MC, Braakenburg BA. Angioplasty of the iliac and femoral arteries. Initial and long-term results in short stenotic lesions. Eur J Radiol 1990;11: 163–167.

62. Rousseau H, Puel J, Joffre F, et al. Self-expanding endovascular prosthesis: an experimental study. Radiology 1987;164:709–714.

63. Palmaz JC, Richter GM, Noeldge G, et al. Intraluminal stents in atherosclerotic iliac artery stenosis: preliminary report of a multicenter study. Radiology 1988;168:727–731.

64. Murphy TP, Webb MS, Lambiase RE, et al. Percutaneous revascularization of complex iliac artery stenoses and occlusions with the use of Wallstents: three-year experience. J Vasc Intervent Radiol 1996;7:21–27.

65. Vorwerk D, Guenther RW. Mechanical revascularization of occluded iliac arteries with use of self-expandable endoprostheses. Radiology 1990;175:411–415.

66. Blum U, Gabelman A, Rececker M, et al. Percutaneous recanalization of iliac artery occlusions: results of a prospective study. Radiology 1993;189:536–540.

67. Yedlicka JW, Ferral H, Bjarnason H, Hunter DW, Castaneda-Zuniga WR, Amplatz K. Chronic iliac artery occlusions: primary revascularization with endovascular stents. J Vasc Intervent Radiol 1994;5:843–847.

68. Toogood GH, Torrie EP, Magee TR, Galland RB. Early experience with stenting for iliac occlusive disease. Eur J Vasc Endovasc Surg 1998;15:165–168.

69. Murphy TP. Complications of arterial stent placement. Reported at the 23rd Annual Scientific Meeting of the Society of Cardiovascular and Interventional Radiology. J Vasc Intervent Radiol 1998;9(suppl):71–75.

70. Long AL, Page PE, Raynaud AC, et al. Percutaneous iliac artery stent: angiographic long-term follow-up. Radiology 1991;180: 771–778.

71. Strecker EP, Boos IB, Hagen B. Flexible tantalum stents for the treatment of iliac artery lesions: long-term patency, complications, and risk factors. Radiology 1996;199:641–647.

72. Cikrit DF, Gustafson PA, Dalsing MC, et al. Long-term follow-up of Palmaz stent for iliac occlusive disease. Surgery 1995;118: 608–614.

73. Long AL, Sapoval MR, Beyssen BM, et al. Strecker stent implantation in iliac arteries: patency and predictive factors for long-term success. Radiology 1995;194:739–744.

74. Sapoval MR, Long AL, Pagny JV, et al. Outcome of percutaneous intervention in iliac artery stents. Radiology 1996;198:481–486.

75. Vorwerk D, Guenther RW, Schurmann K, Wendt G. Late reobstruction in iliac artery stents: percutaneous treatment. Radiology 1995;197:479–483.

76. Bauters C, Banos JL, Van Belle E, et al. Six-month angiographic outcome after successful repeat percutaneous intervention for in-stent restenosis. Circulation 1998;97:318–321.

77. Bosch JL, Hunink MGM. Meta-analysis of the results of percutaneous transluminal angioplasty and stent placement for aortoiliac disease. Radiology 1997;204:87–96.

78. Tetteroo E, van der Graaf Y, Bosch JL, et al. Randomised comparison of primary stent placement versus primary angioplasty followed by selective stent placement in patients with iliac artery occlusive disease. Dutch Iliac Stent Trial Study Group. Lancet 1998;351:1153–1159.

79. Tetteroo E, Haaring C, van der Graaf Y, van Schaik JP, van Engelen AD, Mali WP. Intraarterial pressure gradients after randomized angioplasty or stenting of iliac artery lesions. Dutch Iliac Stent Trial Group. Cardiovasc Intervent Radiol 1996;19:411–417.

80. Bosch JL, Tetteroo E, Mali WP, Hunink MG. Iliac arterial occlusive disease: cost-effectiveness analysis of stent placement versus percutaneous transluminal angioplasty. Dutch Iliac Stent Trial Study Group. Radiology 1998;351:641–648.

81. Labord JC, Palmaz JC, Rivera FJ, Encarnacion CE, Picot MC, Dougherty SP. Influence of anatomic distribution of atherosclerosis on outcome of revascularization with iliac stent placement. J Vasc Intervent Radiol 1995;6:513–521.

82. Vorwerk D, Guenther RW, Schurmann K, Wendt G, Peters I. Primary stent placement for chronic iliac artery occlusions: follow-up results in 103 patients. Radiology 1995;194:745–749.

83. Dyet JF, Gaines PA, Nicholson AA, et al. Treatment of chronic iliac artery occlusions by means of percutaneous endovascular stent placement. J Vasc Intervent Radiol 1997;8:349–353.

84. Reyes R, Maynar M, Lopera J, et al. Treatment of chronic iliac artery occlusions with guide wire recanalization and primary stent placement. J Vasc Intervent Radiol 1997;8:1049–4055.

85. Raza Z, Shaw JW, Stonebridge PA, McCollum PT. Management of iliac occlusions with a new self-expanding endovascular stent. Eur J Vasc Endovasc Surg 1998;15:439–443.

86. Gunther RW, Vorwerk D, Bohndorf K, Peters I, el-Din A, Messmer B. Iliac and femoral artery stenoses and occlusions: treatment with intravascular stents. Radiology 1989;172:725–730.

87. Do-dai D, Triller J, Walpoth BH, Stirnemann P, Mahler F. A comparison study of self-expandable stents vs balloon angioplasty in femoropopliteal artery occlusions. Cardiovasc Intervent Radiol 1992;15:306–312.

88. Sapoval MR, Long AL, Raynaud AC, Beyssen BM, Fiessinger JN, Gaux JC. Femoropopliteal stent placement: long-term results. Radiology 1992;184:833–839.

89. Bergeron P, Pinot JJ, Poyen V, et al. Long-term results with the Palmaz stent in the superficial femoral artery. J Endovasc Surg 1995;2:161–167.

90. Chatelard P, Guibourt C. Long-term results with a Palmaz stent in the femoropopliteal arteries. J Cardiovasc Surg (Torino) 1996;37(3 suppl 1):67–72.

91. Gray BH, Sullivan TM, Childs MB, Young JR, Olin JW. High incidence of restenosis/reocclusion of stents in the percutaneous treatment of long-segment superficial femoral artery disease after suboptimal angioplasty. J Vasc Surg 1997;25:74–83.

92. Rousseau HP, Raillat CP, Joffre FG, Knight CJ, Ginestet MC. Treatment of femoropopliteal stenoses by means of self-expandable endoprostheses: midterm results. Radiology 1989;172:961–964.

93. Zollikofer CL, Antonucci F, Pfyffer M, et al. Arterial stent placement with use of the Wallstent: midterm results of clinical experience. Radiology 1991;179:449–456.

94. Palmaz JC, Kopp DT, Hayashi H, et al. Normal and stenotic renal arteries: experimental balloon-expandable intraluminal stenting. Radiology 1987;164:705–708.

95. Kuhn FP, Kutkuhn B, Torsello G, Modder U. Renal artery stenosis: preliminary results of treatment with the Strecker stent. Radiology 1991;180:367–372.

96. Hennequin LM, Joffre FG, Rousseau HP, et al. Renal artery stent placement: long-term results with the Wallstent endoprosthesis. Radiology 1994;191:713–719.

97. MacLeod M, Taylor AD, Baxter G, et al. Renal artery stenosis managed by Palmaz stent insertion: technical and clinical outcome. J Hypertens 1995;13:1791–1795.

98. Van de Ven PJG, Beutler JJ, Kaatee R, et al. Transluminal vascular stent for ostial atherosclerotic renal artery stenosis. Lancet 1995;346:672–674.

99. Dorros G, Jaff M, Jain A, Dufek C, Mathiak L. Follow-up of primary Palmaz-Schatz stent placement for atherosclerotic renal artery stenosis. Am J Cardiol 1995;75:1051–1055.

100. Rundback JH, Jacobs JM. Percutaneous renal artery stent placement for hypertension and azotemia: pilot study. Am J Kidney Dis 1996;28(2):214–219.

101. Henry M, Amor M, Henry I, et al. Stent placement in the renal artery: three-year experience with the Palmaz stent. J Vasc Intervent Radiol 1996;7:343–350.

102. Iannone LA, Underwood PL, Nath A, Tannenbaum MA, Ghali MGH, Clevenger LD. Effect of primary balloon expandable renal artery stents on long-term patency, renal function, and blood pressure in hypertensive and renal insufficient patients with renal artery stenosis. Cathet Cardiovasc Diagn 1996;37:243–250.

103. Boisclair C, Therasse E, Oliva VL, et al. Treatment of renal angioplasty failure by percutaneous renal artery stenting with Palmaz stents: midterm technical and clinical results. AJR 1997;168: 245–251.

104. Taylor A, Sheppard D, Macleod MJ, et al. Renal artery stent placement in renal artery stenosis: technical and early clinical results. Clin Radiol 1997;52:451–457.

105. White CUJ, Ramee SR, Collins TJ, Jenkins JS, Escobar A, Shaw D. Renal artery stent placement: utility in lesions difficult to treat with balloon angioplasty. J Am Coll Cardiol 1997;30:1445–1450.

106. Blum U, Krumme B, Flugel P, et al. Treatment of ostial renal artery stenoses with vascular endoprostheses after unsuccessful balloon angioplasty. N Engl J Med 1997;336(7):459–465.

107. Fiala LA, Jackson MR, Gillespie DL, O'Donnel S, Lukens M, Gorman P. Primary stenting of atherosclerotic renal artery stenosis. Ann Vasc Surg 1998;12:128–133.

108. Rundback JH, Gray R, Rozenblit G, et al. Renal artery stent placement for the management of ischemic nephropathy. J Vasc Intervent Radiol 1998;9:413–420.

109. Dorros G, Jaff M, Mathiak L, et al. Four-year follow-up of Palmaz-Schatz stent revascularization as treatment for atherosclerotic renal artery stenosis. Circulation 1998;98:642–647.

110. Shannon HM, Gillespie IN, Moss JG. Salvage of the solitary kidney by insertion of a renal artery stent. AJR 1998;171:217–222.

111. Furrer J, Gruntzig A, Kugelmeier J, et al. Treatment of abdominal angina with percutaneous dilatation of an arteria mesenterica superior stenosis. Cardiovasc Intervent Radiol 1980;3:43–44.

112. Hallisey MJ, Deschaine J, Illescas FF, et al. Angioplasty for the treatment of visceral ischemia. J Vasc Intervent Radiol 1995;6: 785–791.

113. Matsumoto AH, Tegtemeyer CJ, Fitzcharles EK, et al. Percutaneous transluminal angioplasty of visceral arterial stenoses: results and long-term clinical follow-up. J Vasc Intervent Radiol 1995;6:165–174.

114. Allen RC, Martin GH, Rees CR, et al. Mesenteric angioplasty in the treatment of chronic intestinal ischemia. J Vasc Surg 1996;24: 415–423.

115. Yamakado K, Takeda K, Nomura Y, et al. Relief of mesenteric ischemia by Z-stent placement into the superior mesenteric artery compressed by the false lumen of an aortic dissection. Cardiovasc Intervent Radiol 1998;21:66–68.

116. Connell DA, Thomson KR, Gibson RN, Wall AJ. Stent placement in coeliac and superior mesenteric arteries to restore perfusion following aortic dissection. Australas Radiol 1995;39:68–70.

117. Waybill PN, Enea NA. Use of a Palmaz stent deployed in the superior mesenteric artery for chronic mesenteric ischemia. J Vasc Intervent Radiol 1997;8:1069–1071.

118. Ozdil E, Krajcer Z, Angelini P. Percutaneous balloon angioplasty with adjunctive stent placement in the mesenteric vessels in a patient with Takayasu's arteritis. Circulation 1996;93:1940–1941.

119. Tyagi S, Verma P, Kumar N, Arora R. Stent angioplasty for relief of chronic mesenteric ischemia in Takayasu arteritis. Indian Heart J 1997;49:315–318.

120. Peene P, Vanrusselt J, Coenegrachts JL, et al. Strecker stent placement in the superior mesenteric artery for recurrent ischemic colitis. J Belge Radiol 1996;79:168–169.

121. Lindblad B, Lindh M, Chuter T, Ivancev K. Superior mesenteric artery occlusion treated with PTA and stent placement. Eur J Vasc Endovasc Surg 1996;11:493–495.

122. Galli M, Goldberg SL, Zerboni S, Almagor Y. Balloon expandable stent implantation after iatrogenic arterial dissection of the left subclavian artery. Cathet Cardiovasc Diagn 1995;7:355–357.

123. Sandison AJ, Panayiotopoulos YP, Carr LA, Reidy JF, Taylor PR. Recurrent coronary-subclavian steal syndrome treated by left subclavian artery stenting. Eur J Vasc Endovasc Surg 1997;34(4): 403–405.

124. Harris NJ, Cameron I, Beard JD, Gaines P. Percutaneous stenting of proximal subclavian artery occlusion. Eur J Vasc Endovasc Surg 1995;34(4):479–480.

125. Martinez R, Rodriguez-Lopez J, Torruella L, Ray L, Lopez-Galarza, Diethrich EB. Stenting for occlusion of the subclavian arteries. Technical aspects and follow-up results. Tex Heart Inst J 1997;24(1):23–27.

126. Burke DR, Gordon RL, Mishkin JD, et al. Percutaneous transluminal angioplasty of subclavian arteries. Radiology 1987;164: 699–704.

127. Breall JA, Grossman W, Stillman IE, et al. Atherectomy of the subclavian artery for patients with symptomatic coronary subclavian steal syndrome. J Am Coll Cardiol 1993;21:1564–1567.

128. Sueoka BL. Percutaneous transluminal stent placement to treat subclavian steal syndrome. J Vasc Intervent Radiol 1996;7: 351–356.

129. North American Symptomatic Carotid Endarterectomy Trial Collaborators. Beneficial effect of carotid endarterectomy in symptomatic patients with high-grade carotid stenosis. N Engl J Med 1991;325:445–453.

130. Executive committee for the asymptomatic carotid atherosclerosis study. Endarterectomy for asymptomatic carotid artery stenosis. JAMA 1995;273:1421–1428.

131. Lattimer CR, Burnand KG. Recurrent carotid stenosis after carotid endarterectomy. Br J Surg 1997;84:1206–1219.

132. Crawley F, Clifton A, Buckenham T, et al. Comparison of hemodynamic cerebral ischemia and microembolic signals detected during carotid endarterectomy and carotid angioplasty. Stroke 1997;28(12):2460–2464.

133. Jordan WD, Voellinger DC, Winfield SF, et al. A comparison of carotid angioplasty with stenting versus endarterectomy with regional anesthesia. J Vasc Surg 1998;28:397–403.

134. Naylor AR, Bolia A, Abbott RJ, et al. Randomized study of carotid angioplasty and stenting versus carotid endarterectomy: a stopped trial. J Vasc Surg 1998;28:326–334.

135. Vitek J, Iyer S, Roubin G. Carotid stenting in 350 vessels: problems faced and solved. J Invas Cardiol 1998;10:311–314.

136. Wholey MH, Wholey M, Bergeron P, et al. Current global status of carotid artery stent placement. Cathet Cardiovasc Diagn 1998; 44:1–6.

137. Mathur A, Roubin GS, Iyer SS, et al. Predictors of stroke complicating carotid artery stenting. Circulation 1998;97:1239–1245.

138. North American symptomatic endarterectomy trial (NASCET) steering committee. North American symptomatic carotid endarterectomy trial: methods, patient characteristics, and progress. Stroke 1991;22:711–720.

139. Ohki T, Marin ML, Lyon RT, et al. Ex vivo human carotid artery bifurcation stenting: correlation of lesion characteristics with embolic potential. J Vasc Surg 1998;27:463–471.

140. DeOcampo J, Brillman J, Levy DI. Stenting: a new approach to carotid dissection. J Neuroimaging 1997;28:187–190.

141. Schwab SJ, Raymond JR, Saeed M, Newman GE, Dennis PA, Bollinger RR. Prevention of hemodialysis fistula thrombosis. Early detection of venous stenoses. Kidney Int 1989;36:707–711.

142. Schwab S, Besarab A, Beathard G, et al. NKF-DOQI clinical practice guidelines for vascular access. Am J Kidney Dis 1997;30(suppl 3):S150–S191.

143. Safa AA, Valji K, Roberts AC, Ziegler TW, Hye RJ, Oglevie SB. Detection and treatment of dysfunctional hemodialysis access grafts: effect of a surveillance program on graft patency and the incidence of thrombosis. Radiology 1996;199:653–657.

144. Turmel-Rodrigues L, Pengloan J, Blanchier D, et al. Insufficient dialysis shunts: improved long-term patency rates with close hemodynamic monitoring, repeated percutaneous balloon angioplasty, and stent placement. Radiology 1993;187:273–278.

145. Robers AB, Kahn MB, Bradford S, et al. Graft surveillance and angioplasty prolongs dialysis graft patency. J Am Coll Surg 1996;183:486–492.

146. Beathard GA. Percutaneous transvenous angioplasty in the treatment of vascular access stenosis. Kidney Int 1992;42:1390–1397.

147. Kanterman RY, Vesely TM, Pilgram TK, Guy BW, Windus DW, Picus D. Dialysis access grafts: anatomic location of venous stenosis and results of angioplasty. Radiology 1995;195:135–139.

148. Gray RJ, Horton KM, Dolmatch BL, et al. Use of Wallstents for hemodialysis access-related venous stenoses and occlusions untreatable by balloon angioplasty. Radiology 1995;195:479–484.

149. Vesely TM, Hovsepian DM, Pilgram TK, Coyne DW, Shenoy S. Upper extremity central venous obstruction in hemodialysis patients: treatment with Wallstents. Radiology 1997;204:343–348.

150. Quinn SF, Schuman ES, Demlow TA, et al. Percutaneous transluminal angioplasty versus endovascular stent placement in the treatment of venous stenoses in patients undergoing hemodialysis: intermediate results. J Vasc Intervent Radiol 1995;6:851–855.

151. Turmel-Rodrigues LA, Blanchard D, Penglaon J, et al. Wallstents and Craggstents in hemodialysis grafts and fistulas: results for selective indications. J Vasc Intervent Radiol 1997;8:975–982.

152. Funaki B, Szymski GX, Leef JA, Rosenblum JD, Burke R, Hackworth GA. Wallstent deployment to salvage dialysis graft thrombolysis complicated by venous rupture: early and intermediate results. AJR 1997;169:1435–1438.

153. Rundback JH, Leonardo R, Rozenblit G, Poplausky MR. Vein rupture complicating hemodialysis access angioplasty: percutaneous treatment and outcomes in seven patients. AJR 1998; 171:1081–1084.

154. Hurlbert SN, Rutherford RB. Primary subclavian-axillary vein thrombosis. Ann Vasc Surg 1995;9:217–223.

155. Rutherford RB. Primary subclavian-axillary vein thrombosis: the relative roles of thrombolysis, percutaneous angioplasty, stents, and surgery. Semin Vasc Surg 1998;11(2):91–95.

156. Hall LD, Murray JD, Boswell GE. Venous stent placement as an adjunct to the staged, multimodal treatment of Paget-Schroetter syndrome. J Vasc Intervent Radiol 1995;6:565–569.

157. Rutherford RB, Hurlbert SN. Primary subclavian-axillary thrombosis: consensus and commentary. Cardiovasc Surg 1996;4: 420–423.

158. Meier GH, Pollack JS, Rosenblatt M, et al. Initial experience with venous stents in exertional axillary-subclavian vein thrombosis. J Vasc Surg 1996;24:974–981.

159. Perez CA, Presant CA, Van Amburg AL. Management of superior vena cava syndrome. Semin Oncol 1978;5:123–124.

160. Irving JD, Dondelinger RF, Reidy JF, et al. Gianturco self-expanding stents: clinical experience in the vena cava and large veins. Cardiovasc Intervent Radiol 1991;15:328–333.

161. Gaines PA, Belli AM, Anderson PB, et al. Superior vena caval obstruction managed by the Gianturco Z stent. Clin Radiol 1994;49:202–208.

162. Watkinson AF, Hansell DM. Expandable Wallstent for the treatment of obstruction of the superior vena cava. Thorax 1993; 48:915–920.

163. Dyet JF, Nicholson AA, Cook AM. The use of the Wallstent endovascular prosthesis in the treatment of malignant obstruction of the superior vena cava. Clin Radiol 1993;48:381–385.

164. Elson JD, Becker GJ, Wholey MH, Ehrman KO. Vena caval and central venous stenoses: management with Palmaz balloon-expandable intraluminal stents. J Vasc Intervent Radiol 1991;2: 215–223.

165. Kee ST, Kinoshita L, Razavi MK, Nyman URO, Semba CP, Dake MD. Superior vena cava syndrome: treatment with catheter-directed thrombolysis and endovascular stent placement. Radiology 1998;206:187–193.

166. Hochrein J, Bashore TM, O'Laughlin MP, Harrison JK. Percutaneous stenting of superior vena cava syndrome: a case report and review of the literature. Am J Med 198;104:78–84.

167. Crowe MT, Davies CH, Gaines PA. Percutaneous management of superior vena cava occlusions. Cardiovasc Intervent Radiol 1995;18:367–372.

168. Dondelinger RF, Goffette P, Kurdziel J, Roche A. Expandable metal stents for stenosis of the venae cavae and large veins. Semin Intervent Radiol 1991;8:252–263.

169. Rosch J, Uchida BT, Hall DL, et al. Gianturco-Rosch expandable Z-stents in the treatment of superior vena cava syndrome. Cardiovasc Intervent Radiol 1992;15:319–327.

170. Rosenblum J, Leef J, Messersmith R, et al. Intravascular stents in the management of acute superior vena cava obstruction of benign etiology. J Parenter Enteral Nutr 1994;18:362–366.

171. Rilinger N, Gorich J, Mickley V, et al. Endovascular stenting in patients with iliac compression syndrome. Experience in three cases. Invest Radiol 1996;31(11):729–733.

172. Juhan CM, Alimi YS, Barthelemy PJ, Fabre DF, Riviere CS. Late results of iliofemoral venous thrombectomy. J Vasc Surg 1997;25(3): 417–422.

173. Semba CP, Dake MD. Iliofemoral deep venous thrombosis: aggressive therapy with catheter-directed thrombolysis. Radiology 1994;191:487–494.

174. Bjarnason H, Druse JR, Asinger DA, et al. Iliofemoral deep venous thrombosis: safety and efficacy outcomes during 5 years of catheter-directed thrombolytic therapy. J Vasc Intervent Radiol 1997;8(3):405–418.

175. Nazarian GK, Bjarnason H, Dietz CA, Bernadas CA, Hunter DW. Iliofemoral venous stenoses: effectiveness of treatment with metallic endovascular stents. Radiology 1996;200:193–199.

176. Palmaz JC. Intravascular stents: tissue-stent interactions and design considerations. AJR 1993;160:613–618.

177. Schurmann K, Vorwerk D, Kulisch A, et al. Neointimal hyperplasia in low-profile nitinol stents, Palmaz stents, and Wallstents: a comparative experimental study. Cardiovasc Intervent Radiol 1996;19:248–254.

178. Newman VS, Berry JL, Routh WD, Ferario CM, Dean RM. Effects of vascular stent surface area and hemodynamics on intimal thickening. J Vasc Intervent Radiol 1996;7:387–393.

179. Vorwerk D, Redha F, Neuerburg J, Clerc C, Gunther RW. Neointima formation following arterial stent placement of self-expanding stents of different radial force: experimental results. Cardiovasc Intervent Radiol 1994;17:27–32.

180. Seeger JM, Ingegno MD, Bigatan E, et al. Hydrophilic surface modification of metallic endoluminal stents. J Vasc Surg 1995;21: 327–335.

181. Serruys PW, Emanuelsson H, van der Giessen W, et al. Heparin-coated Palmaz-Schatz stent in human coronary arteries: early outcome of the Benestent-II pilot study. Circulation 1996;93:412–422.

182. Srivatsa SS, Fitzpatrick LA, Tsao PW, et al. Selective alpha v beta 3 integrin blockade potently limits neointimal hyperplasia and lumen stenosis following deep coronary arterial stent injury: evidence for the functional importance of integrin alpha v beta 3 and osteopontin expression during neointima formation. Cardiovasc Res 1997;26:408–428.

183. Carter AJ, Fischell TA. Current status of radioactive stents for the prevention of in-stent restenosis. Int J Radiat Oncol Biol Phys 1998;122:127–133.

184. Hehrlein C, Kubler W. Advantages and limitations of radioactive stents. Semin Intervent Cardiol 1997;122:109–113.

2

Polymeric Vascular Graft Materials

JULIO C. PALMAZ

Information about properties of vascular graft materials has traditionally been in the domain of scientists and engineers who specialize in vascular endoprosthetics or catheter manufacturing. But with the evolution of endovascular techniques, medical professionals have become increasingly interested in the technical aspects of implantable materials, as well. For example, a physician placing an endovascular stent-graft for correction of an aortic abdominal aneurysm needs a device that promotes thrombosis on its outer surface to avoid endoleaks yet prevents thrombosis on its inner surface to support long-term patency. While a single material with dual surface properties is not yet available, it is important for the medical practitioner to recognize that a great deal of development and testing of vascular polymeric bypass materials has already been done. With insight from this work, it may be possible to develop modified polymeric materials for stent-graft use. Therefore, it is important for medical professionals, as well as scientists and engineers, to understand the composition and structure of polymeric materials that are being developed for endovascular applications.

Different properties are required from vascular substitute materials with regard to target vessel size (Table 2–1). While antithrombogenic properties are desirable at the lumen surface of vascular conduits of all sizes, resistance to thrombosis is especially important in conduits of small diameter. However, mechanical endurance is a problem for large conduits but not small ones. Difficulties arise in the design of intermediate-sized conduits, where properties such as thromboresistance and durability are both required.

Polymeric materials that are currently available differ in regard to thromboresistance, durability, and physical characteristics. For instance, expanded polytetrafluoroethylene (ePTFE) conduits are relatively plastic. For this reason, tubular ePTFE conduits that have been manufactured for use as surgical bypass conduits can be mounted on the outside of a balloon-expandable stent and stretched to a much greater diameter. Because of the plasticity of ePTFE, once it has been stretched there is minimal elastic recoil, and it remains implanted with very little residual stress (Table 2–2).

Polyethylene terephthalate (PET) is a rigid polymeric fabric that has been used extensively for vascular repair and bypass grafting. Because it is rigid, it can only be used in a textile form—woven or knitted. While PET is rigid and ePTFE is plastic, once these materials are implanted in vivo they both remain relatively free from residual stress. Polyurethanes (PUs) are elastomeric and, unlike ePTFE and PET, when stretched by a stent they remain stress-loaded.

Vascular polymers are also quite different with regard to surface energy, which in turn may be loosely correlated with thrombogenicity. For example, ePTFE has low surface energy and low thrombogenicity (Table 2–3). Metals typically have high surface energy and high thrombogenicity. PET and PU are somewhere in between on these two parameters.

While surface energy is an important factor, it is nevertheless only one of many parameters that defines surface reactivity. Although surface reactivity is incompletely understood, it is important in both early and late biological interactions (Table 2–4). Increased sur-

Stent-Grafts: Current Clinical Practice. Edited by Dolmatch and Blum. Thieme Medical Publishers, Inc., New York © 2000.

TABLE 2–1. Relevance of the Main Biological Properties of Biopolymers in Regard to Endovascular Conduit Diameter

	Large Diameter	Small Diameter
Thromboresistance	+	++
Mechanical endurance	++	+
Tissue reaction	+	++

+, mild to moderate; ++, moderate to marked.

TABLE 2–3. Surface Free Energy and Thrombogenicity of Vascular Polymers

	Surface Free Energy (dynes/cm)	Thrombogenicity (Subjective)
PTFE	1.8	Low
PET	18.9	Moderate
PU	20.6	Moderate
316-L SS	31.5	High

face reactivity potentiates acute thrombosis, but induces tissue incorporation that may provide long-term patency. In contrast, low surface reactivity reduces thrombogenicity in the early phase, but may lead to poor tissue ingrowth and late thrombosis. These considerations are critical when considering materials for use in stent-grafts and pose many challenges for future development.

It is also important to recognize that the combination of a stent and polymeric graft material may produce a device with mechanical and biological properties of both materials. Furthermore, a composite device of stent and graft may ultimately heal differently from graft alone. However, this chapter considers only polymeric graft materials, focusing on the physicochemical and biological properties of the three materials that are being used or considered for endovascular stent-grafts: PET, ePTFE, and PU.

■ Chemical Structure of Vascular Polymers

PET is composed of long chains of alternating units of glycol and terephthalic acid (Fig. 2–1). The tensile strength of PET is derived from the high dissociation energies of the covalent bonds along the polymer chain. Weaker hydrogen and van der Waals forces determine the spatial conformation of the chains that are characteristically disposed as alternating segments of tangled and parallel arrangement at 10-nm intervals. This gives PET fibers the microscopic appearance

of concentric dark and light bands surrounding nuclei or spherulites.[1]

ePTFE is chemically composed of carbon chains saturated with fluorine (Fig. 2–1). The chain twists 180 degrees every 13 carbon atoms. Because of the large size of fluorine atoms in comparison to carbon atoms, the former arrange themselves as a sheath completely covering the carbon chain.[2] This arrangement provides conformational rigidity and chemical stability that may explain some of the characteristics of this polymer such as low friction coefficient and high melting point.[3] These physical aspects of ePTFE correlate with some of the biological properties such as low thrombogenicity and modest tissue reaction. Microscopically, ePTFE shows bands with width and length depending on the molecular weight and conditions of crystallization. These bands have perpendicular striations resulting from repeating crystalline and noncrystalline zones. In the crystalline portions or striae, the ePTFE molecules are arranged in a parallel fashion, perpendicular to the long axis of the bands, and chain folding occurs in the noncrystalline areas.[4]

PUs are a chemically complex and diverse group of related compounds. PUs can be rigid or soft, depending on their composition. Current vascular PUs are elastomeric and, like other related compounds, have polymeric chains with alternating aliphatic soft segments and urethane derivative or hard segments (Fig. 2–2). While the urethane portion of the chain tends to form hydrogen bonds with adjacent similar moieties forming crystals, the aliphatic segments are randomly oriented.[5] PUs have been tried in the past,

TABLE 2–2. Endovascular Materials Mechanics

	During Deployment	After Deployment
ePTFE	Plastic	Minimal residual stress
PET	Rigid	Nonstressed
PU	Elastic	Stressed

ePTFE, expanded polytetrafluoroethylene; PET, polyesterterephthalate; PU, polyurethane.

TABLE 2–4. Thrombogenicity, Healing and Risk of Occulsion of Vascular Polymers

Magnitude	Early Outcome	Late Outcome	Risk to Manage
High	Thrombogenic	Healing potential	Early occlusion
Low	Nonthrombogenic	No healing potential	Delayed occlusion

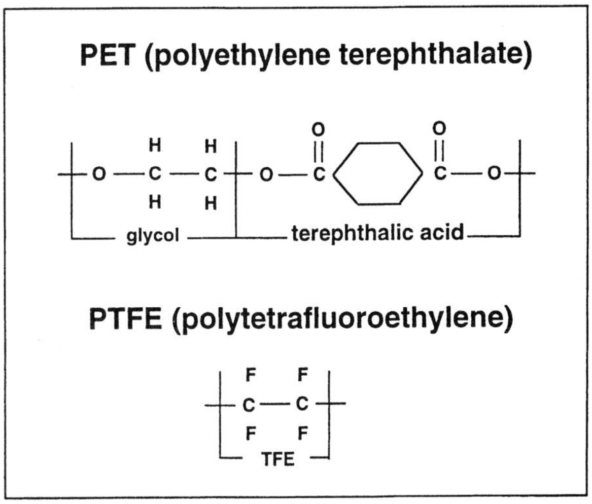

PET (polyethylene terephthalate)

PTFE (polytetrafluoroethylene)

FIGURE 2–1. Basic backbone units of PET (top) and PTFE (bottom).

■ Physical Properties of Vascular Polymers

Among the various physical properties of the vascular polymers, surface energy influences both early (Table 2–3) and late biocompatibility phenomena. Surface energy is a physical parameter that defines, among other things, the behavior of fluids on the material's surface. For example, the lower the energy, the lower the water affinity for the surface. Although the ideal energy in regard to vascular biocompatibility is debatable,[7,8] there is a rough correlation between high energy levels and increased thrombogenicity among the materials relevant to this subject.

The three vascular polymers under consideration have very different mechanical properties. PET is relatively rigid and is manufactured as bundled fibers, and therefore the vascular prosthetic applications of PET are largely in textile forms. Of the two most common fabrics, knitted and woven, the latter is the most commonly used for endovascular applications because it can be made in very thin profiles (Fig. 2–3). However, woven PET fabrics do not stretch, tend to wrinkle and pleat easily, and have limited ability to conform to sinuous tubular shapes. Knitted PET is classified as warp or weft depending on the predominant orientation of the fibers in the transverse or longitudinal axis of the conduit, respectively.[9] Knitted fabrics are more pliable than woven ones, particularly when crimped with transverse ridges. However, the greater wall thickness of knitted PET compared to woven PET precludes the use of knitted material for endovascular applications where low profile is

as vascular substitutes, but have failed because of biodegradation. Early PUs such as polyether and polyester polyurethanes were susceptible to hydrolytic degradation at the ester linkages in the soft segments.[6] In recently developed PUs, such as polycarbonate polyurethane (Corethane, Corvita, Inc., Miami, FL; ChronoFlex, PolyMedica, Woburn, MA), the polymer chain sites deemed to be at risk of cleavage were replaced with chemical groups resistant to degradation. These modifications in the chemical structure are claimed to have solved the biodegradation problem of PU.[6]

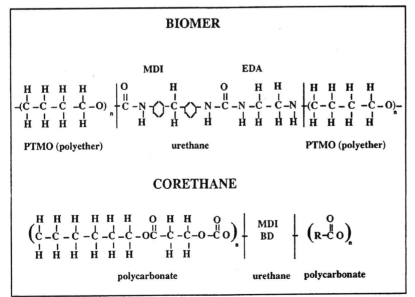

FIGURE 2–2. Basic backbone units of polyether polyurethane (Biomer) and polycarbonate polyurethane (Corethane).

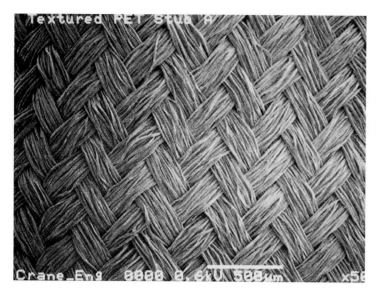

FIGURE 2–3. Scanning electron micrograph of woven PET. Each fiber bundle consists of many individual strands of PET. This woven material can be made very thin while retaining its relative inelasticity.

necessary. Woven PET can be manufactured in thicknesses of 0.1 mm or less.[10]

Since PET fabric, particularly in woven form, is dimensionally rigid after placement, it only remains stressed by the stretching effect of the anchoring stents or the supportive skeleton used to maintain tubular shape. ePTFE is substantially plastic and after deployment carries a small residual elastic load against the anchoring apparatus that does not seem to disappear with time.[11]

PUs, in the durometer grade used for vascular applications, are elastomeric and therefore have full elastic recovery within the stress limits imposed. This means that the material after deployment remains significantly stressed. This may be of some concern for PUs because permanent elastic loading accelerates degradation.[5] For this reason mechanical endurance of these polymers is commonly evaluated under stressed conditions.[12]

The mechanical endurance and structural integrity of any endovascular material is a matter of concern in large vessels because as the wall tension increases proportionately with the diameter so does the mechanical load to the device. Just as it happens with stents, stent-grafts need to remain mechanically and structurally sound through the survival of the host because any degree of tissue encapsulation of the material cannot be expected to bear the mechanical loads imposed. Pseudoaneurysm formation and possible rupture should be expected if the stent-graft disrupts or detaches itself from the point of anchorage. PET and ePTFE materials are approved vascular surgical materials, but if modifications are introduced to meet the needs for endovascular application, new tests may be required to assure that biological and mechanical endurance is not decreased. Both PET and ePTFE thin wall conduits need to be proven to resist dilatation or any other form of failure after long-term implant. Tensile strength of ePTFE, radially dilated for endovascular use, was found slightly decreased in the radial direction and significantly decreased longitudinally.[11] Similar observations were made in samples explanted 1 year after placement in dogs.[13]

Expansion is part of the manufacturing process that modifies solid PTFE material into a porous lattice. Unlike PET, PTFE cannot be formed by melt extrusion. Tubular extrusion of a mixture of PTFE powder and a mineral spirit followed by heating produces partial coalescence of the particles. Longitudinal expansion at this point results in separation of the particles and formation of longitudinal strands or fibrils (Fig. 2–4). Therefore, PTFE for vascular prosthetic applications is known as "expanded" polytetrafluoroethylene (ePTFE). The particles remain as solid plates or nodes disposed perpendicularly to the longitudinal axis of the tubing. After expansion, this structure is set in a stable form by an additional heating process called sintering.[3,11] The large proportion of air in the material following longitudinal expansion of extruded tubing accounts for its white color.

The ePTFE vascular conduits are manufactured as simple or composite materials. In the latter, two layers are disposed at a 90 degree angle to each other to reinforce their hoop strength. Single-layer tubing is preferred for endovascular applications because it is amenable to radial expansion, which can be done before or during an endovascular procedure. When ePTFE is used to cover a balloon-expandable metal stent, the material dilates simultaneously with the stent, with a resulting decrease in the material's wall thickness.[11] Stents are intended to serve as anchoring devices, reinforcing skeleton, or both. Radial expansion of ePTFE tubing is possible because of the plastic elongation of the circumferentially oriented nodes. As the nodes elongate, the insertion points of the

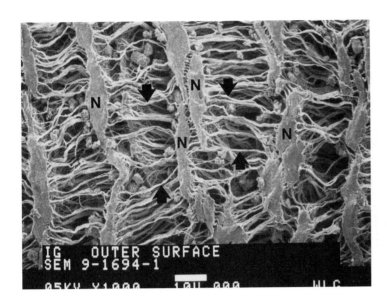

FIGURE 2–4. Scanning electron micrograph of expanded polytetrafluoroethylene (ePTFE). Note the dense PTFE bands, called nodes (N), and the filamentous cross-bridging fibrils (arrows). One measure of ePTFE porosity is the distance between the nodes, which is called the internodal distance (IND).

fibrils spread, but the fibril length remains unchanged. The radial force needed to radially expand ePTFE is relatively low in small diameter tubing, but it may be significant at large diameters. Therefore, most authors prefer to expand ePTFE simultaneously with the stent at the target site, for a final diameter of 12 mm or smaller. For these diameters, 3-mm ePTFE tubing can be used, which is easily dilated with currently available high pressure balloons. For larger target diameters, ePTFE can be preexpanded prior to insertion and folded around the longitudinal axis of the balloon prior to insertion in the delivery sheath. Although ePTFE can be dilated five to six times the original diameter, three to four times expansion is practical and probably safe.[11] Radial dilatation affects some physical properties of ePTFE more than others. Both the longitudinal and radial tensile strength are significantly decreased after expansion, and the ability of the material to hold sutures is significantly decreased. Therefore, if sutures are used to anchor the material to stents, it is possible that a tear may develop at the suture site during deployment, causing the material to fall out of the stent-graft assembly.[11] Anchoring of ePTFE to the stent should be done with a noncutting tapered needle with a diameter matched to the suture thread.[11] Preferred suture material is 6–0 polyester coated with polybutilate (Ethibond, Ethicon, Inc., Sommerville, NJ) or ePTFE (Goretex, WL Gore & Associates, Elkton, MD).

Porosity of ePTFE, measured as the pressure required to promote transmural fluid leak, is actually decreased after radial dilatation because the distance between nodes does not change. The decreased porosity may be related to crowding of the fibrils as the material loses thickness by radial expansion.[11] Fortunately, radially expanded ePTFE does not lose a significant amount of its tensile strength following implantation in animals.[13]

A relevant practical consideration is the tendency of ePTFE tubing to shorten longitudinally during balloon dilatation, if the coaxial balloon is longer than the segment of ePTFE to be dilated. This is caused by the tendency of the balloon to inflate first at the noncovered ends. This causes the ePTFE to retract toward the center, tearing the sutures away from the material. Also, radial expansion of the retracted material becomes more difficult because the unyielding fibrils orient themselves along the circumference as the ePTFE tube shortens. To avoid disruption of the ePTFE during deployment, the total balloon length, including the tapered ends, should match the length of ePTFE. Cutting of ePTFE tubing to a desired length can be done with a sharp scalpel blade against a firm background. This helps to avoid fraying of the edges.

PUs are not yet approved by the U.S. Food and Drug Administration (FDA) as a vascular substitute material and are currently undergoing clinical evaluation studies. One device (Corvita, Inc., Miami, FL) combines a braided elastic stent made of chromium-cobalt-nickel alloy with Corethane, a PU elastomer that is believed to be more biostable than many other PUs. The polymer is spun woven around a rotating mandrel in the form of monofilaments that are extruded in liquid form from fine nozzles. Corethane solidifies by evaporation of the solvent.[14] Porosity is determined by the angle of winding (pitch angle), the thickness of each filament, and number of layers of Corethane (Fig. 2–5). Expansion of the Corvita stent-graft, up to six times its constrained diameter,[15] is accomplished by elastic recovery of the braided metallic stent with its Corethane cover. Change in the pitch angle of the composite stent tines and spun woven cover partially accounts for the increase in diameter as the device shortens.

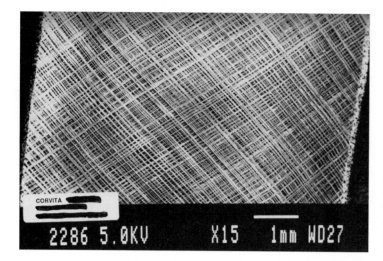

FIGURE 2–5. Scanning electron micrograph of the flow surface of a Corethane graft. The individual fibers have been created by a spray/evaporation technique that allows variation of fiber thickness and crossing angle relative to other deposited fibers. Using this method, the porosity of the graft material can be altered.

■ Choice of Polymer for Endovascular Applications

Because thrombogenicity is most relevant for small-caliber conduits, ePTFE seems to be the material of choice for target site diameters up to 10 mm. There is clinical and laboratory evidence of decreased thrombus formation on the surface of ePTFE as compared with PET when used as surgical bypass conduit.[16,17] A neointimal layer is minimal or absent, except at the transition with the adjacent vessel surface. Endothelium has been found scattered through the lumen of animal and human endovascular ePTFE,[11,18] but often not confluent or complete. Since a neointimal layer seems to be necessary for firm attachment of endothelium, it is not unexpected to find some degree of neointimal formation in endovascular ePTFE.[19]

The ideal porosity of polymeric materials is a matter of debate. Porosity of PET fabrics is difficult to define, as it depends on the cross section of the filament, bundling of the yarn, and type of weave. In ePTFE, a structural correlate to porosity is the mean internodal distance (IND) between adjacent nodes. However, the distance between fibrils is usually not considered despite the fact that it should also affect porosity. ePTFE material for surgical bypass commonly has an IND of 30 μm. However, ePTFE can be manufactured with larger INDs and perhaps this should be a feature of ePTFE material for dedicated endovascular use. Some authors believe that pore size should be small enough to prevent tissue penetration that may lead to exuberant neointimal growth.[20] Others advocate large pore size to stimulate myofibroblastic and capillary penetration. Capillary growth through the interstices of the material wall could provide a source of endothelialization as the vessels reach the luminal surface.[21] However, pore size is not the only factor determining the ability of tissue to grow through the prosthetic material. PET fabrics have large pore size

but tissue penetration does not consistently reach the luminal surface. Because altering porosity does not seem to alter the healing pattern of PET,[9] it is possible that the surface characteristics of this material, rather than the structure, may determine tissue response.

Largely because of its thrombogenicity, PET conduits are reserved for endovascular implants 10 mm or larger. The flow magnitude in vessels of these diameters usually prevents thrombus formation. However, thrombogenicity may not be a disadvantage for certain applications, such as endovascular grafting of aortic aneurysms, because it may assist in the thrombosis of the stagnant blood flow in the excluded aneurysmal lumen. Failure of thrombosis to occur leads to a leak between the graft material and the aneurysmal wall. Lower leak rates reported with PET-covered devices[10] as compared with ePTFE-covered devices[22] (15% versus 50%, respectively) suggests an advantage of the former material in this application. It is therefore conceivable that a dual layer cover, consisting of a low thrombogenicity material such as ePTFE on the inside of the stent-graft and a thrombogenic material such as PET on the outside surface, may be practical. In addition, a fibroblastic tissue reaction to an outer layer of PET may be beneficial in large vessel applications because it may promote adherence of the device to the vessel wall or thrombus. This is of critical importance in aortic aneurysms where the potential for dilatation of the aorta at the points of anchor of the device implies a risk for development of an attachment site leak and subsequent rupture.

■ Conclusion

None of the materials considered in this brief review are ideal for vascular endoprosthetic use. Selection of any one polymeric graft material at the present time is a compromise between its advantages and limitations.

However, it is expected that engineering modifications of both the structure and basic chemistry of the current materials or development of entirely new ones may result in better endovascular stent-grafts.

REFERENCES

1. Hastings GW, Ducheyne P. Macromolecular Biomaterials. CRC Series in Structure-Property Relationship of Biomaterials. Boca Raton, FL: CRC Press, 1984.

2. ICI Advanced Materials. Physical properties of "fluon" unfilled and "fluorocomp" filled ePTFE. Technical Service Note F12/13. 2nd ed. Wekwyn Garden, Herts, England: Imperial Chemical Industries PLC Advanced Materials Business Group.

3. McClurken ME, McHaney JM, Colone WM. Physical properties and test methods for expanded polytetraflouroethylene (ePTFE) grafts. Authorized reprint from Special Technical Publication 898. Philadelphia: American Society for Testing Materials, 1986.

4. Speerschneider CJ, Li CH. Some observations on the structure of polytetrafluoroethylene. J Appl Physics 1962;33:1871–1874.

5. Stokes K, McVenes R. Polyurethane elastomer biostability. J Biomater Appl 1995;9:321–354.

6. Pinchuck L. A review of the biostability and carcinogenicity of polyurethanes in medicine and the new generation of "biostable" polyurethanes. J Biomater Sci Polymer Edn 1994;6:225–267.

7. Baier RE, Dutton RC. Initial events in interaction of blood with a foreign surface. J Biomed Mater Res 1969;3:191–206.

8. Ruckenstein E, Gourisankar SV. A surface energy criterion of blood compatibility of foreign surfaces. J Colloid Interface Sci 1984;101:436–451.

9. Snyder WR. Fabrication and testing of textile vascular prostheses. In: Wright CB, Hobson RW, Hiratka LF, Lynch TG, eds. Vascular Grafting. Clinical Applications and Techniques. pp. 13–22. Boston: John Wright-PSG, 1983.

10. Blum U, Voshage G, Lammer J, et al. Endoluminal stent-grafts for infrarenal abdominal aortic aneurysms. N Engl J Med 1997;336: 13–20.

11. Palmaz F, Sprague E, Palmaz JC. Physical properties of polytetrafluoroethylene bypass material after balloon dilatation. J Vasc Intervent Radiol 1996;7:657–663.

12. Szycher M, Reed A, Siciliano AA. In vivo testing of a biostable polyurethane. J Biomat Appl 1991;6:110–130.

13. Palmaz JC, Tio FO, Laborde JC, et al. Use of stents covered with polytetrafluoroethylene in experimental abdominal aortic aneurysm. J Vasc Intervent Radiol 1995;6:879–885.

14. Leidner J, Wong EWC, McGregor DC, Wilson GJ. A novel process for the manufacturing of porous grafts: process description and product evaluation. J Biomed Mater Res 1983;17:229–247.

15. Dereume JPE, Ferreira J. The Corvita system. In: Hopkinson B, Yusuf W, Whitaker S, Veith F, eds. Endovascular Surgery for Aortic Aneurysms. pp. 122–139. London: WB Saunders, 1997.

16. Hamlin GW. Evaluation of the thrombogenic potential of three types of arterial grafts in an artificial circulation. Br J Surg 1978;65: 272–276.

17. Kalman PG, Rotstein OD, Niven J, Glynn MFX, Romaschin AD. Differential stimulation of macrophage procoagulant activity by vascular grafts. J Vasc Surg 1993;17:531–537.

18. Marin ML, Veith FJ, Cynamon J, et al. Human transluminally placed endovascular stented grafts: preliminary histopathologic analysis of healing grafts in aortoiliac and femoral occlusive disease. J Vasc Surg 1995; 21:595–604.

19. Palmaz JC. Lifeline Foundation Research Initiatives in Vascular Disease Conference, "How to Build a Blood Vessel," Bethesda, MD, Feb. 28, 1997.

20. Marin ML, Veith FJ, Cynamon J, et al. Effect of polytetrafluoroethylene covering of Palmaz stents on the development of intimal hyperplasia in human iliac arteries. J Vasc Intervent Radiol 1996;7:651–656.

21. Clouse AW, Kirkman TR, Reidy MA. Mechanisms of arterial graft healing. Rapid transmural capillary ingrowth provides a source of intimal endothelium and smooth muscle in porous ePTFE prostheses. Am J Pathol 1986;123:220–230.

22. Kato N, Dake MD, Semba CP, et al. Treatment of aortoiliac aneurysms using single-piece tapered stent-grafts. J Vasc Intervent Radiol 1998;9:41–49.

3

Healing Response to Vascular Stent-Grafts

BART L. DOLMATCH, YONG HUA DONG, AND LUCAS H. BRENNECKE

The molecular and cellular processes that contribute to healing of endovascular stent-grafts are complex. Nevertheless, the final response consists of a varying combination of four tissue types: thrombus, neointima, endothelium, and inflammatory cell infiltrates. Schatz[1] characterized the earliest response to metallic stent implantation in a canine model, noting early thrombus formation, with subsequent development of a cellular neointima that matures into a relatively fibrotic neointima. Endothelialization of the mural thrombus begins within the first few days of thrombus deposition, and a monolayer of endothelial cells usually covers the luminal surface of this neointima within a few weeks. The healing response to various stent-grafts in canine and porcine models, as well as in humans, has been studied recently. While the time frame of healing parallels that seen with metallic stents, the degree of proliferation and the location of each of the four tissue types is influenced by a number of factors: the type of polymeric graft, microstructure and porosity of the graft material, location of the metal stent struts, and mechanical factors related to placement of the stent-graft. This chapter reviews the endovascular healing response related to three synthetic polymeric materials that have been used in stent-grafts—expanded polytetrafluoroethylene (ePTFE), polyethylene terephthalate (PET), and polyurethanes (PUs)—focusing on those healing characteristics that are relevant to stent-graft use in humans. A brief overview of bioabsorbable graft materials and biological stent-graft coverings such as collagen and autologous vein is also presented.

■ Bare Stents

Within the first few seconds following implantation, fibrin and other plasma proteins are deposited upon the metallic struts of a stent.[2] This, in effect, passivates the electronegative stent surface and prepares it for cellular colonization. Within the first 15 minutes following stent implantation, platelets and leukocytes adhere to the fibrin-covered stent surface and contribute to early thrombus formation. The degree of thrombus that forms on the stent struts influences the proliferation of subsequent neointimal growth.[1] After several days, the earliest myointimal cells and some inflammatory cells (polymorphonuclear leukocytes and macrophages) are seen within the thrombus. This cellular response proceeds with deposition of a collagenous matrix, proliferation of myointimal cells, and development of a monocellular endothelial layer. Although this process is focused upon the stent struts (Fig. 3–1A), it typically becomes generalize to include the entire surface within 3 months (Fig. 3–1B). The degree of neointimal proliferation will ultimately determine the degree of stent-related or in-stent restenosis.

Inflammation is occasionally seen after metallic stent implantation, often in association with disruption of the internal elastic media, compression of the substent arterial media, or the presence of thrombus that is undergoing organization. There is no evidence that metal stents are particularly inflammatory. This is probably owing to the early deposition of fibrin and plasma proteins that reduces the exposure of the stent to blood flow. When it is seen, stent-related inflammation is

Stent-Grafts: Current Clinical Practice. Edited by Dolmatch and Blum. Thieme Medical Publishers, Inc., New York © 2000.

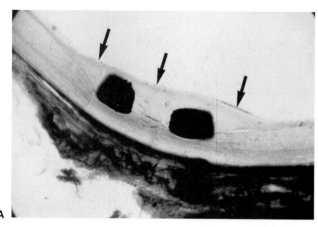
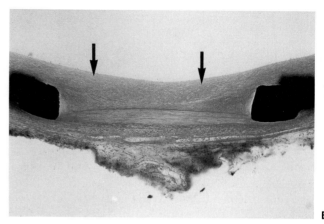

A   B

FIGURE 3–1. Photomicrograph of canine iliac artery stent implants. **(A).** At 1 month there is a focal mound of organized thrombus around the stent struts (arrows). **(B).** At 3 months, organized thrombus (arrows) has evolved into a generalized neointimal covering of the entire vascular lumen.

characterized by mononuclear cell infiltrates and rarely by multinucleated giant cell formation. It is unusual to see signs of inflammation beyond 1 month in animal models.

Injury to the vessel wall following vascular stent placement occurs predominantly at the ends of the stent (Fig. 3–2). We believe it is caused by forceful expansion (or even overexpansion) of the noncompliant stent ends within the artery (during Palmaz stent deployment or balloon dilatation following Wallstent deployment). This can lead to disruption of the internal elastic lamina and media, and even transmural perforation by the ends of the stent struts. A recent report by Farb et al[3] confirmed the importance of avoiding stent-related

arterial wall trauma. They described stent-induced trauma to the media of human coronary arteries, with an associated increase of inflammation and in-stent restenosis. The recommendation from that study, as well as our conclusion from the laboratory, is that any dilation of a stent should be performed gently, taking care to avoid unnecessary trauma to the vessel wall particularly at the ends of the stent. Similar vascular wall injury has been noted in our lab in association with postimplantation balloon dilation of various stent-grafts. We therefore believe that care should be used when balloon dilating stents and stent-grafts in an effort to limit neointimal stenosis adjacent to the ends of the implant.

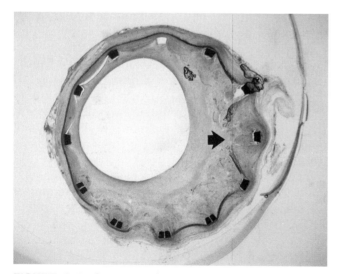

FIGURE 3–2. Cross section through the end of a stent placed in a pig iliac artery 6 weeks earlier. The internal elastic lamina has been ruptured (arrow) and there is proliferative neointima related to this traumatic event.

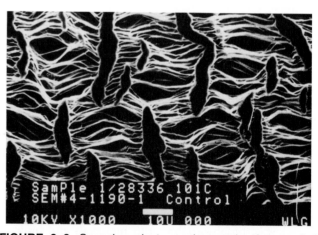

FIGURE 3–3. Scanning electron micrograph of expanded polytetrafluoroethylene (ePTFE). The dark vertical bands are nodes and the thin white filaments that bridge the nodes are fibrils. The length of the fibrils is the internodal distance (IND).

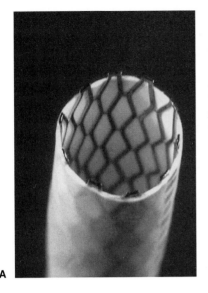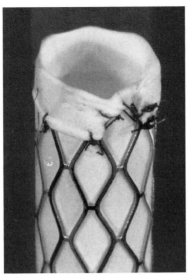

FIGURE 3–4. Prototypes of the ePTFE stent-grafts used in our canine experiments. (**A**). Outer-covered stent-graft, with both metal stent and ePTFE graft exposed on the inside. (**B**). Inner-covered stent-graft, with only ePTFE exposed on the inside.

■ Expanded Polytetrafluoroethylene (ePTFE)

Expanded polytetrafluoroethylene (ePTFE) has a complex microstructure consisting of parallel nodes and cross-bridging fibrils (Fig. 3–3). This design has been optimized to yield a synthetic conduit that has acceptable handling and healing characteristics for surgical bypass grafting. Most clinical experience has been obtained using ePTFE stent-grafts made by suturing this graft material to the outside of a Palmaz stent. These homemade ePTFE stent-grafts, therefore, have a composite luminal surface of ePTFE graft and metallic stent. We looked at healing of this type of device, comparing it to two other types of implants: an ePTFE

stent-graft with the stent on the outside and only the ePTFE graft faced the luminal flow surface, and a bare Palmaz stent (Fig. 3–4).[4] Our first observation was that the bare Palmaz stent outperformed the two ePTFE stent-grafts in terms of having the least amount of neointimal formation (in a healthy canine iliac artery model). For the ePTFE stent-grafts with both stent and graft exposed to the luminal surface, there was a fairly exuberant neointima that began as strut-associated thrombus and matured over 6 months into a relatively acellular neointima consisting of mostly collagen extracellular protein matrix (Fig. 3–5). A confluent endothelial layer was seen at 3 and 6 months by scanning electron microscopy.

The second type of ePTFE stent-graft, with only ePTFE on the luminal surface, had a scant and delicate

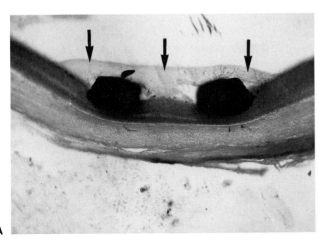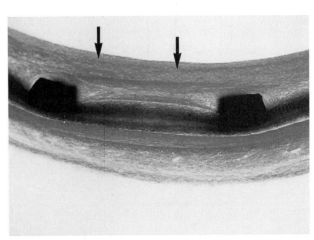

FIGURE 3–5. Cross-sections of outer-covered ePTFE stent-grafts at 1 and 3 months. (**A**). There is focal organized thrombus surrounding the metal stent struts (arrows). (**B**). The neointimal response has generalized into a complete luminal covering that blankets both the stent and the ePTFE graft material (arrows).

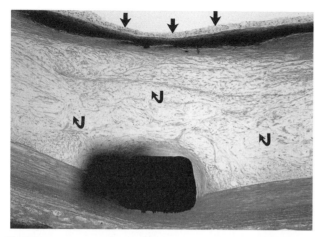

FIGURE 3–6. Cross section of the inner-covered ePTFE stent-graft at 3 months. A very thin layer of neointima is seen on the luminal surface (straight arrows). There is proliferative neointima in the subgraft layer, in association with the metal stent strut (curved arrows).

neointima that was incomplete in the 3-month explants and most of the 6-month explants. There was, however, substantial subgraft neointima seen in association with the subgraft metal stent struts (Fig. 3–6). When the stent struts are exposed to blood flow, the neointima forms predominantly on the luminal surface. When the stent struts are underneath the ePTFE, a subgraft neointima predominantly forms with only a thin, fragile, incomplete luminal neointima. These findings suggest that the metal of the stent directs the proliferation of neointima in composite ePTFE-stent implants. The importance of the metallic stent in directing the location of neointima related to ePTFE graft material has also been supported by the work of Chalmers et al.[5,6] They found that a stent placed across the anastomosis of an interposition ePTFE arterial graft shifted neointimal proliferation from the anastomosis into the stented segment of graft.

Many investigators report that endoluminal ePTFE stent-grafts develop a more complete endothelial lining than surgically placed interposition grafts.[7–9] However, Ohki et al[7] also found a greater degree of neointimal hyperplasia on the luminal surface of ePTFE stent-grafts compared to conventional bypass grafts in a canine model, whereas Ombrellaro et al[8] and Weatherford et al[9] noted an attenuated neointimal response for the stent-grafts. It is important to note that each of these studies was performed in a canine artery model, where there is a relatively poor tissue response following placement of polymeric graft materials.[10] This closely mimics the response in humans. Therefore, the finding of enhanced endothelialization for ePTFE stent-grafts compared to surgically placed ePTFE in a canine model is probably predictive of a similar response

in humans. The disparity of observations regarding the degree of neointimal proliferation, however, may be explained by difference in the experimental method or stent-graft design.

The time for an endothelial lining to form is also considerably shorter for ePTFE stent-grafts than for surgically placed ePTFE grafts. In dogs,[11] pigs,[12] and humans,[13] ePTFE stent-grafts of varying designs develop neointimal healing with a complete endothelial monolayer at 4 to 6 weeks. This is different from results for surgically placed interposition ePTFE bypass grafts, in which the endothelial covering is usually incomplete after many months.[14,15]

During our early stent-graft research we noted that balloon dilatation of ePTFE occasionally compressed the spaces between the nodes of graft material, resulting in a compacted, dense graft with scant neointimal infiltration (Fig. 3–7A). In a later experiment, we specifically used ePTFE with very large spaces between the nodes and found a highly cellular neointimal infiltration into the graft interstices (Fig. 3–7B). This ultimately led to work in a porcine model of neointimal proliferation where ePTFE stent-grafts of different pore sizes were placed in balloon-injured iliac arteries. In ePTFE with small pores, the luminal neointima consisted of a poorly adherent rind of organized thrombus that easily separated from the graft surface (Fig. 3–8A). In fact, the neointima was so poorly adherent to the graft surface that seromas were seen in vivo with intravascular ultrasound and later confirmed by histology. ePTFEs with larger pores developed less neointima that was better incorporated onto the graft surface (Fig. 3–8B). We therefore believe that there is a lower limit of pore size that allows the development of a durable and limited neointima. To date, however, this lower limit of pore size has not been adequately characterized, in part because there are no reporting standards regarding the microstructure of ePTFE graft materials besides internodal distance (IND) and water permeability. We believe that to understand the optimal microstructure for ePTFE stent-graft factors such as the interfibril distance, percent graft versus open space (related to thickness of the nodes and fibrils), graft thickness, and three-dimensional graft geometry must be considered.

The degree of inflammation associated with polymeric vascular implants correlates with neointimal proliferation, and the fact that ePTFE is less inflammatory than a number of other polymers, including PET, is an important attribute of this material.[11] In animal models of noncoronary vascular implants, macrophage infiltrates may be seen, but giant cells are rare. Overall, ePTFE stent-grafts in peripheral arteries are relatively inert. There are data, however, that show this is not true in the coronary arteries. Virtually all poly-

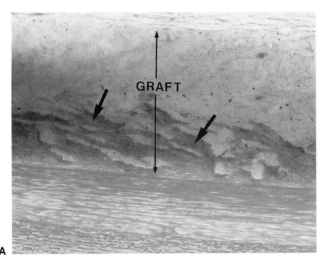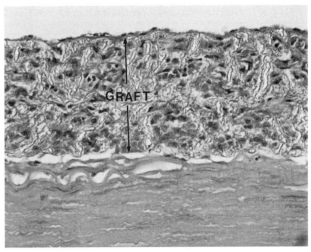

FIGURE 3–7. Photomicrographs of dense and porous ePTFE materials that have been implanted as stent-grafts into canine iliac arteries after several months. (**A**). There is little cellular infiltration of the dense ePTFE, and only a small amount of collagenous matrix within the graft interstices (arrows). (**B**). Extensive cellular infiltration into the ePTFE graft interstices has occurred in this highly porous ePTFE.

meric implants in the coronary arteries incite inflammation,[16] and the development of coronary artery stent-grafts may be limited by these findings.

In summary, we believe that ePTFE is an excellent polymeric barrier that can be optimized for endovascular use. Certain fundamentals, however, must be respected. For example, dense ePTFE of low porosity will not develop a stable neointima and in fact may lead to a greater neointimal thickness than stents alone (Fig. 3–8A). Very porous ePTFEs have not been adequately evaluated, but may be too leaky for use in the treatment of aneurysms. Metallic stent struts play an important role in directing the proliferation of neointima. Modified accordingly, ePTFE can probably be tailored for different stent-graft applications and may be the most acceptable material for use in small and medium-sized vessels with diameters between 4 and 10 mm.

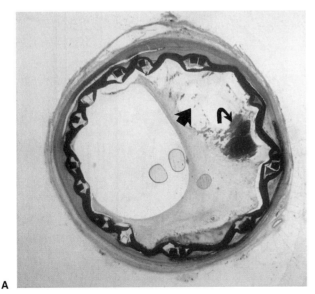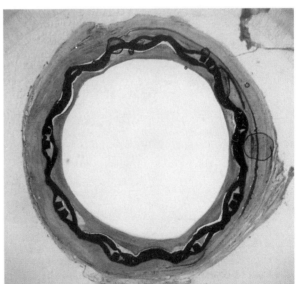

FIGURE 3–8. Low and medium porosity ePTFE stent-grafts in the pig iliac artery. (**A**). At 6 weeks there neointima has detached from the graft surface of the low porosity ePTFE. This has resulted in formation of a seroma (straight arrow) containing thrombus (curved arrow). (**B**). Medium porosity ePTFE with a stable neointimal lining (arrow) at 6 weeks. For both medium and high porosity ePTFE, there were no signs of neointimal detachment or seroma formation.

■ Polyethylene Terephthalate (PET)

Used historically as an aortic and iliac artery bypass conduit, PET is a medical-grade textile that has proven to be a durable and reliable vascular bypass graft material. Although the success of PET can be attributed to the development of this polymeric material through years of research, Wesolowski et al[17] demonstrated the relatively high tolerance to a number of materials when surgically implanted as an aortic replacement in dogs and pigs. Both woven glass and perforated metallic lead pipe remained patent for many months in the aorta, a high-flow vessel of large caliber that rarely develops occlusive thrombus or neointimal stenosis. Yet while many materials may serve as an aortic substitute, PET has been adopted as a first-line synthetic aortic graft material. It is easily handled by the surgeon and well tolerated by the patient.

PET aortic stent-grafts in animal and humans are similarly well tolerated from a healing and hemodynamic perspective. Stenosis of the aortic cuff has not been reported, and occlusion of the bifurcating iliac limbs of these stent-grafts is an uncommon event. PET implants, however, are not free from clinical problems. Following PET stent-graft implantation for treatment of abdominal aortic aneurysms, there may be an associated postimplantation syndrome in up to 25 to 35% of patients.[18–20] This syndrome, characterized by fever, pain, and leukocytosis is believed related to either the PET polymer itself or adsorbed contaminants from the manufacturing process. While no long-term adverse effects have been reported in association with this clinical syndrome, it is nevertheless uncomfortable for the patient and a cause for concern regarding the possibility that the stent-graft has become infected. There are no doubt many additional tests performed to rule out infection, including repeated complete blood counts, blood cultures, chest radiographs, and even computed tomography (CT) scans.

Despite the postimplantation syndrome, PET will probably continue to be a widely used polymeric graft material for aortic stent-grafting. The real challenge with this material, however, remains in designing stent-grafts for use in vessels 5 to 10 mm in diameter. We have characterized PET-covered Wallstents (Boston Scientific Vascular, Watertown, MA), called Wallgrafts, in a canine arterial model.[11] Inflammation related to PET Wallgrafts at 1 month was seen in gross specimens as mild to moderate adventitial swelling with enlargement of adjacent lymph nodes (Fig. 3–9). Histological evaluation revealed macrophages and foreign-body giant cells around the individual fibers and fiber bundles (Fig. 3–10A). Within 3 to 6 months, this inflammatory response had become quiescent, adventitial swelling was not seen, and there were only small infiltrates of macrophages and giant cells around the graft fibers (Fig. 3–10B). In place of the inflammatory response seen at 1 month was a diffuse fibrotic neointima at the luminal surface of the graft, often producing a diffuse in-stent stenosis of up to 50% (Fig. 3–11). Similar reports of inflammation and neoin-

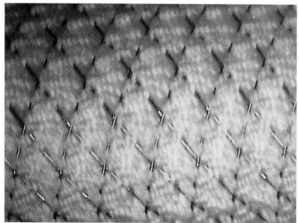

A

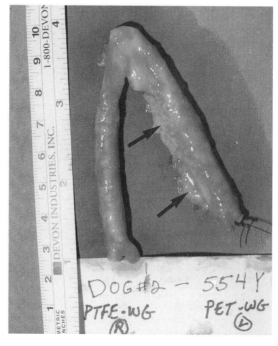

B

FIGURE 3–9. Co-braided polyethylene terephthalate (PET) Wallstent implants in the canine iliac artery. (**A**). This prototype stent-graft consists of metal Wallstent wires co-braided with PET fiber bundles. (**B**). The co-braided PET-Wallstent was placed in the right iliac artery and an ePTFE covered Wallstent in the left. This specimen was obtained after 1 month. Note the swelling and adherent adventitial fat (arrows) related to the PET implant, whereas the ePTFE stent-graft adventitia is normal in appearance and size.

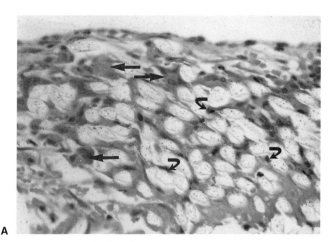
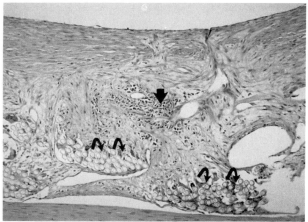

FIGURE 3–10. Findings of inflammation following implantation of PET stent-grafts. (**A**). High-power magnification of a PET stent-graft after 1 month in the canine iliac artery. The PET fibers are seen as round clear "holes." There are multinucleated giant cells (straight arrows) and macrophages (curved arrows) in between individual PET fibers. (**B**). Stable late inflammatory changes at 3 months in the canine iliac artery. A small infiltrate of macrophages is seen in the middle of the specimen (arrow). The graft fibers are noted toward the bottom of the specimen, and are surrounded by multinucleated giant cells and macrophages (curved arrows).

timal proliferation have been described in sheep iliac arteries,[21] rabbit aortae,[22] and the human aorta, iliac, and femoral arteries.[19–21,23,24]

In our experience, both the inflammatory response to PET stent-grafts and the degree of luminal narrowing seem related and cannot be ignored in small and medium-sized vessels 5 to 10 mm in diameter. In dogs, these findings are most pronounced in the femoral artery, less apparent in the iliac artery, and relatively minor in the aorta. In an intriguing clinical series of PET stent-grafts, Sapoval and colleagues[25] treated stenoses at the venous anastomosis and outflow veins of arteriovenous dialysis shunts with the Cragg PET-covered stent-grafts. Clinical signs of inflammation

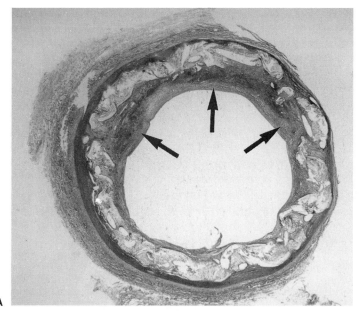
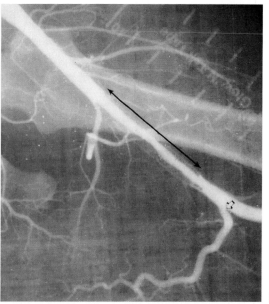

FIGURE 3–11. Fibrotic neointimal formation associated with healing of PET stent-grafts. (**A**). This cross-section shows luminal narrowing due to fibrotic neointima (arrows) after 6 months of implantation in the canine iliac artery. (**B**). Luminal narrowing 1 month after placement of a PET stent-graft in the canine femoral artery (double-headed arrow). Histology confirmed that the narrowing was due to the growth of a fibrotic neointima similar to that in **A.** A small branch vessel remains patent distal to the stent-graft (small open arrow).

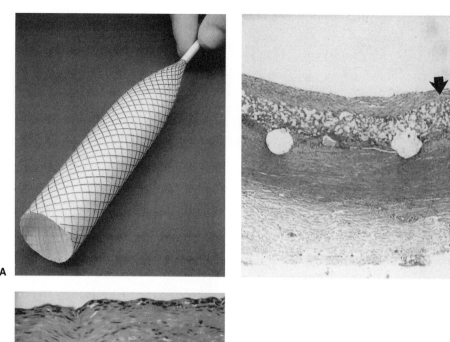

FIGURE 3–12. The Corvita polyurethane (Corethane) endoluminal graft. (**A**). A partially deployed self-expanding Corethane endoluminal stent-graft. (**B**). There is a thin luminal neointima attached to the stent-graft surface (arrow). (**C**). High-powered light micrograph of the neointimal response to the Corethane endoluminal stent-graft. The PU fibers have been removed during the process of specimen preparation and are seen as clear "holes." The neointima consists of a collagenous matrix and myointimal cells.

were seen in all three cases where the stent-graft was placed in forearm shunts. In fact, one of these stent-grafts was removed at 15 days because of severe inflammation and adjacent hematoma leading to skin necrosis. Patency was poor, as well, with 28.5% primary patency at 6 months.

Because of inflammation and neointimal stenosis, we doubt that PET will be useful in human vessels much smaller than 10 mm. While the relationship between vessel size and PET stent-graft performance is unclear, it is likely that PET use will be limited to the aorta and iliac arteries, and that clinical manifestations of the postimplantation syndrome will be unavoidable for some patients in whom PET stent-grafts are placed.

■ Polyurethanes (PUs)

This broad class of elastomers has been under evaluation as a surgical bypass graft material for nearly 40 years,[26] but only recently incorporated into stent-grafts. Most of the early polyurethanes proved to be bio-unstable, developing brittleness that led to microfissures in the graft wall of vascular implants.[27] Recent modifications have led to polycarbonate polyurethanes such as Corethane (Corvita, Inc., Miami, FL) that are believed to be resistant to degradation in vivo. Corethane serves at the polymeric graft material for the Corvita endoluminal vascular prosthesis. In dogs, the Corvita endoluminal graft develops a fibrous

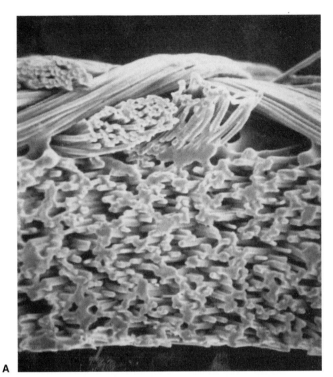

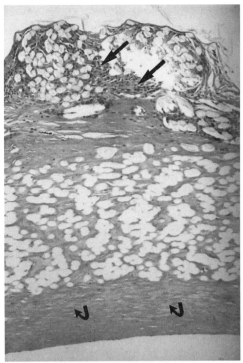

FIGURE 3–13. Composite PET-PU bypass conduit. (**A**). The woven PET fiber mesh is on the outside of the graft (top of the photograph) and the Corethane material lies beneath. (Cross section 100×.) (**B**). The PET fiber bundles are surrounded by a typical cellular inflammatory response (straight arrows). There is virtually no inflammation associated with the PU material (the clear "holes" at the middle of the specimen). Only a relatively acellular neointima covers the surface of the Corethane (curved arrows).

collagenized neointima with little inflammation or myointimal cell proliferation (Fig. 3–12A,B) similar to earlier reports of healing related to microporous polyester polyurethanes implanted as bypass conduits.[28] An interesting comparison between the relative lack of inflammation for Corethane and the inflammatory nature of PET is shown in Figure 3–13. Here, a PET-wrapped Corethane bypass graft has been removed and studied by histology. There is a great deal of inflammation associated with the PET and very little with the Corethane. Excellent patency rates for this surgically placed 4-mm composite Corethane/PET bypass conduits in dogs has been reported.[29,30]

While patency for a Corethane/PET composite is better than for similar-diameter ePTFE bypass grafts, not all reports of PU bypass graft patency are as good. Working upon prior data that showed microporous PU has a more rapid healing response and better neointimal incorporation than PET in large-caliber prostheses,[28] Geeraert and Callaghan[31] looked at PU as a small vessel replacement. They implanted 3-mm internal-diameter PU conduits in various locations in dogs and noted an exceedingly high rate of early thrombosis. Similarly, van der Lei et al[32] implanted short interposition PU grafts in

the rabbit carotid artery. They prepared half of the grafts with heparin bonding and half without, hoping that bonded heparin would reduce early thrombosis. None of their grafts, however, remained patent at 14 days. It therefore seems that the theoretical advantages of PUs, such as compliance, lack of an associated inflammatory response, and versatility of fabrication, do not confer any benefit regarding patency when PUs are used as a small-artery substitute.

The above data suggest that PU may be a useful bypass material for use in medium-size and large diameter vessels. There are virtually no data regarding the possible use of PU stent-grafts in humans. The Corvita endoluminal stent-graft trial in human iliac and femoral arteries in the United States was halted in part due to early implant occlusion. The reasons for these occlusions are not clear, and it is possible that there were early technical problems associated with device implantation. Nevertheless, at this time there are no plans to restart this clinical trial. The Corvita abdominal aortic aneurysm trial has similarly been halted, but for nonmedical reasons. While biostable polyurethanes are conceptually attractive for use in medium-size and large endovascular stent-grafts, there are no clinical studies planned in the foreseeable future. The role of PUs for endovascular treatment of aneurysms and occlusive vascular disease may not be known for many years.

■ Materials in Development

Beyond the three materials discussed so far, the history of surgical bypass conduit development includes research on a number of polymers that are poor vascular substitutes such as nylon, Vinyon-N, orlon, Ivalon, and silicone.[27,33] Biodegradable materials have been studied as well. One interesting approach has been the development of a composite graft prepared from a mixture of polyurethane and poly-L-lactic acid.[34,36] The goal was to develop a graft that would become partially replaced by the patient's own tissue, producing a stable and viable endothelium. This was achieved in the lab but unfortunately not tested in clinical practice.

Collagen has been considered as a biological polymeric covering for stent-grafts. Different properties can be obtained by selecting specific types of collagen and cross-linking them to various degrees. This affords a final material that may have different rates of biodegradation. This is attractive when considering different stent-grafts applications. For instance, if used to treat occlusive vascular disease, biodegradation of a stent-graft covering could release entrapped medications aimed at preventing neointimal hyperplasia. Meanwhile, endogenous tissues would replace the collagen. A preliminary report[37] demonstrated the feasibility of a collagen-covered stent-graft placement in a pig model (Fig. 3–14), but there are no clinical trials planned at this time.

The only biological covering that has been used in humans has been autologous vein.[38–42] The potential benefits of autologous vein are related to its natural properties, such as compliance, tolerance to radial dilation, resistance to infection, and its thin wall that makes delivery into small blood vessels feasible. In addition, there are theoretical advantages regarding thromboresistance and long-term healing, since it is the patient's own tissue. Autologous vein, however, is not a problem-free material. It must be harvested from the patient at the time of stent-graft placement, therefore necessitating a surgical procedure. The quality of the vein may vary depending on the condition of the vein and the technique used to harvest it. Finally, unlike commercially prepared synthetic stent-grafts where the stent and graft are integrally related, preparation of a vein stent-graft requires suturing vein to the stent. Therefore, there is no way to assure that the vein has not contracted on the stent or detached from the stent entirely, since the vein segment cannot be seen fluoroscopically.

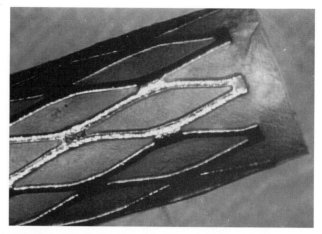

FIGURE 3–14. Early prototype of a collagen-covered Palmaz stent. Preliminary work demonstrated that collagen can function as a biodegradable graft-type barrier.

In one report using a pig model, autologous vein stent-grafts placed in the iliac arteries were thromboresistant and healed with minimal hyperplasia.[43] In another porcine experiment, patency of vein-covered stent-grafts in the iliac and carotid arteries was poor, and a significant number of implants migrated.[44] Dilatation of these implants is clearly an important component of the procedure that may limit migration and thrombosis. While all of this work is intriguing, the ultimate patency of vein stent-grafts in humans is not known. To date, most of the published literature consists of case reports without follow-up.

■ Summary

There are three polymeric vascular graft materials that have the potential for successful use in vascular stent-grafts. While ePTFE and PET are being incorporated into stent-grafts for treatment of aneurysmal and occlusive vascular disease, neither has been optimized for endovascular use. PET induces an inflammatory response that may be seen clinically as fever, leukocytosis, and pain. As the degree of inflammation increases, the tendency to develop a fibrotic neointimal stenosis within the stent-graft increases as well. Regarding inflammation and neointimal proliferation, PET is best tolerated in the aorta and iliac arteries where it is predominantly used to treat aneurysms. ePTFE is far less inflammatory than PET, and may offer advantages in treating arteries from 4 to 10 mm in diameter. Because of its microstructure, there are a number of modifications that can be made to customize ePTFE for different applications such as for treatment of occlusive peripheral vascular disease. PUs are still in a developmental phase and may not progress further as a viable option for use in endovascular stent-grafts. A number of other synthetic polymers, evaluated decades earlier for surgical use, have not been assessed as stent-graft coverings.

Biological barriers such as autologous vein and perhaps even collagen can be incorporated into stent-grafts. Stent-grafts covered with vein have been used successfully in humans. While they must be custom-made at the time of the procedure, vein-covered stent-grafts offer certain advantages that synthetic polymers cannot, such as resistance to infection, low profile, excellent compliance, and tissue compatibility during the healing phase. It is apparent that as the application of stent-grafts becomes more diverse, many of the materials that have been evaluated for surgical bypass conduit during the past decades will need to be revisited.

REFERENCES

1. Schatz RA. A view of vascular stents. Circulation 1989;79:445–457.
2. Palmaz JC. Intravascular stents: tissue-stent interactions and design considerations. AJR 1993;160:613–618.
3. Farb A, Sangiorgi G, Carter AJ, et al. Pathology of acute and chronic coronary stenting in humans. Circulation 1999;99:44–52.
4. Dolmatch BL, Tio RO, Li XD, Dong YH. Patency and tissue response related to two types of polytetrafluoroethylene-covered stents in the dog. J Vasc Intervent Radiol 1996;7:641–649.
5. Chalmers RTA, Hoballah JJ, Sharp WJ, et al. The effect of an intraluminal stent on neointimal hyperplasia at an end-to-side polytetrafluoroethylene graft arterial anastomosis. Am J Surg 1994;168:85–90.
6. Chalmers RTA, Hoballah JJ, Sharp WJ, Kresowik TF, Corson JD. Effect of an endovascular stent on healing of an end-to-end polytetrafluoroethylene-artery anastomosis in a canine model. Br J Surg 1994;81:1443–1447.
7. Ohki T, Marin ML, Veith FJ, et al. Anastomotic intimal hyperplasia. A comparison between conventional and endovascular stent graft techniques. J Surg Res 1997;69:255–267.
8. Ombrellaro MP, Stevens SL, Sciarrotta J, et al. Effect of balloon-expandable and self-expanding stent fixation on endoluminal polytetrafluoroethylene graft healing. Am J Surg 1997;173:461–466.
9. Weatherford DA, Ombrellaro MP, Schaeffer DO, et al. Healing characteristics of intraarterial stent grafts in an injured artery model. Ann Vasc Surg 1997;11:54–61.
10. Sauvage LR, Berger KE, Wood SJ, Yates SG, Smith JC, Mansfield PB. Interspecies healing of porous arterial prostheses. Arch Surg 1974;109:698–705.
11. Dolmatch BL, Dong YH, Trerotola SO, et al. Tissue response to covered Wallstents. J Vasc Intervent Radiol 1998;9:471–478.
12. Yee DC, Williams SK, Salzmann DL, et al. Stent versus endovascular graft healing characteristics in the porcine iliac artery. J Vasc Intervent Radiol 1998;9:609–617.
13. Marin ML, Veith FJ, Cynamon J, et al. Human transluminally placed endovascular stented grafts: preliminary histopathologic analysis of healing grafts in aortoiliac and femoral artery occlusive disease. J Vasc Surg 1995;21:595–604.
14. Clowes AW, Gown AM, Hanson SR, Reidy MA. Mechanisms of arterial graft failure. Am J Pathol 1985;118:43–54.
15. Golden MA, Hanson SR, Kirkman TR, Schneider PA, Clowes AW. Healing of polytetrafluoroethylene arterial grafts is influenced by graft porosity. J Vasc Surg 1990;11:838–845.
16. van der Giessen WJ, Lincoff AM, Schwartz RS, et al. Marked inflammatory sequelae to implantation of biodegradable and non-biodegradable polymers in porcine coronary arteries. Circulation 1996;94:1690–1697.
17. Wesolowski SA, Fries CC, Karlson KE, De Bakey M, Sawyer PN. Porosity: primary determinant of ultimate fate of synthetic vascular grafts. Surgery 1961;50:91–96.
18. Blum U, Langer M, Spillner G, et al. Abdominal aortic aneurysms: preliminary technical and clinical results with transfemoral placement of endovascular self-expanding stent-grafts. Radiology 1996;198:25–31.
19. Blum U, Voshage G, Lammer J, et al. Endoluminal stent-grafts for infrarenal abdominal aortic aneurysms. N Engl J Med 1997;336(1):13–20.
20. Norgren L, Swartbol P. Biological responses to endovascular treatment of abdominal aortic aneurysms. J Endovasc Surg 1997;4:169–173.
21. Schurmann K, Vorwerk D, Bucker A, et al. Perigraft inflammation due to Dacron-covered stent-grafts in sheep iliac arteries: correlation of MR imaging and histopathologic findings. Radiology 1997;204:757–763.
22. Tepe G, Duda SH, Hanke H, et al. Covered stents for prevention of restenosis: experimental and clinical results with different stent designs. Invest Radiol 1996;31:223–229.
23. Sapoval MR, Gaux JC, Long AL, et al. Transient periprosthetic thickening after covered-stent implantation in the iliac artery. AJR 1995;164:1271–1273.
24. Hayoz D, Do DD, Mahler F, Triller J, Spertini F. Acute inflammatory reaction associated with endoluminal bypass grafts. J Endovasc Surg 1997;4(4):354–360.
25. Sapoval MR, Turmel-Rodrigues LA, Raynaud AC, et al. Cragg covered stents in hemodialysis access: initial and midterm results. J Vasc Intervent Radiol 1996;7:335–342.
26. Dreyer B, Akutsu T, Kolff JW. Aortic grafts of polyurethane in dogs. J Appl Physiol 1960;15:18.
27. Hiratzka LF, Goeken JA, White RA, Wright CB. In vivo comparison of replamineform silastic and bioelectric polyurethane arterial grafts. Arch Surg 1979;114:698–702.
28. Berkowitz HD, Perloff LJ, Roberts B. Pseudointimal development on microporous polyurethane lattices. Surgery 1972;72(6):888–896.
29. Wilson GJ, MacGregor DC, Clement P, et al. The composite Corethane/Dacron vascular prosthesis. Canine in vivo evaluation of 4 mm diameter grafts with 1 year follow-up. ASAIO Trans 1991;37:M475–476.
30. Wilson GJ, MacGregor DC, Clement P, et al. A compliant Corethane/Dacron composite vascular prosthesis. Comparison with 4 mm ePTFE grafts in a canine model. ASAIO J 1993;39:M526–531.
31. Geeraert AJ, Callaghan JC. Experimental study of selected small caliber arterial grafts. J Cardiovasc Surg 1977;18:155–162.
32. van der Lei B, Bartels HL, Dijk F, Wildevuur RH. The thrombogenic characteristics of small caliber polyurethane vascular prostheses after heparin bonding. ASAIO Trans 1985;31:107–108.
33. Wesolowski SA, Fries CC, Karlson KE, DeBakey M, Sawyer PN. Porosity: primary determinant of ultimate fate of synthetic vascular grafts. Surgery 1961;50(1):91–96.
34. Lommen E, Gogolewski S, Pennings AJ, et al. Development of a neo-artery induced by a biodegradable polymeric vascular prosthesis. Trans ASAIO 1983;29:255.
35. van der Lei B, Nieuwenhuis P, Molenaar I, Wildevuur CRH. Long-term biologic fate of neoarteries regenerated in microporous, compliant, biodegradable, small-caliber vascular grafts in rats. Surgery 1987;101(4):459–467.
36. van der Lei B, Wildevuur CRH. From a synthetic, microporous, compliant, biodegradable small-caliber vascular graft to a new artery. Thorac Cardiovasc Surg 1989;37:337–347.
37. Hicks ME, Burmeister P, Tio FO, Stejskal BA, Del Toro C. Evaluation of collagen-covered nitinol stents in a swine model. J Vasc Intervent Radiol Suppl 1996;7(1; part 2):214(abstr).

38. Derns DB, Darcy MD, Baumann DS, Allen BT. Autologous vein-covered stent for the endovascular management of an iliac artery-ureteral fistula: case report and review of the literature. J Vasc Surg 1996;24(4):680–686.

39. McGraw JK, Patzik SM, Gale SS, Dodd JT, Boorstein JM. Autogenous vein-covered stent for the endovascular management of a superior mesenteric artery pseudoaneurysm. J Vasc Intervent Radiol 1998;9(5):779–782.

40. Van Nieuwenhove Y, van den Brande P, van Tussenbroek F, Debing E, von Kemp K. Iatrogenic carotid artery pseudoaneurysm treated by an autologous vein-covered stent. Eur J Vasc Endovasc Surg 1998;16(3):262–265.

41. Colombo A, Itoh A, DiMario C, et al. Successful closure of a coronary vessel rupture with a vein graft stent: case report. Cathet Cardiovasc Diagn 1996;38(2):172–174.

42. Urban P, Bednarkiwicz M, Bruschweiler I, Frangos A. Percutaneous sealing of a coronary aneurysm. Circulation 1999; 99: 973–974.

43. Stefanadis C, Toutouzas K, Vlachopoulos C, et al. Stents wrapped in autologous vein: an experimental study. J Am Coll Cardiol 1996; 28(4):1039–1046.

44. Byer A, Ussia G, Galleti G. Autologous vein lined and vein covered stent in swine arteries. An experimental study to assess and compare patency and intimal hyperplastic response. J Cardiovasc Surg 1998; 39(4):393–398.

4

Abdominal Aortic Aneurysm: Natural History and Surgical Treatment

PATRICK L. WYFFELS

Since the original management of an abdominal aortic aneurysm (AAA) by nongrafting and nonresectional treatment, many modifications and refinements in the operative treatment and in the perioperative patient management have occurred. These have progressively and significantly decreased the mortality and morbidity of elective aortic aneurysm surgical repair to less than 2% in low-risk patients and 8% in high-risk patients,[1,2] with overall mortalities less than 5%.[3] Unfortunately, the operative mortality of ruptured AAA has continued to range between 40 and 70%.[4–6] Prehospital deaths from ruptured AAAs are as high as 62%,[7] making the overall death rate over 90%. Endoaneurysmorrhaphy remains the only definitive prevention for aneurysm rupture, with estimates of 2,000 lives saved and $50 million saved annually with operative intervention prior to rupture.[8] Long-term follow-up has shown operative grafting to be durable, with low complication rates and excellent long-term survival rates.[9–11]

As our surgical techniques have matured and become less disruptive to the patient's physiology, overall hospital stay and cost have also decreased. Minimally invasive endovascular techniques[12] are being developed that may eventually supplant the traditional operative management of an abdominal aneurysm in many patients.

This chapter reviews our current knowledge of the natural history of this disease and the surgical treatment that continues to serve as the "gold standard" in the care of the patient with an AAA.

■ Natural History

Definitions

A precise and uniformly accepted definition of an aneurysm has always been difficult to achieve and continues to be lacking. The variations that exist cause reporting inconsistencies and make accurate comparisons of data impossible. Changing definitions alters the prevalence ratio (risk of disease) in both magnitude and direction.[13] The normal size and variation of the aorta with relationship to age and gender have added to the difficulty. The aorta gradually decreases in size from the aortic root to its bifurcation. Abdominal aortic size changes with age (increasing size with age) and gender (larger in males than in females). The size can be determined by applying nomograms that use the patient's gender and body surface area. In general, the female aorta ranges from 14 to 20 cm, whereas the male aorta ranges from 18 to 24 cm.[14,15]

Ectasia refers to vessels that are dilated but not to the extent of an aneurysm. In the past, an aneurysm has been defined as the portion of a vessel that is twice the diameter of the normal proximal vessel. This has been well accepted. Additional refinements in aortic measuring have led to definitions such as a 50% increase from the normal proximal aorta.[14] Collin[16] proposed that an aneurysm is present when the maximum external diameter of the infrarenal aorta is either greater than 4.0 cm or exceeds the maximum diameter of the aorta between the origin of the superior mesenteric and left renal arteries by at least 0.5 cm. The current recommended reporting practice is to define an aneurysm as a dilation of the aorta involving an increase in diameter of at least 50% as compared with the expected normal diameter.[17] An aneurysm may be *fusiform,* in which most or all of the artery is abnormally enlarged with tapering at the ends of the aneurysm, or *saccular,* with localized dilation of the circumference of the aorta. Saccular protrusions, which involve only a portion of the aortic wall, may also be present.[18] In addition, arteries may have very localized areas, or *blisters,* representing a weakened arterial wall site.[19] These may not be identified by preoperative evaluations but rather at the time of operative management of another problem. A uniform definition is intuitively necessary to make reports of frequency, prevalence, and prevalence ratio accurate and comparable. Treatment results can then be accurately evaluated.

Pathophysiology

The aortic wall is a heterogeneous structure composed of elastin, which is easily stretched, and collagen, which resists stretch. The extensile and tensile properties of the aortic wall are due to the elastin and collagen fibers found in the media. The basic structural unit of the media comprises smooth muscle cells sandwiched by concentric lamellae of elastin and collagen within the extracellular matrix. Elastin is synthesized and deposited in early childhood and no further significant synthesis occurs in adult life. The smooth muscle cell phenotype is responsible for the amount of elastin and collagen synthesized.[20] It has been well documented that the majority of AAAs occur in the infrarenal aorta.[21] Multiple factors are involved. The loss of elasticity as the aorta enters the abdomen is due to the relative increase in collagen fibers and a decrease in elastin fibers, when compared with the thoracic aorta.[22,23] Less arterial wall blood supply,[24] increased systolic pressure, and increased pulse pressure wave enhance the potential for mechanical injury and subsequent aneurysm formation.

Many AAA etiologies have been identified, including cystic medial necrosis, mycotic infections, trauma, arteritis, connective tissue disease, anastomotic disruption, and atherosclerosis. The most common cause of aneurysm formation has been considered to be atherosclerotic. Recent extensive research, however, has revealed that the pathophysiological changes in the infrarenal aortic wall leading to aneurysm formation are much more complex.

Smooth muscle cell cellular kinetics are different between AAA disease and atherosclerosis.[25] *Elastin degradation* is believed to lead to initial infrarenal aortic dilation, with changes in the collagen structure predisposing

to aneurysm rupture.[26] During this interval a complex remodeling process involving many constituents occurs in an aneurysm but not in the atherosclerotic aorta. Activated lymphocytes secrete polypeptide products called *cytokines.*[27,28] They serve within the immune system as molecular signals between immunocompetent cells. In certain states they are released within the circulation and exert systemic effects.[29] Cytokines participate in the pathophysiology of aneurysm development. The main cytokines that participate in the pathogenesis of an abdominal aortic aneurysm are tumor necrosis factor, interleukin -1b, -2, -6, and -8, platelet growth factor, and endothelin 1 and 2.[30,31] AAAs are characterized by both increases in proteolysis and changes in the biosynthesis of the extracellular matrix proteins.[32,33]

Proteoglycans are important components of the extracellular matrix, particularly the small proteoglycans, biglycan, and decorin. Biglycan and decorin regulate cell proliferation and collagen assembly. The marked decrease in biglycan messenger ribonucleic acid (mRNA) levels is unique to aneurysmal disease of the aorta. By contrast, in atherosclerosis and stenosis, biglycan expression is increased in comparison with the normal artery. The decrease in biglycan expression may reflect important regulatory changes specific for the AAA. Furthermore, a decrease in the biglycan gene expression and biosynthesis could have broad impact on the physiology and matrix architecture of the aorta.[34]

Protease activity in the form of *matrix metalloproteinase* appears to play a prominent role in the formation of infrarenal aortic aneurysms. *Macrophages* participate in the delivery, expression, and possible activation of matrix destructive proteases during AAA pathogenesis, and thus suggests a role for the activation of metalloproteinases in the progression of this disease.[35] The association between proteolysis and chronic inflammation in AAA disease suggests a possible immune-mediated mechanism. The inflammation may be induced by the chemotactic properties of elastin-derived peptides.[36] Understanding the interaction between aortic mesenchymal cells (smooth muscle cells and fibroblasts) and inflammatory cells (lymphocytes and macrophages) should allow for the identification of genetic factors that predispose to AAA.[37] Autoimmunity has been proposed to play a role in the pathogenesis of the nonspecific AAA,[38–40] and an association between North American black patients and human leukocyte antigen (HLA) alleles[41] and between these alleles and Japanese patients[42] has been demonstrated. These associations suggest an important genetic risk factor for the development of an AAA.

Environmental factors have been implicated as well. Nicotine induces neutrophil elastase activity release and is playing an active role in the development of vascular disease by inducing neutrophils to release elastase activity.[43] A link between smoking and increased proteolytic

activity in the human aortic wall exists and implicates smoking in the etiology of aortic aneurysms.[44] In addition, infectious etiologies are possibly involved, as *Chlamydia pneumoniae* has been detected at a significantly higher frequency in the walls of infrarenal AAAs than in the walls of nonaneurysmal infrarenal abdominal aortas.[45] Therefore, the atherosclerotic process that is occasionally associated with infrarenal aortic aneurysms is more likely coincidental, and the actual process present is a degenerative and inflammatory one with a possible autoimmune background modulated further by environmental factors.

Enlargement/Rupture Risks

Abdominal aneurysms represent several potential complications. Intraluminal thrombus may be well organized (Fig. 4–1A) or may be fragile debris (Fig. 4–1B) prone to distal embolization with resultant tissue ischemia. Infrequent but real considerations include aortoenteric fistula, thrombosis, dissection, infection, and adjacent organ obstruction. The major risk of an AAA is rupture. Typically, rupture results in rapid exsanguinating hemorrhage with its associated high prehospitalization mortality as well as high operative mortality and morbidity. Occasionally, slower bleeding can present with back pain and require preoperative confirmation in the hemodynamically normal patient. Even slower bleeding can present with atypical pain and cutaneous signs of hemorrhage. To have an impact on the incidence of complications and prevent death, we must first identify that an AAA exists.

Most AAAs are identified on physical exam or incidentally during diagnostic testing (sonography, computed tomography [CT], magnetic resonance imaging, arteriography) performed for another problem. Large patient size can obscure the physical findings of an aneurysm, and physical exams can be incomplete. Aneurysm size is not well established by arteriography due to associated thrombus. Ultrasound screening for AAA disease is a reliable and useful method.[46,47] Although measuring aneurysm size can be precise by CT, which is superior to ultrasound, this precision may not be obtainable in practice because of differences in measurement techniques. Difference in imaging modalities increase variability further.[48] Intra- and interobserver variability occurs as well.[49] Screening patient populations at risk continues to be prudent. Patient populations at risk for development of an AAA include smokers,[50–53] male patients with hypertension,[50,54] patients with peripheral vascular occlusive disease,[55–57] siblings with brothers who have aneurysmal disease,[58,59] offspring of patients dying from aneurysm rupture,[60] patients older than 60 years of age,[61] and patients with bronchiectasis.[62]

Once an AAA is present, it is necessary to determine if that aneurysm is at risk for rupture and to repair it electively. Risk of rupture has been typically associated with the size, as determined by the maximum diameter. The larger the aneurysm, the more likely it is to rupture. It has been reported that the annual incidence of rupture is approximately 4% for 5-cm aneurysms, 7% for those approaching 6 cm, and 19% for those 7 cm in diameter.[63] Five-year risk of rupture for aneurysms 4 to 5 cm have been reported as 3 to 12%.[64–66] Small aneurysms can also rupture. Scott et al[67] reported a 7-year-risk of rupture of 2.1% for aneurysms originally found to be 3.0 to 4.4 cm, and a 5-year cumulative risk of rupture of 4%

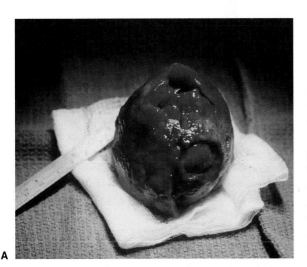
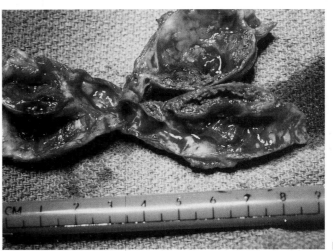

FIGURE 4–1. (A). Well-organized thrombus peeled from within a large infrarenal aortic aneurysm, emphasizing that the arteriographic opacified lumen does not necessarily represent true aneurysm size. **(B)**. Aneurysm segments with loose, friable debris, and potential for embolization.

for presenting aneurysms less than 4.0 cm in diameter was reported by Galland et al.[68]

Many reviews have dealt with the issue of aneurysm expansion rates. An average expansion rate of 0.4 cm per year has been reported but should only be used as a rough guideline because the course of the individual aneurysm is unpredictable, with intervals of stability and slow and rapid expansion.[69] Aneurysms expand at different rates based on original size at the time of detection. In a series of 233 aneurysm patients followed with serial ultrasound examinations, mean expansion rates of 2.6 mm per year, 4.1 mm per year, and 6.5 mm per year were found for aneurysms measuring less than 41 mm, 41 to 60 mm, and greater than 60 mm, respectively.[70] The authors emphasize that aneurysms were seen to expand at an erratic rate both in terms of time and size. It is currently recommended that aneurysms larger than 4.0 cm in diameter be repaired in good-risk patients.[71]

The challenge resides in identifying small aneurysms at risk for rupture. It is known that well-organized thrombus reduces the effect of the pressure load on the aneurysmal aortic wall,[72] and that thrombus area is nearly constant over the cardiac cycle,[73] perhaps decreasing the rate of expansion and rupture. The presence of a blister or lack of continuity of the aortic wall outside its thrombus are considered to be findings of high risk for rupture.[74] Flattening of the curvature of the aneurysm wall, which can be determined on CT, was significantly associated with an increased rate of expansion of small aneurysms.[75] Computer models have shown that the magnitude of stress within an AAA increases with size and with asymmetry, so that the potential for rupture may be dependent on the shape of the aneurysm.[76] Asymmetry is a frequent finding in AAAs.

Aortic compliance, as measured by the pressure-strain elastic modulus and stiffness, may allow a more precise estimate of AAA rupture risk than size alone. Baseline AAA compliance is significantly related to rupture and the future requirement for operative repair. The failure of compliance to increase with size may be a marker for rapid growth, development of symptoms, and rupture.[77] Cytokines participate in the pathophysiology of aneurysms. The rising and declining levels of some plasma cytokines can serve as markers of the growth and symptomatology of AAAs.[31] Experimentally, hypertension causes disruption and inflammatory cell infiltration within the wall of the aorta and increases the growth rate of an AAA.[78] The presence of β-adrenergic blockade appeared to have an independent effect on aneurysm growth rate, suggesting a possible role for β-adrenergic blockade as a therapeutic strategy in controlling expansion rates of small AAAs.[79]

Rapid expansion has also been reported in patients with advanced age, severe cardiac disease, previous stroke, and history of cigarette smoking.[80] A 15-year retrospective review at a major cardiovascular referral center has suggested that aortic aneurysms grow biexponentially. Aortic aneurysms began to grow faster at about 3 months before rupture. It is important to determine at what point the growth of aortic aneurysm changes its rate faster than before, and once that point is observed, elective repair should be considered.[81] Clearly, the law of Laplace, indicating that less pressure is necessary to distend a cavity as the radius increases, does not conform to the many factors currently being identified in aneurysm growth and rupture risk. Lack of knowledge among practitioners of even straightforward gender-related aortic size differences and overreliance on simplistic clinical paradigms that dictate operations for 5-cm-diameter aneurysms and watchful waiting for 4- to 5-cm AAAs may result in unintended bias in patient selection and increase the risk of rupture and death. It may be that a 5-cm-diameter aneurysm in a woman with a predicted normal aortic size of 1.4 cm represents a more advanced stage of disease than a 5-cm-diameter aneurysm in a man with a normal aortic diameter of 2.5 cm. More precise and detailed algorithms are needed to permit clinicians to tailor decisions to patients' size, sex, and risk factors. Development of such algorithms requires expansion of clinical and epidemiological studies to include enough women to make precise risk estimates.[82] The challenge, then, remains to stratify the risk of death and complication based on the size and morphology of the aneurysm, the age and gender of the patient, and the presence of associated risk factors for rupture.

Operative Mortality and Morbidity Risk

The operative mortality rates have steadily fallen to rates of 1.4 to 4.8%.[3] There has been a clear distinction between patients who are considered to be high risk and those who are low risk with operative mortality rates of 1 to 2%. High-risk criteria for patients undergoing repair of an AAA have been well established and include advanced age (85 years of age and older), marked renal insufficiency (serum creatinine greater than 3 mg/dL), severe pulmonary disease, cirrhosis with ascites, and severe cardiac disease (class III or IV angina, recent episode of congestive heart failure, large ventricular aneurysm, severe valvular disease, angina after coronary artery bypass grafting, severe coronary artery disease).[83] As the number of high-risk factors increases, so does the mortality. In a recent series of 110 consecutive high-risk patients, the operative mortality was 2.2% in the one-risk group, 5.9% in the two-risk group, and 11.1% in the three-risk group.[2] The common risk factor in patients who died after aneurysmectomy was pulmonary insufficiency, which induced prolonged periods of assisted ventilation. The ability to have successful outcomes with high-risk patients is dependent on identifying the risk factors present, optimizing the patient's preoperative hemodynamic status, and providing aggressive perioperative care.

Associated medical diseases include coronary artery disease (asymptomatic angina, myocardial infarction), chronic obstructive pulmonary disease, cardiac valvular disease, hypertension, smoking, peripheral vascular occlusive disease, renal insufficiency, diabetes mellitus, and cholelithiasis. These have a significant impact on operative mortality as well as the potential for operative morbidity. Elective postoperative complications include cardiac events with ischemia, arrhythmia, and congestive heart failure (15%), pulmonary insufficiency (8%), renal damage (6%), bleeding (4%), distal thromboembolism (3%), and wound infection (2%).[84] Ischemic colitis, stroke, and paraplegia or paraparesis are distinctly uncommon complications.

■ Management

General/Medical

The general management of all aneurysm patients remains medical, including treatment of lipid and cholesterol abnormalities. In addition, treatment of associated medical problems, such as hypertension, is pursued. Counseling and alternatives in smoking cessation are provided. Encouragement in exercise programs is emphasized. Associated surgical lesions, such as peripheral aneurysms, are excluded or treated.

Assessment of the patient's age, quality of life, and the severity of associated medical diseases should provide a rational determination of the course of treatment. This will allow patients to be classified into operative and nonoperative categories. Contraindications to elective aortic reconstruction (no treatment) include myocardial infarction within the past 6 months, intractable congestive heart failure, intractable angina pectoris, severe pulmonary insufficiency with dyspnea at rest, severe chronic renal insufficiency, incapacitating residual effects from stroke, and a life expectancy of less than 2 years.[3] Although theoretical at present, future nonoperative treatments may include modulation of the patient's immune status,[38] beta blockers to decrease aneurysm size independent of lowered blood pressure,[85] modification of metalloproteinases by nonantibiotic tetracyclines,[86] and treatment with antiangiogenic agents.[87] In patients who are operative candidates, the size of the aneurysm has been pivotal. In addition, the patient's age and gender as well as the aneurysm's morphology are considered to identify aneurysms at increased risk of rupture. In patients with low-risk small aneurysms long-term follow-up with serial examinations by an accurate, inexpensive modality such as sonography is prudent. Repair of asymptomatic aneurysms larger than 4 cm in diameter or twice the diameter of the normal infrarenal aorta is recommended by an ad hoc committee of the Society for Vascular Surgery and the North American chapter of the International Society for Cardiovascular Surgery.[71] The standard in aneurysmal disease treatment is surgical endoaneurysmorrhaphy.

Surgical Management of Infrarenal Abdominal Aortic Aneurysm

Thorough preoperative evaluation and preparation, including a detailed interview and physical examination to identify concomitant abnormalities, remain the foundation for an excellent surgical outcome. A cervical bruit mandates noninvasive carotid evaluation and endarterectomy for hemodynamic lesions. Abdominal bruits suggest mesenteric or renal artery stenosis. Decreased lower extremity pulses require Doppler evaluation. Prominent popliteal artery pulses should precipitate duplex scanning to exclude aneurysmal disease involving these vessels. Pulmonary testing is tailored to the severity of the patient's disease. Coronary artery disease is common in patients undergoing AAA repair, with 35.7% having preoperative coronary revascularization at some point. Selective preoperative coronary artery disease screening achieves excellent perioperative and late results in this population.[88] As cardiac complications remain a significant cause of mortality, symptomatic patients should be intensively evaluated to stratify risk and identify remediable lesions.

The preoperative period allows time to identify, modify, and subsequently optimize the patient's physiological state. Carotid endarterectomy and/or coronary artery angioplasty or bypass may be done prior to aneurysm treatment. Diagnostic multiplane arteriography is performed to evaluate the mesenteric (especially the inferior mesenteric artery), renal, and internal iliac artery flow, allowing better operative planning.

Surgical endoaneurysmorrhaphy remains the gold standard in the operative treatment of an AAA. The first successful aortic reconstruction for an aneurysm was performed by Dubost et al[89] in 1951 with a homologous arterial graft. The current approach to endoaneurysmorrhaphy was suggested by Matas and subsequently described by Creech[90] in 1966. The iliac arteries are occluded followed by clamping of the infrarenal aorta. A prosthetic graft is secured in place with the aortic anastomosis sutured first, followed by the iliac anastomosis. The technique involves leaving the back wall of the aneurysm intact to decrease dissection and the blood loss associated with it. This approach was modified as reported by Purdy et al[91] in 1986 for high-risk patients. This "reverse insertion" of a bifurcated graft has been my standard operation for the infrarenal AAA since that time. It effectively decreases aortic cross clamp time, thereby limiting the physiological changes that occur in all patients. In addition, it decreases the amount of bleeding from the proximal suture line.

Intraoperative Procedure

The patient enters a prewarmed operative suite. The patient's temperature is monitored throughout the procedure and the environment adjusted to maintain the protective effects of normothermia.[92] A preoperative intravenous antibiotic has been administered. Because deep-vein thrombosis can occur even in patients who receive intraoperative anticoagulation, pulsatile sequential stockings are placed on the lower extremities prior to induction of general endotracheal anesthesia. These are stopped before aortic cross-clamping and resumed at the end of the operative procedure. If acceptable to the patient, an epidural catheter is placed for postoperative pain management and to potentially shorten the intensive care and hospital stay.[93]

A midline transperitoneal (retroperitoneal if multiple previous procedures) approach is made to the aorta. Operative exposure is maximized, the number of assistants minimized, and operative time decreased with the use of fixed retractors. Gentle circumferential dissection of the infrarenal aorta is performed to allow proximal control while minimizing the potential for distal embolization of aneurysmal contents[94] (Fig. 4–2). The iliac arteries may require minimal dissection for control depending on their consistency. Care has to be taken to prevent an iliac vein injury, which can lead to significant blood loss and risk to the patient. The inferior mesenteric artery flow is assessed with an intraoperative Doppler probe. A tube graft (Fig. 4–3) is selected, if ap-

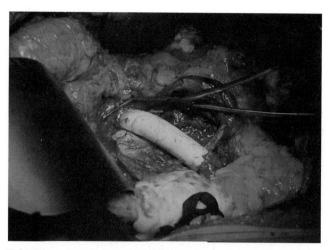

FIGURE 4–3. Tube graft has been sewn in place and flow restored. The large aneurysm sac will be trimmed and wrapped around the graft. Inferior mesenteric arterial flow was excellent from the superior mesenteric and internal iliac arteries and did not require implantation on the graft (head, upper left; feet, lower right).

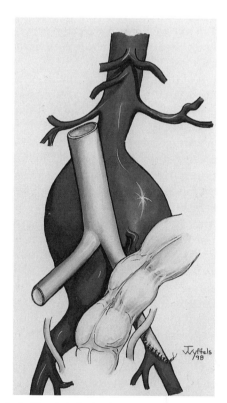

FIGURE 4–4. The left limb of the bifurcated graft has been sewn to the distal common iliac artery. The limb of the graft is tunneled behind the left ureter. During suturing, arterial flow was continuous to the left external iliac artery and left leg from pelvic collateral vessels.

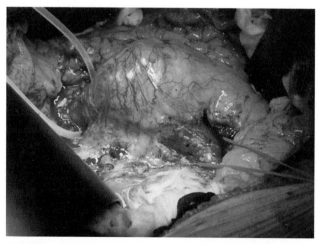

FIGURE 4–2. Large infrarenal aortic aneurysm that does not involve the iliac arteries. Proximal (thick clear Silastic) and distal (thin red Silastic) control through gentle dissection prevents distal embolization (head, upper left; feet, lower right).

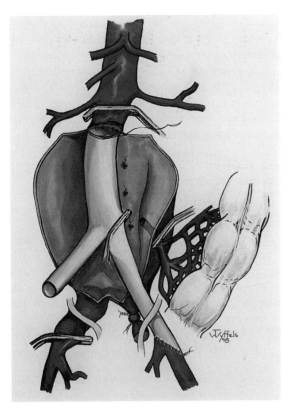

FIGURE 4–5. Proximal (aortic) anastomosis is now sewn. The graft is then flushed out the open graft limb and flow returned to the ipsilateral leg as well as the contralateral leg through pelvic collaterals. Total aortic cross-clamp time has been limited to only the aortic suturing time.

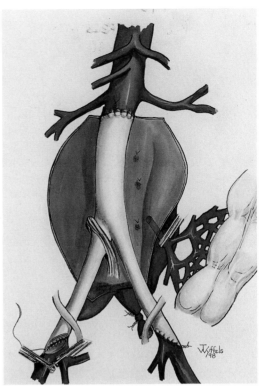

FIGURE 4–6. The remaining graft limb is sutured while flow to the ipsilateral leg is temporarily interrupted. Care is taken to ensure a retroureter position of the limb of the prosthetic vascular graft.

plicable, as it shortens the operative time and decreases operative blood loss.[95,96] However, the iliac arteries are frequently involved in the aneurysm and a bifurcated graft is required. Bifurcated graft placement follows the technique of Purdy et al.[91] This essentially reverses the sequence of anastomotic suturing.

Systemic heparin is given to decrease the incidence of intraoperative myocardial infarction[97] and limit other small vessel thrombosis. The infrarenal aorta is measured and a bifurcated polytetrafluoroethylene (PTFE) graft of an appropriate size is selected for implantation. One of the distal iliac artery anastomoses is secured first (Fig. 4–4) while maintaining perfusion to both lower extremities (ipsilateral flow by way of pelvic collateral vessels) and, if patent, through the inferior mesenteric artery. With this accomplished, the graft limb is temporarily occluded with a clamp or balloon occlusion catheter. Intravenous mannitol is given. The contralateral iliac artery is occluded, followed by slow cross-clamping of the infrarenal aorta. The aneurysm is opened on its anterior surface, the thrombus extracted, the inferior mesenteric artery occluded (if patent), and

back bleeding lumbar artery orifices oversewn. The proximal graft to the infrarenal aortic anastomosis is then sutured (Fig. 4–5), the aorta flushed through the open graft limb, which is then clamped, and the aorta slowly opened to the previously sutured iliac graft limb.

With the opposite graft limb occluded, the remaining distal common iliac artery anastomosis is completed (Fig. 4–6). Prior to ligature of the suture, the graft, and vessels are flushed. Once flow is established to that leg, Doppler flow to the iliac and the inferior mesenteric artery is examined. Attention is directed to revascularize the inferior mesenteric artery (carrel patch) and to maintain or revascularize at least one internal iliac artery to prevent colorectal ischemia.[98] Although it is preferred to place the vascular graft entirely in the abdomen, reducing the incidence of graft infection, extensive iliac occlusive disease may require bypass grafting to the common femoral arteries (Fig. 4–7). In those cases, inferior mesenteric artery implantation is necessary. Prior to operative completion, lower extremity perfusion is assessed with a sterile Doppler probe. The aneurysm wall is sutured around the trunk of the vascu-

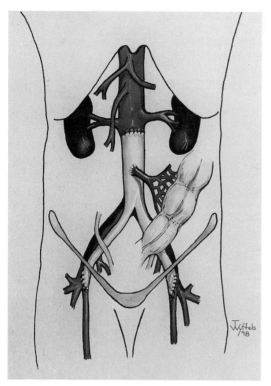

FIGURE 4–7. Aortic reconstruction of elderly man with extensive iliac occlusive disease with implantation of inferior mesenteric artery to trunk of graft to prevent colorectal ischemia.

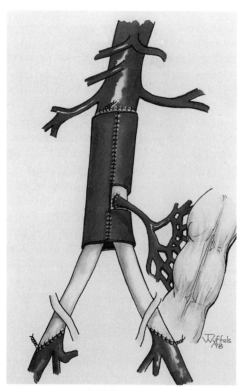

FIGURE 4–8. The completed endoaneurysmorrhaphy with excess portions of the aneurysm wall affixed around the graft.

lar graft (Fig. 4–8) and the peritoneum closed over the retroperitoneal structures. If cholelithiasis is present, a cholecystectomy is completed before abdominal wall closure. The patient is awakened, extubated, and transferred to the postoperative recovery room. If cardiac or pulmonary status dictate, the patient is transferred directly to the surgical intensive care unit for continuation of aggressive perioperative care.

Postoperative Care

The focus of postoperative care is on maintaining a normal hemodynamic status, optimizing pulmonary function, controlling pain, allowing early mobilization, and providing nutritional support. An organized approach among caregivers facilitates a patient's postoperative progress. The use of clinical pathways and case management can be helpful in both providing excellent patient care with excellent patient outcomes and reducing inpatient hospital stays and hospital costs.[99] These pathways aid in identifying patients who may require prompt and efficient discharge planning, early consultation with a home care nurse, or transfer to a convalescent facility.[100]

■ Conclusions

Abdominal aortic aneurysms continue to cause significant mortality and morbidity. Extensive research has demonstrated that the most common cause of an infrarenal aortic aneurysm is a degenerative and inflammatory process with autoimmune and environmental modulation. Decisions regarding patient management cannot be made until the aneurysm has been identified. Screening programs of patients at risk need to be utilized. Operative candidates with aneurysms larger than 4.0 cm should undergo elective endoaneurysmorrhaphy. Smaller aneurysms need to be evaluated for those at high risk for rupture and repaired. The challenge, then, remains to stratify the risk of death and complication based on the size and morphology of the aneurysm, the age and gender of the patient, and presence of associated risk factors for rupture. Elective operative mortality of less than 5% is currently commonplace. Preoperative optimization of the patient leads to favorable postoperative results that are durable with few long-term complications. Patients with aneurysm disease need to be followed closely to identify and manage additional aneurysm development as well as to manage associated medical problems. Although minimally invasive endovascular techniques are developing, endoaneurysmorrhaphy remains the "gold standard" of care for the patient with an infrarenal abdominal aortic aneurysm.

REFERENCES

1. Golden MA, Whittemore AD, Donaldson MC, et al. Selective evaluation and management of coronary artery disease in patients undergoing repair of abdominal aortic aneurysms: a 16-year experience. Ann Surg 1990;212:415–423.

2. Morishita Y, Toyohira H, Yuda T, et al. Surgical treatment of abdominal aortic aneurysm in the high-risk patient. Jpn J Surg 1991;21:595–599.

3. Ernst CB. Abdominal aortic aneurysm. N Engl J Med 1993;328(16):1167–1172.

4. Campbell WB, Collin J, Morris PJ. The mortality of abdominal aortic aneurysm. Ann R Coll Surg Engl 1986;68:275–278.

5. Johansen K, Kohler TR, Nocholls SC, et al. Ruptured abdominal aortic aneurysm: the Harborview experience. J Vasc Surg 1991;13:240–247.

6. Dardik A, Burleyson GP, Bowman H, et al. Surgical repair of ruptured abdominal aortic aneurysms in the state of Maryland: factors influencing outcome among 527 recent cases. J Vasc Surg 1998;28:413–420.

7. Ingoldby CJH, Wujanto R, Mitchell JE. Impact of vascular surgery on community mortality from ruptured aortic aneurysms. Br J Surg 1986;73:551–553.

8. Pasch AR, Ricotta JJ, May AG, et al. Abdominal aortic aneurysm: the case for elective repair. Circulation 1984;70(suppl 1):1–4.

9. Cronenwett JL. Factors influencing the long-term results of aortic aneurysm surgery. In: Yao J, Pearce W, eds. Long-Term Results in Vascular Surgery. Appleton & Lange, 1993:171–179.

10. Hallett JW, Naessens JM, Ballard DJ. Early and late outcome of surgical repair for small abdominal aortic aneurysms: a population-based analysis. J Vasc Surg 1993;18:684–691.

11. Geroulakos G, Lumley JS, Wright JG. Factors influencing the long-term results of abdominal aortic aneurysm repair. Eur J Vasc Endovasc Surg 1997;13:3–8.

12. Moore WS, Rutherford RB. Transfemoral endovascular repair of abdominal aortic aneurysm: results of the North American EVT phase 1 trial. J Vasc Surg 1996;23:543–553.

13. Moher D, Cole CW, Hill GB. Epidemiology of abdominal aortic aneurysm: the effect of differing definitions. Eur J Vasc Surg 1992;6:647–650.

14. Lanne T, Sandgren T, Sonesson B. A dynamic view on the diameter of abdominal aortic aneurysms. Eur J Vasc Endovasc Surg 1998;15:308–312.

15. Ouriel K, Green RM, Donayre C, et al. An evaluation of new methods of expressing aortic aneurysm size: relationship to rupture. J Vasc Surg 1992;15:12.

16. Collin J. A proposal for a precise definition of abdominal aortic aneurysm. A personal view. J Cardiovasc Surg Torino 1990;31:168–169.

17. Johnston KW, Rutherford RB, Tilson, et al. Suggested standards for reporting on arterial aneurysms. J Vasc Surg 1991;13:452–458.

18. Iwai T, Sato S, Muraoka Y, et al. Atherosclerotic abdominal aorta saccular protrusion. Int Surg 1996;81:189–194.

19. Faggioli GL, Stella A, Gargiulo M, et al. Morphology of small aneurysms: definition and impact on risk of rupture. Am J Surg 1994;168:131–135.

20. Patel MI, Hardman, David TA, et al. Current views on pathogenesis of abdominal aortic aneurysms. J Am Coll Surg 1995;181:371–382.

21. Feibleib M, Thom T, Havlik RJ. Decline in the coronary heart disease mortality in the United States. Atherosclerosis Rev 1982;9:29–41.

22. Harkness MLR, Harkness RD, McDonald DA. The collagen and elastin content of the arterial wall in the dog. Proc R Soc Lond 1957;146(B):531–541.

23. Zatina MA, Zarinis CK, Gewertz BL, et al. Role of median lamellar architecture in the pathogenesis of aortic aneurysms. J Vasc Surg 1984;1:442–448.

24. Roberts WC. Pathology of arterial aneurysms. In: Bergan JJ, Yao JST, eds. Aneurysms Diagnosis and Treatment. New York: Grune & Stratton, 1982:17–44.

25. Patel MI, Ghosh P, Melrose J, et al. Smooth muscle cell migration and proliferation is enhanced in abdominal aortic aneurysms. Aust NZ J Surg 1996;66(5):305–308.

26. Satta J, Juvonen T, Haukipuro K, et al. Increased turnover of collagen in abdominal aortic aneurysms, demonstrated by measuring the concentration of the aminoterminal propeptide of type III procollagen in peripheral and aortal blood samples. J Vasc Surg 1995;22:155–160.

27. Deschepper CF, Ganong WF. Renin and angiotensin in endocrine glands. In: Martini L, Ganong WF, eds. Frontiers in Neuroendocrinology, vol 10. New York: Raven Press, 1988.

28. Ziegler EJ. Tumor necrosis factor in human cells. N Engl J Med 1988;318:1533.

29. Dinarello CA, Mier JW. Lymphokines. N Engl J Med 1987;317:940.

30. Hingorani A, Ascher E, Scheinman M, et al. The effect of tumor necrosis factor binding protein and interleukin-1 receptor antagonist on the development of abdominal aortic aneurysms in a rat model. J Vasc Surg 1998;28:522–526.

31. Treska V, Topolcan O, Wenham PW, et al. Cytokine metabolism in aneurysm of the abdominal aorta. Rozhl Chir 1998;77:225–229.

32. Anidjar S, Kieffer E. Pathogenesis of acquired aneurysms of the abdominal aorta. Ann Vasc Surg 1992;6:298–305.

33. Reilly JM, Brophy CM, Tilson MD. Characterization of an elastase from aneurysmal aorta which degrades intact aortic elastin. Ann Vasc Surg 1992;6:499–502.

34. Tamarina NA, Grassi MA, Johnson DA, et al. Proteoglycan gene expression is decreased in abdominal aortic aneurysms. J Surg Res 1998;74:76–80.

35. Newman KM, Jean Claude J, Li H, et al. Cellular localization of matrix metalloproteinases in the abdominal aortic aneurysm wall. J Vasc Surg 1994;20:814–820.

36. Satta J, Laurila A, Paakko P, et al. Chronic inflammation and elastin degradation in abdominal aortic aneurysm disease: an immunohistochemical and electron microscopic study. Eur J Vasc Endovasc Surg 1998;15:313–319.

37. Halloran BG, Baxter BT. Pathogenesis of aneurysms. Semin Vasc Surg 1995;8:85–92.

38. Gregory AK, Yin NX, Capella J, et al. Feature of autoimmunity in the abdominal aortic aneurysm. Arch Surg 1996;131:85–88.

39. Koch AE, Haines GK, Rizzo RJ, et al. Human abdominal aneurysms: immunophenotypic analysis suggesting an immune mediated response. Am J Pathol 1990;137:1199–1219.

40. Brophy CM, Reilly JM, Smith GJW, et al. The role of inflammation in nonspecific abdominal aortic aneurysm disease. Ann Vasc Surg 1991;5:229–233.

41. Tilson MD, Ozsvath KJ, Hirose H, et al. A genetic basis for autoimmune manifestations in the abdominal aortic aneurysm resides in the MHC class II locus DR-beta-1. NY Acad Sci 1996;800:208–217.

42. Hirose H, Takagi M, Miyagawa N, et al. Genetic risk factor for abdominal aortic aneurysm: HLA-DR2(15), a Japanese study. J Vasc Surg 1998;27:500–503.

43. Murphy EA, Danna-Lopes D, Sarfati I, et al. Nicotine-stimulated elastase activity release by neutrophils in patients with abdominal aortic aneurysms. Ann Vasc Surg 1998;12:41–45.

44. Parra JR, Canbria RA, Freischlag JA, et al. Smoking increases proteolytic activity in the human abdominal aorta. Vasc Surg 1998;32(6):595–602.

45. Petersen E, Boman J, Persson K, et al. *Chlamydia pneumoniae* in human abdominal aortic aneurysms. Eur J Vasc Endovasc Surg 1998;15:138–142.

46. Krohn CD, Kullmann G, Kvernebo K, et al. Ultrasonographic screening for abdominal aortic aneurysm. Eur J Surg 1992;158:527–530.

47. Simoni G, Pastorino C, Perrone R, et al. Screening for abdominal aortic aneurysms and associated risk factors in a general population. Eur J Vasc Endovasc Surg 1995;10:207–210.

48. Lederle FA, Wilson SE, Johnson GR, et al. Variability in measurement of abdominal aortic aneurysms. J Vasc Surg 1995;21:945–952.

49. Singh K, Bonaa KH, Solberg S, et al. Intra- and interobserver variability in ultrasound measurements of abdominal aortic diameter. The Tromso Study. Eur J Vasc Endovasc Surg 1998;15:497–504.

50. Thurmond AS, Semler HJ. Abdominal aortic aneurysm: incidence in a population at risk. Cardiovasc Surg Torino 1986;27:457–460.

51. Krupski WC. The peripheral vascular consequences of smoking. Ann Vasc Surg 1991;5:291–304.

52. van Laarhoven SJ, Borstlap AC, van Berge-Henegouwen DP, et al. Chronic obstructive pulmonary disease and abdominal aortic aneurysms. Eur J Vasc Surg 1993;7:386–390.

53. Franks PJ, Edwards RJ, Greenhalgh RM, et al. Risk factors for abdominal aortic aneurysms in smokers. Eur J Vasc Endovasc Surg 1996;11(4):487–492.

54. Williams IM, Hughes OD, Townsend E, et al. Prevalence of abdominal aortic aneurysm in a hypertensive population. Ann R Coll Surg Engl 1996;78:501–504.

55. MacSweeney ST, O'Meara M, Alexander C, et al. High prevalence of unsuspected abdominal aortic aneurysm in patients with confirmed symptomatic peripheral or cerebral arterial disease. Br J Surg 1993;80:582–584.

56. Wolf YG, Otis SM, Schwend RB, et al. Screening for abdominal aortic aneurysms during lower extremity arterial evaluation in the vascular laboratory. J Vasc Surg 1995;22:417–421, discussion 421–423.

57. Galland RB, Simmons MJ, Torrie EP. Prevalence of abdominal aortic aneurysm in patients with occlusive peripheral vascular disease. Br J Surg 1991;78:1259–1260.

58. Webster MW, Ferrell RE, St. Jean PL, et al. Ultrasound screening of first-degree relatives of patients with an abdominal aortic aneurysm. J Vasc Surg 1991;13:9–13, discussion 13–14.

59. van der Graaf Y, Akkersdijk GJ, Hak E, et al. Results of aortic screening in the brothers of patients who had elective aortic aneurysm repair. Br J Surg 1998;85:778–780.

60. Bengtsson H, Sonesson B, Lanne T, et al. Prevalence of abdominal aortic aneurysm in the offspring of patients dying from aneurysm rupture. Br J Surg 1992;79:1142–1143.

61. Boll AP, Verbeek AL, van de Lisdonk EH, et al. High prevalence of abdominal aortic aneurysm in a primary care screening programme. Br J Surg 1998;85:1090–1094.

62. Sterpetti AV, Cavallaro A, Cavallari N, et al. Factors influencing the rupture of abdominal aortic aneurysms. Surg Gynecol Obstet 1991;173:175–178.

63. Taylor LM, Porter JM. Basic data related to clinical decision-making in abdominal aortic aneurysms. Ann Vasc Surg 1986;1:500.

64. Limet R, Sakalihassen N, Albert A, et al. Determination of the expansion rate and incidence of rupture of abdominal aortic aneurysms. J Vasc Surg 1991;14:540–548.

65. Johansson G, Nydahl S, Olofsson P, et al. Survival of patients with abdominal aortic aneurysm: comparison between operative and nonoperative management. Eur J Vasc Surg 1990;4:497–502.

66. Glimaker G, Holmberg L, Elvin A, et al. Natural history of patients with abdominal aortic aneurysm. Eur J Vasc Surg 1991;5:125–130.

67. Scott RA, Tisi PV, Ashton HA, et al. Abdominal aortic aneurysm rupture rates: a 7-year follow-up of the entire abdominal aortic aneurysm population detected by screening. J Vasc Surg 1998;28:124–128.

68. Galland RB, Whiteley MS, Magee TR. The fate of patients undergoing surveillance of small abdominal aortic aneurysms. Eur J Vasc Endovasc Surg 1998;16:104–109.

69. Berstein EF, Chan EL. Abdominal aortic aneurysm in high risk patients: outcome of selective management based on size and expansion rate. Ann Surg 1984;200:255–263.

70. Stonebridge PA, Draper T, Kelman J, et al. Growth rate of infrarenal aortic aneurysms. Eur J Vasc Endovasc Surg 1996;11:70–73.

71. Hollier LH, Taylor LM, Ochsner J. Recommended indications for operative treatment of abdominal aortic aneurysm: report of a subcommittee of the Joint Council of the Society for Vascular Surgery and the North American Chapter of the International Society for Cardiovascular Surgery. J Vasc Surg 1992;15:1046–1056.

72. Di Martino E, Mantero S, Inzoli F, et al. Biomechanics of abdominal aortic aneurysm in the presence of endoluminal thrombus: experimental characterisation and structural static computational analysis. Eur J Vasc Endovasc Surg 1998;15:290–299.

73. Vorp DA, Mandarino WA, Webster MW, et al. Potential influence of intraluminal thrombus on abdominal aortic aneurysm as assessed by a new non-invasive method. Cardiovasc Surg 1996;4:732–739.

74. Faggioli GL, Stella A, Gargiulo M, et al. Morphology of small aneurysms: definition and impact on risk of rupture. Am J Surg 1994;168:131–135.

75. Veldenz HC, Schwarcz TH, Endean ED, et al. Morphology predicts rapid growth of small abdominal aortic aneurysms. Ann Vasc Surg 1994;8:10–13.

76. Vorp DA, Raghavan ML, Webster MW. Mechanical wall stress in abdominal aortic aneurysm: influence of diameter and asymmetry. J Vasc Surg 1998;27(4):632–639.

77. Wilson K, Bradbury A, Whyman M, et al. Relationship between abdominal aortic aneurysm wall compliance and clinical outcome: a preliminary analysis. Eur J Vasc Endovasc Surg 1998;15:472–477.

78. Gadowski GR, Ricci MA, Hendley, et al. Hypertension accelerates the growth of experimental aortic aneurysms. J Surg Res 1993;54:431–436.

79. Englund R, Hudson P, Hane K, et al. Expansion rates of small abdominal aortic aneurysms. Aust NZ J Surg 1998;68:21–24.

80. Chang JB, Stein TA, Liu JP, et al. Risk factors associated with rapid growth of small abdominal aortic aneurysms. Surgery 1997;121:117–122.

81. Hirose Y, Takamiya M. Growth curve of ruptured aortic aneurysm. J Cardiovasc Surg Torino 1998;39:9–13.

82. Katz DJ, Stanley JC, Zelenock GB. Abdominal aortic aneurysms. Semin Vasc Surg 1995;8:289–298.

83. Hollier LH, Reigel MM, Kazmier FJ, et al. Conventional repair of abdominal aortic aneurysm in the high-risk patient: a plea for abandonment of nonresectional treatment. J Vasc Surg 1986;3:712–717.

84. Johnston KW. Multicenter prospective study of nonruptured abdominal aortic aneurysms. II. Variables predicting morbidity and mortality. J Vasc Surg 1989;9:437–447.

85. Slaiby JM, Ricci MA, Gadowski GR, et al. Expansion of aortic aneurysms is reduced by propranolol in a hypertensive rat model. J Vasc Surg 1994;20:178–183.

86. Curci JA, Petrinec D, Liao S, et al. Pharmacologic suppression of experimental abdominal aortic aneurysms: a comparison of doxycycline and four chemically modified tetracyclines. J Vasc Surg 1998;28:1082–1093.

87. Thompson MM, Jones L, Nasim A, et al. Angiogenesis in abdominal aortic aneurysms. Eur J Vasc Endovasc Surg 1996;11:464–469.

88. Won A, Acosta JA, Browner D, et al. Validation of selective cardiac evaluation prior to aortic aneurysm repair. Arch Surg 1998;133: 833–838.

89. Dubost C, Allary M, Oeconomos N. Resection of an aneurysm of the abdominal aorta: reestablishment of the continuity by a preserved human arterial graft, with result after five months. Arch Surg 1952;64:405–408.

90. Creech O Jr. Endoaneurysmorrhaphy and treatment of aortic aneurysm. Ann Surg 1966;164:935.

91. Purdy RT, Beyer FC 3d, McCann WD, et al. Reduced aortic cross-clamp time in high-risk patients with abdominal aortic aneurysm. J Vasc Surg 1986;3:820–823.

92. Elmore JR, Franklin DP, Youkey JR, et al. Normothermia is protective during infrarenal aortic surgery. J Vasc Surg 1998;28: 984–994.

93. Major CP Jr, Greer MS, Russell WL, et al. Postoperative pulmonary complications and morbidity after abdominal aneurysmectomy: a comparison of postoperative epidural versus parenteral opioid analgesia. Am Surg 1996;62:45–51.

94. Kuhan G, Raptis S. "Trash foot" following operations involving the abdominal aorta. Aust NZ J Surg 1997;67:21–24.

95. Snellen JP, Terpstra OT, van Urk H. The use of a straight tube graft decreases blood loss and operation time in patients with an abdominal aortic aneurysm. Neth J Surg 1984;36:45–47.

96. Agus GB, De Angelis R, Mondani P, et al. Optimal site for proximal and distal anastomoses in AAAs repair. J Cardiovasc Surg Torino 1995;36:465–467.

97. Thompson JF, Mullee MA, Bell PR, et al. Intraoperative heparinization, blood loss and myocardial infarction during aortic aneurysm surgery: a Joint Vascular Research Group study. Eur J Vasc Endovasc Surg 1996;12:86–90.

98. Shigematsu H, Nunokawa M, Hatakeyama T, et al. Inferior mesenteric and hypogastric artery reconstruction to prevent colonic ischaemia following abdominal aortic aneurysmectomy. Cardiovasc Surg 1993;1:13–18.

99. Muluk SC, Painter L, Sile S, et al. Utility of clinical pathway and prospective case management to achieve cost and hospital stay reduction for aortic aneurysm surgery at a tertiary care hospital. J Vasc Surg 1997;25:84–93.

100. Kalman PG, Johnston KW. Sociologic factors are major determinants of prolonged hospital stay after abdominal aneurysm repair. Surgery 1996;119:690–693.

5

Endovascular Grafts for the Treatment of Abdominal Aortic Aneurysms: Development of Stent-Grafts, Design of Devices, and Technical Results

MARK M. DAVIDIAN, JAMES F. BENENATI, AND ALEX POWELL

Abdominal aortic aneurysms (AAAs) present a significant cost to society as a whole. Approximately 46,000 open repairs were performed in the United States in 1992, up from 40,000 in 1988.[1] The incidence of AAAs has been rising, with a report from the Mayo clinic citing a frequency of 36.2 per 100,000.[2] Common complications of AAAs include rupture and distal embolization, with approximately 90% of patients dying after rupture. A study estimated that 2,000 lives and $50 million could be saved if aneurysms had been treated before rupture.[3] Aneurysms, defined as an increase of the diameter of the aorta by 50% of the expected diameter, are generally treated if symptomatic. There has been a historical cutoff point of 5 cm for elective repair of asymptomatic aneurysms. This has been challenged, however, and many aneurysms are electively operated upon at 4 cm. These analyses assume a constant and low operative morbidity and mortality ranging from 4–6% for elective surgical repair, from 50–60% for emergent repair of rupturing or ruptured aneurysms.[1] The natural history of AAAs is derived from historical data with a 5-year survival of only 19%, with 63% of the deaths from rupture of the aneurysm in 102 patients.[4] There has been no controlled prospective study ever performed comparing operative repair to no repair.

Katz and Cronenwett found that elective repair of small (4cm) aneurysms was cost-effective if used in carefully selected patients based upon an assumed operative mortality of 4.6% for elective repair and an annual rupture rate of 3.3%.[5,6] However, there is a significant difference of opinion as to the annual rate of rupture of 4 cm aneurysms in the literature, varying from zero to 5.4%.[1] Practice guidelines now recommend repair of aneurysms as small as 4 cm in selected patients.[7]

■ Rationale for Endograft Treatment of Abdominal Aortic Aneurysms

Endoprostheses have been developed to avoid major abdominal surgery and the related morbidity and mortality. Potential advantages of endograft treatment of AAA over open surgery are its less invasiveness associated with a shorted hospital stay and recovery time, and particularly the therapeutic option for patients who are not surgical candidates. Some of these have already been realized in the literature.

Endografts have developed these recent years as a logical outgrowth of the combination of stent and graft technology. Stainless steel and nitinol stents, respectively, have been used in conjunction with various graft materials, such as polyester (Dacron), polytetrafluoroethylene (PTFE), or polycarbonate. The earliest endografts were simply fashioned by hand suturing graft material to the stent.

Guidelines for the development and use of endografts were written by the Endovascular Graft Committee, with input from the Society for Vascular Surgery and the International Society for Cardiovascular Surgery, and the Society of Cardiovascular and Interventional Radiology in 1995.[8] Reporting standards were later published in 1997.[9]

■ Anatomic Factors Influencing Placement of Endografts

Specific anatomic requirements need to be fullfilled and evaluated prior to performing an endograft repair of an AAA. Each device has anatomic inclusion and exclusion criteria. The following anatomic factors are heavily influencing the indication for endografting and its technical results.

Proximal Attachment Site or Infrarenal Neck

The segment of aorta below the lowest renal artery to the origin of the aneurysm is referred to as the proximal neck. This is the proximal deployment site for all infrarenal attachments. This segment should be relatively disease free and tubular in configuration. Atheroma, calcification, and thrombus in the proximal neck can influence the ability to achieve a complete seal. Significant disease in the proximal neck may be a contraindication to infrarenal attachment. Flaring of the proximal neck is not ideal and in some trials it is a contraindication to deployment. The diameter of the proximal neck is of critical importance. Each device has a specific range of diameters that can be accommodated. Undersizing obviously leads to leaks, and significant oversizing may lead to kinking and infolding of the device. This may result in endoleaks and may be a nidus for thrombus formation within the endograft. The length of the neck is one of the most important measurements. Sufficient neck length must be present to fully anchor the device. Generally, 15 mm is the length of neck required to anchor safely most devices being used at this time.

Some newly developed devices allow for suprarenal attachment (see below). In this situation 5 mm of infrarenal neck is still required. Suprarenal attachment is advantageous because the suprarenal aorta is usually disease free compared with the infrarenal segment. This theoretically allows for better sealing and decreases the possibility of migration and leaking.

Angulation of either the neck or aneurysm from the vertical plane of the aorta may cause difficulties in implantation. Kinking and downward migration during deployment are 2 potential complications of severe angulation. Many devices use an angulation of 60 degrees as a contraindication to endograft placement.

Patency of Aortic Branches

Patency of the inferior mesenteric artery (IMA) and superior mesenteric artery (SMA) must be carefully evaluated on both computerized tomography (CT) and angiography prior to endograft deployment. An occluded SMA with a hypertrophied IMA supplying flow to all of the SMA branches would be a contraindication to endograft placement. Endograft placement in this situation risks significant bowel ischemia. Patients with a chronically occluded IMA present the most favorable anatomy, as they have had time to develop SMA collaterals to IMA territory. They also will not be at risk for collateral en-

doleak from the IMA. Situations often arise, however, where both the SMA and the IMA are patent. In this case coil embolization of the proximal IMA prior to endograft placement when the IMA was large may be indicated. This reduces the chances that perfusion from SMA collaterals (Arch of Riolan, or marginal artery of Drummond) will form the basis of an endoleak.

The presence of accessory renal arteries also must be sought for carefully on preoperative angiography and CT. As is well known, these vessels can originate from as low as the iliac arteries. The decision to place the endograft across an accessory vessel is a difficult one, as there are potential risks of potentiating renal insufficiency and hypertension. Currently, most of the Food and Drug Administration (FDA) trials leave this decision in the hands of the investigator.

Lumbar arteries are commonly identified on preprocedural angiography and CT. These form the basis of the most common endoleak encountered. These endoleaks, however, have a high rate of spontaneous closure, and there is still controversy about prophylactic embolization of lumbar collaterals.

Distal Attachment Sites

Aneurysms involving both common iliac arteries to the level of the internal iliac are not suitable for endovascular repair with bifurcated devices because both internal iliac arteries would need to be embolized for aneurysm exclusion. This poses a high risk of pelvic ischemia. There are currently no FDA trials that will allow exclusion of both internal iliac arteries. There are patients in published series in which both internal iliacs were covered with no sequelae, but there are also reports of fatal pelvic ischemia from this maneuver. It has been acceptable practice to exclude and embolize one internal iliac artery. This is done in cases where the aneurysm extends the length of one common iliac, but not the other. Embolization with coils is done before device deployment across the internal iliac origin into the external iliac artery. This prevents the internal iliac from filling the aneurysm sac in a retrograde fashion. Buttock claudication may occur after successful endograft repair of AAAs where one internal iliac was embolized, and this complication should be discussed with the patient before the procedure. The ideal situation exists where there is normal caliber common iliac arteries bilaterally for obtaining a complete seal.

Aneurysms involving both hypogastric arteries cannot be treated by "traditional" stent grafts. However, there are some high-risk trials for poor surgical candidates where an aorto-unilateral device can be placed and then a crossed femoral bypass be performed. In this procedure, the contralateral iliac artery is either surgically ligated or occluded with coils. Although this particular procedure involves an extraanatomic bypass, it does avoid the more complex and risky intraabdominal or retroperitoneal approach necessary for traditional repair.

Condition of the Iliac Arteries for Accepting the Delivery Device

Careful inspection of the iliac and common femoral arteries is crucial for deciding upon candidacy for endograft repair of AAAs. Because the placement of the endograft is through femoral arteriotomy and percutaneously placed sheaths, the diameter, tortuosity, and presence of atherosclerotic occlusive disease is of paramount concern. Most cases of failure to deploy the endograft in the literature are due to inability to pass the device up the iliac arteries. Forceful pushing can lead to iliac rupture and subsequent emergent conversion to open repair. Angioplasty and stenting can be used preoperatively to treat atherosclerotic occlusive disease of the iliac system, but care must be taken to avoid dislodging the stent when pushing the delivery device into the aorta. In general, women have significantly smaller iliac arteries than men and careful measurement must be done to ensure that a given device can be accommodated by the iliac arteries. Diseased and tortuous iliacs can also cause problems with deployment.

Accompanying advanced age, hypertension, and atherosclerosis is vessel tortuosity. Severe iliac artery tortuosity can make safe passage of the device difficult. The use of a stiff wire can help in these situations, but iliac rupture can occur with relatively minor force in the presence of significant tortuosity. In some cases, tortuosity may be overcome by gaining a broader exposure to the common femoral artery and manually pulling down to straighten out the external iliac artery. Alternatively, a retroperitoneal exposure of the external iliac artery may facilitate device passage into the aorta. Finally, one could attempt to pass a guidewire into the brachial artery from the common femoral artery and pin it both at the groin and arm, thus increasing the rigidity of the guidewire and possibly making it easier to pass the device. However, this has been associated with avulsion of the subclavian artery and it also predisposes the patient to potential cerebrovascular events.

Preprocedural Evaluation

It should be evident from the discussion above that preprocedural evaluation is crucial for successful patient selection and treatment. As a rule, contrast-enhanced spiral CT with three-dimensional (3D) reconstructions and catheter-based angiography with a marking catheter for patient evaluation is used. Both modalities are reliable for complementary information. In general, aortic diameters are more reliably obtained with CT, whereas lengths of the neck, total aneurysm, and iliac system are more reliably obtained with angiography. Some centers use 3D MR-angiography as well for preprocedural testing.

■ Device Design—General Considerations

Characteristics of the ideal endograft for AAA are low profile, high flexibility, ability to be placed suprarenal, kink resistance, easy and precise deployment mechanism, permanent fixation, and ability to tailor limb length. No ideal device exists at the present time, and in order to achieve certain characteristics, others must be sacrificed. Several different design strategies have been employed. Each has advantages and disadvantages.

Unibody Versus Modular Design

The earliest endografts designed by Parodi were unibody in design, meaning they were made of one piece of endograft. These unibody designs are primarily for aorto-iliac repair of AAAs requiring the surgical creation of a crossed femoral bypass, and surgical or endovascular ligation of the contralateral common iliac artery.

Another use of the unibody design, however, has been in creating bifurcated endografts. This is the design used by the EVT device (Endovascular Technologies, Menlo Park, CA). The use of one piece without fitted components eliminates the endoleaks seen originating in "joints" between components of modular endografts. The difficulty with this design is the delivery system, which must allow the entire bifurcated endograft to pass through one delivery sheath and iliac artery, requiring to snare a deployment wire from the contralateral groin for contralateral limb delivery.

To decrease the profile of the delivery system and improve the ease of delivery, most manufactured endografts today employ a modular design. This allows lower profile, as the contralateral limb of the graft is deployed in a retrograde fashion from the contralateral groin. This also increases the flexibility of the delivery system, allowing the passage through more tortuous arteries as compared to the unibody design. While a snaring maneuver is sometimes needed for contralateral limb deployment, the open pants leg of the main endograft piece can often be intubated from the contralateral groin with an angled catheter and wire. In many instances, deployment of these modular devices is accomplished simply by unsheathing the outer jacket on the delivery catheter. Perhaps one of the most appealing features of the modular design is the ability to easily use proximal and distal extender pieces to fix endoleaks and recover from device placement that is either too distal from the renal arteries or not seated far enough into the common or external iliac artery.

Supported Versus Unsupported

Devices can be further separated into supported versus unsupported. This describes whether or not the endograft has stent material throughout its length, or only at the attachment sites. The original Parodi device was routinely supported only by a proximal Palmaz stent. Most hand-fashioned aorto-iliac unibody endografts are unsupported in this fashion. Advantages include easier pushability through the iliac arteries, disadvantages the propensity for unsupported endografts to kink and to become narrowed in areas of atherosclerotic disease. Most manufactured devices today come fully supported, with the exception being the EVT device.

Attachment Mechanism

Attachment to the arterial wall is achieved by several different methods. Small hooks are employed by the EVT, the Vanguard (Boston Scientific Corp., Natick, MA), and Excluder (Gore & Associates, Flagstaff, AZ) device to anchor the proximal end of the device into the aorta. Barbed Gianturco stents are used by the Zenith device (Cook Inc., Bloomington, IN). Most devices use some degree of radial force, and some use this as the sole method of attachment. Examples are the Vanguard, the Talent (World Medical, Sunrise, FL), the AneuRx (Medtronic, Sunnyvale, CA), and the Excluder devices.

Supporting Skeleton

Various types of stent design and material have been used for endografts. Many production endografts use nitinol stents as the framework for a supported endograft. This is seen in the Vanguard, Talent, and Excluder devices. Gianturco Z-stents line the Zenith and Chuter endografts as well as many hand-fashioned devices.

As device profile decreases, these procedures continue to evolve toward a completely percutaneous delivery system. Many of the devices now have contralateral limbs that can be deployed through percutaneous access (Vanguard and Excluder devices). Cordis/Johnson & Johnson Endovascular is soon to bring a low-profile system to clinical trials that brings the promise of a device that is deployed entirely through percutaneous access. With these systems comes the realization of the less invasive promise of these devices.

■ Description of Devices

Parodi Device and Similar Hand-Fashioned Devices

Dotter first proposed endoprostheses in 1969.[10] Becker et al were the first to describe the deployment of a covered stent in a human.[11] Animal studies of percutaneous exclusion and treatment of AAAs began with Parodi's work in 1976. He used a knitted Dacron (polyester) tube graft mounted on the outside of Palmaz stents. Since that time, animal work has continued, again mainly in dogs. Some of the focus of this research has been to investigate new materials, histologic changes in the aorta after endograft placement, the significance of lumbar and mesenteric artery filling of the sac, and monitoring pressures in the residual aneurysm sac.[12–26]

Parodi et al's work then continued in humans, first published in 1991.[15] Three of the first five patients received stent-grafts with only cephalic-end stent placement, and two received grafts with both ends of the graft supported by Palmaz stents. Four of five patients were treated successfully, and the fifth was misdeployed, requiring open surgery. An endoleak was noted in a patient with only proximal stent placement, but this was treated successfully with use of an additional stent at the distal attachment. Since that time, Parodi et al have published their more recent experience with endograft placement associated with a 30-day mortality of 9%, including two patients with delayed aortic rupture (both had proximal endoleaks).[27–29] Overall, 75% of the grafts placed for AAA were technically successful.

The Stanford experience with an aorto-iliac handmade device in 15 patients was published in 1998.[30] These were all high-risk patients with short distal necks considered to be unsuitable for tube grafts. The authors fashioned the endografts from Z-stents (Cook, Bloomington, IN) covered with a PTFE graft. The contralateral iliac artery was embolized with an occluder device. Leaks were noted in 53% of patients.

Silberzweig and colleagues reported their experience of 36 patients with aorto-iliac aneurysm repair.[31] They used an 8-mm thin-walled PTFE graft dilated to 30 mm proximally. A large Palmaz stent was sutured into the proximal end of the graft with 2 cm of bare stent above the graft. These were all aorto-iliac devices with occlusion of the contralateral iliac artery with use of an occlusive endovascular device and surgical fem-fem crossover grafting. Overall, 31% of their endografts required iliac stenting to correct for intra-graft stenosis. This prompted them to conclude that a fully supported graft was necessary to prevent these complications.

Chuter Device

The first bifurcated endograft used in humans was designed by Chuter et al.[32–35] Their experience in 14 dogs was published in 1993.[32] Of note is that the technical success of the bifurcated endograft improved dramatically over time as the device improved from a 50% to a 100% technical success rate for the last 17 endografts.[36] A recent publication covers their experience in 50 high-risk patients with a tubular aorto-aortic and an aorto-iliac design.[37–38] The endograft for this cohort was made of Cooley Verisoft fabric (Meadox Medicals, Oakland, NJ) with Gianturco Z-stents both proximally and distally. Most of the devices deployed were aorto-iliac (42/50) with an occluder used for the contralateral iliac and a surgical femoral-femoral bypass created to restore flow. The remaining 8 patients were treated with tube grafts. The initial success rate was 88% with 4 of the endoleaks treated by endovascular means and 2 sealing spontaneously. A bifurcated device could not be fashioned due to the size constraints of the delivery system. Most of the complications were local wound and/or vascular with one femoral to femoral bypass occlusion and 4 groin hematomas requiring reoperation. A recent review details the insertion technique of this family of devices.[38]

Endovascular Technologies Endoprosthesis (EVT)

One of the first production endografts to enter clinical trials, the EVT device (Endovascular Technologies, Menlo Park, CA) will most likely be the first to meet FDA approval for clinical use. The proximal and distal attachment mechanisms consist of a self-expanding zigzag attachment mechanism with hooks for penetration of the aortic wall (Fig. 5–1). The fabric is Dacron and the graft is fitted into a jacketed delivery device that is 24-Fr (ID). While some early attachment wire fractures occurred early in the phase I and II FDA clinical trials, the problem was corrected quickly by the manufacturer. Deployment of the device requires a surgical arteriotomy on the primary side of deployment for the main trunk and ipsilateral limb. The contralateral limb is deployed through a percutaneously placed 12-Fr (ID) sheath, while a surgical arteriotomy is an option for those cases in which greater control is desired. The drawback of the arteriotomy is more ischemia time for the limb and greater infection rate.

Much data has been gained with the EVT device. Its use (tube design) was reported by Moore and Rutherford in 46 patients.[39] Seven procedures had to be converted to open repair. Most of these were caused by deployment problems in the iliac artery. Endoleaks were initially detected in 17 of the remaining 39 patients; nine of these resolved spontaneously; six were treated expectantly with no increase in aneurysm size, and one required delayed conversion to open repair due to continued expansion; and one was treated successfully by balloon angioplasty. A metallic attachment fracture that led to removal of implant in one patient, and recognized in eight additional patients, caused a voluntary and temporary suspension until redesign was carried out.

Subsequently, Edwards et al described their experience with the EVT device after phase I and early phase II results of the tube graft and phase I of the bifurcated system.[40] Their phase I experience with the tube graft included five patients, one of which required open surgery due to iliac artery rupture during device deployment. Another patient went on to thrombose the access iliac artery and required a crossover fem-fem graft. The phase II trial of the tube grafts involved randomization to endograft or open surgical repair. Four patients were randomized to tube grafts. Two patients had endoleaks,

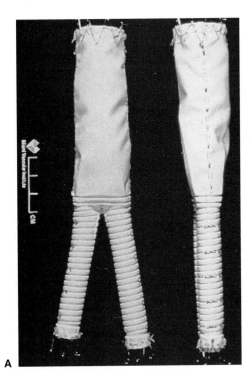

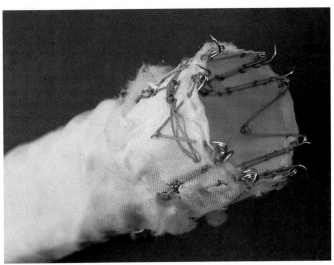

FIGURE 5–1. EVT endograft (Endovascular Technologies, Menlo Park, CA). (**A**). EVT device: unibody, unsupported design with attachment hooks at both proximal and distal ends. (**B**). Close-up view of the attachment mechanism of the proximal endograft which consists of a self-expanding zigzag attachment mechanism with hooks for penetration of the aortic wall.

A

with one requiring operative repair due to enlargement of the aneurysm and one resolving without treatment. There were only three patients in the phase I trial of the bifurcated system. One of these patients developed both a proximal and distal leak. The distal leak persisted and the aneurysm continued to enlarge. Another patient required stenting of an intragraft stenosis or kink in the iliac segment.

Balm et al reported their experience in the phase I trial of the EVT device in 31 patients in 1996.[41] One patient was converted to open repair after the patient complained of back pain and a postoperative CT showed a proximal leak. One patient died after reexploration of the groin for limb ischemia. One patient experienced a stroke and another temporary renal insufficiency. One toe amputation was performed for atheroembolism and two had petechiae, which resolved without amputation.

Moore and Colburn reported the UCLA experience with the EVT device in 1994 and 1996.[42,43] They placed 16 tube and 3 bifurcated grafts. Two of these patients were converted to open surgery early. One patient was converted late after attachment pin fractures caused migration of the device. They described five endoleaks, only two of which persisted without enlargement of the aneurysm sac.

The most recent published data on the EVT device comes from Brewster et al.[44] They reported their experience with 25 EVT devices under the phase I and II FDA. These were compared to a concurrent nonrandomized cohort of surgical patients who appeared to be fairly well matched in regard to anatomic and systemic parameters. No deaths have occurred in either group, and the rate of complications in the two groups seemed equal in occurrence. The types of complications, however, differed dramatically between the endovascular and open surgical groups; 16 of 28 endovascular patients had local or vascular complications as opposed to 2 of 28 patients treated with open repair. There were 4 systemic or remote complications in the endovascular group and 18 in the open surgical group. This clearly shows that endovascular repair has a very different postoperative as well as intraoperative course.

White-Yu Device

The White-Yu device consists of wire forms embedded into polyester fabric and is designed in a straight or bifurcated fashion. May, White, and Yu published several reports of their experience with endograft placement for the treatment of AAA.[45–51] In 1996 they reported their experience with 100 endografts, most of which were White-Yu devices (n=63), and EVT devices (n=15).[49] Their results with this device in 93 patients was published in 1997.[37] Seventy-six of these patients were

treated for AAA with 39 tube grafts, 20 tapered aortoiliac, and 20 bifurcated devices placed. Success rates were 81% for tube grafts, 95% for aortoiliac, and 75% for bifurcated devices. The overall 30-day mortality rate (including the thoracic, iliac, and popliteal procedures) was 3.1%. They had five primary endoleaks with two patients converted to open repair, two further being treated by additional covered stents, and one that healed without treatment. The three secondary endoleaks were treated by percutaneous means. One patient is described as having a secondary endoleak that ruptured, requiring emergent surgery.

This group also published a comparison of endoluminal repair of AAA to open surgery. In this report, 108 patients receiving endografts for elective repair of AAA were compared to 195 elective operative repairs.[51] Again, there was a majority of tubular grafts deployed. There were 68 White-Yu grafts, 15 EVT devices, and 14 Vanguard devices deployed. Thirteen of the 108 patients required immediate conversion to open repair, and five additional patients delayed conversion for endoleak and renal artery obstruction by the endograft. There were a total of 13 endoleaks, six of which were delayed. Three of these endoleaks sealed spontaneously. Of note is that the perioperative mortality rate was the same for both groups (5.6%), with half of the mortality in the endoluminal repair group occurring in patients requiring emergent conversion to open repair. Remote and systemic complications were also not significantly different (17% for endoluminal group versus 20% for open repair), which is at odds with most other studies.

Vanguard Device

The Vanguard device (Boston Scientific Corp., Natick, MA) comprises tube and bifurcated designs. First implanted in a patient in May 1994, this endograft is a fully supported thin weave of polyester surrounding an endoskeleton of nitinol (Fig. 5–2). There is bare stent on the top end of the endograft. The endograft comes prefabricated in aortic component diameters of 22–30 mm and iliac component diameters of 10–12 mm. It can also be custom made. The delivery device is 18-Fr (ID) for the deployment of the main graft and iliac limb, requiring a surgical arteriotomy. The contralateral iliac limb is delivered with use of a 10-Fr (ID) sheath via a percutaneous approach. A proximal neck lengths of at least 15 mm is needed.

Blum et al reported their experience with the Vanguard (formerly known as the Mialhe/Stentor) device in 1996.[52] The initial report in 1996 covered 26 men, three of whom received tube grafts, and the other 23 patients received bifurcated devices. The three tube grafts were deployed successfully without immediate complications.

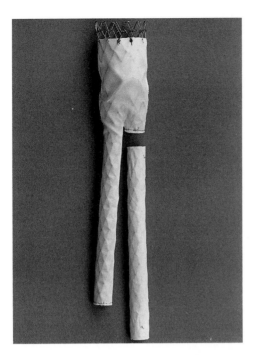

FIGURE 5–2. Vanguard bifurcated endograft (Boston Scientific Corp., Natick, MA). This endograft is a fully supported thin weave of polyester surrounding an endoskeleton of nitinol. There is bare stent on the top end of the endoprosthesis.

The 23 patients with bifurcated grafts experienced technical difficulties including the following: four patients required extension covered grafts to fully exclude the iliac artery aneurysm; three distal endoleaks had sealed without treatment by 4 to 7 days following deployment; and one patient had a major distal leak from improper sizing of the iliac limb (this was treated successfully by deploying a covered stent at 3 months). Complications included distal embolization in two patients, surgical groin hematoma in one, death from hepatorenal syndrome in one, and embolic occlusion of the graft from a cardiac source in another. Of note is that no patients required conversion to open surgery.

This report was followed up by Blum et al in 1997.[53] At this time, 154 patients had been collected (out of 331 referred for AAA evaluation), with 133 bifurcated grafts, and 21 tube grafts placed; 134 of the 154 patients had primary technical success (86% for tube grafts and 78% for bifurcated grafts). The group had one death, and only 3 procedures converted to open repair. Fourteen other complications had occurred, most of which were minor. The two other major complications were foot amputation and iliac artery rupture. Fourteen immediate leaks occurred, three in the patients with tube grafts and 11 in the bifurcated cohort. The leaks in most patients were treated by additional covered stents. There were 7 late leaks detected, all treated by coil embolization.

This experience was again published in 1998 when 228 patients had been enrolled.[54] The authors reported an initial success rate of 96% and an endoleak type II-rate for the patients treated with the most recent design of the bifurcated Vanguard device (100 patients).

Dorffner et al also reported their experience of 28 patients (11 tube grafts and 17 bifurcated grafts) with the Vanguard device in 1997;[55] 32% of patients referred to them were eventually endograft candidates, lower than that reported by Blum et al. In this series, there was one conversion to open repair when a bifurcated endograft migrated and showed a proximal leak on postprocedural angiography. In one patient, an arteriotomy of the external iliac was performed to gain access to the aorta proximal to a stenosis of the distal external iliac artery. Immediate distal leaks were seen in half of their bifurcated grafts, but almost all were treated successfully by placing additional covered stents; 14 out of 17 bifurcated grafts required additional covered stents to exclude leaks. In the group with tube grafts, four of 11 had leaks detected at CT by 1 week. Three of these leaks sealed spontaneously. One of these recurred and was treated successfully along with the other leak, with one also requiring embolization of a lumbar artery. This study therefore had a high eventual success (93%), but the majority of patients required additional percutaneous intervention for complete exclusion of their aneurysm.

Mialhe et al also reported their experience of the Stentor device (MinTec, La Ciotat, France) in 79 patients.[56] This group consisted of eight tube grafts and 71 bifurcated grafts. The primary technical success rate was 78%. There were 13 immediate leaks and six delayed leaks. Seven of those were treated successfully by the placement of an additional straight covered stent. There were no conversions to open repair. A considerable number of local, remote and systemic complications was observed: four immediate postoperative deaths, four pulmonary complications, one cholesterol embolization to the kidneys, and colonic ischemia in a further three patients. In addition, five pelvic thromboses and one embolic occlusion of the popliteal artery occurred, eventually treated with a Fogarty balloon catheter.

Talent Device

The Talent Endoprosthesis (World Medical, Sunrise, FL) is a fully supported graft with a nitinol frame and a polyester covering on both inner and outer surfaces (Fig. 5–3A). The device can be custom made for each patient and is also available in off-the-shelf sizes of 22 mm–32 mm. It is available as a tube or bifurcated graft. It is one of two endografts that is available in an "open-weave" configuration in the proximal aortic component with bare wire

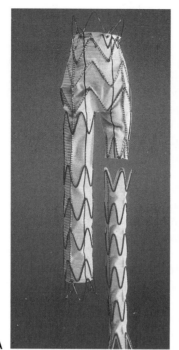
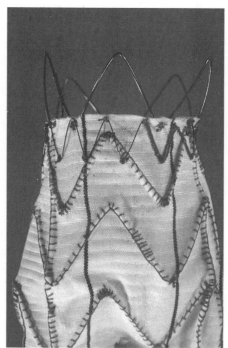

FIGURE 5–3. Talent Endoprosthesis (World Medical, Sunrise, FL). (**A**). Talent endograft device. This is an example of a modular supported, bifurcated device. (**B**). Close-up view of the bare spring portion of the proximal endograft, which is available for suprarenal deployment.

that can be deployed across the origin of the renal arteries (Fig. 5–3B). Because of this configuration, the requirement for proximal neck length for deployment is lessened to 5 mm. Most other endografts require 10–15 mm of nonaneurysmal proximal aortic neck length for safe deployment. Another significant advantage of this graft is the ability to accommodate proximal aortic diameters of up to 34 mm. The delivery system of most of the Talent endografts is 22–24-Fr (OD) on the ipsilateral and 18-Fr (OD) for the contralateral delivery device with need of a bilateral surgical femoral access. To accommodate aortic diameters up to 34 mm, a 24-Fr (OD) sheath is needed. The delivery catheter is a type of pusher with a balloon for deployment and for postdeployment "tamping." The manufacturer is now starting to enroll patients in a trial of a newer, lower profile system.

First placed in humans in December 1995, it has quickly gained clinical experience with over 5000 grafts placed for AAAs as of August 1999.[57–60] In a review of the device to date, Machan and Fry reviewed the world experience with the Talent endograft in 394 patients with AAAs.[59] These were all performed in patients who were not surgical candidates. There were 327 bifurcated and 67 tube grafts deployed. Of 301 patients available for follow-up, there were 29 (9.6%) conversions to open repair, a somewhat higher figure than quoted for other en-

dografts. Three of these patients who needed conversion to open repair subsequently died. There were 42 perigraft endoleaks (14%), but no comment upon their management or outcome was made in the review.

AneuRx Device

The AneuRx device is a bifurcated, modular nitinol frame lined by a thin-walled Dacron prosthesis at the inside (Medtronic, Sunnyvale, CA) (Fig. 5–4). The stent graft is available in varying diameters (20–28mm), lengths (135 and 165 mm) and configurations (straight or bifurcated) as well as the optional extension cuffs to ensure complete aneurysm exclusion. The endograft is delivered via a 21-Fr (ID) sheath, whereas the contralateral groin is initially catheterized with an 16-Fr (ID) sheath, requiring a bilateral surgical cutdown.

White et al published their experience in 16 patients with the AneuRx device as part of the phase I FDA trial in 1997.[61] There were no conversions to open repair. There was one endoleak detected at the 6-month CT exam, presumably from a tear in the fabric during insertion, but the aneurysm has decreased in cross-sectional area by 44%. There was one perioperative death due to cholecystitis. Of note is that this group uses intravenous ultrasound (IVUS) for every placement, with the

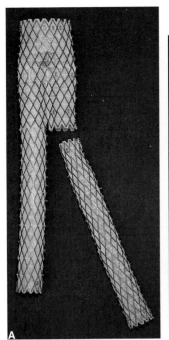
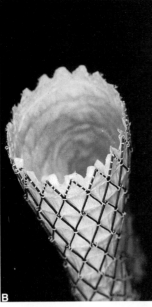

FIGURE 5–4. AneuRx device (Medtronic, Sunnyvale, CA). **(A).** This device is a bifurcated, modular nitinol frame lined by a thin-walled Dacron prosthesis at the inside. **(B).** No fixation system at the top of the endoprosthesis.

thought that this offers more precise measurements than angiography or CT.

These results were followed up with a report by Zarins et al in 1999.[62] They reported on the AneuRx experience in 190 patients in comparison to 60 nonrandomized surgical controls. This covered their FDA phase I and II trials with 40 and 150 patients, respectively. Each center enrolled a small number of surgical controls before they were allowed to perform the endograft deployments. They reported a primary success rate of 78% in the endograft group, defined as a patient alive, with no endoleak, and no reoperation, repeat procedure, or major complication. The rate of endoleaks was 21% at time of discharge, 9% at 6 months, and 6% at 12 months. There were 39 leaks detected at the initial CT scan broken down as follows: seven at the proximal attachment site, 12 from collateral refilling, 10 at the distal attachment site, and 10 from "transgraft" flow. Six (50%) of the collateral leaks sealed spontaneously. Ten endovascular procedures were used to seal endoleaks. Only one patient with a persistent endoleak had enlargement of the aneurysm. There was a significant difference in the need for major reoperation in the two groups (10% in the surgical group versus 1% in the endograft group). There was, interestingly, no difference in the need for local groin exploration in the 2 groups. The rate of medical complications was higher in the surgical group (12% vs 3%). The 30-day mortality rate was 2.6% in the

endograft group and 0% in the surgical group. Two deaths were associated with chronic obstructive pulmonary disease (COPD), one from cholecystitis as described above, one from myocardial infarction (MI) during coronary intervention 3 weeks after successful endograft placement, and one from colon ischemia from covering a patent IMA and internal iliac artery.

Excluder Device

The Excluder endograft (Gore and Assoc., Flagstaff, AZ) is a fully supported graft with a PTFE covering on the inner surface of a nitinol skeleton (Fig. 5–5). The endograft has a low profile and is modular, with both aortic and iliac extenders available. The iliac diameters are available in 12 and 14.5 mm to accommodate iliac arteries 10 to 13.5 mm in diameter. The main trunk and ipsilateral limb comes in 16- and 18-cm lengths. The aortic end of the endograft in 23-, 26-, and 28.5-mm diameters to accommodate aortic diameters of 19 to 26 mm.

The ipsilateral groin sheath is 18-Fr (ID), with the contralateral sheath being 12-Fr (ID). The 18-Fr sheath is placed through a surgical arteriotomy, with the contralateral sheath being placed percutaneously. The graft is unique in its deployment. The device is deployed by pulling off a rip-cord arrangement to unjacket the device and deploy it quickly (identical to the Hemobahn endograft). Appropriately sized balloons are then used to model fully the proximal graft attachment of the main body of the graft and the ipsilateral iliac limb.

Blum et al recently communicated a series of 62 patients treated with the Excluder device.[63] The primary technical success rate was 90%, the rate of type II-endoleaks with lumbar refilling 10%. Apart from one local problem at the access site (laceration of the femoral artery, requiring a patch repair) no further complications occurred. A phase II FDA trial is ongoing in Europe and the USA. Enrollment in this phase of FDA testing should be completed in the fall of 1999.

Zenith Endograft

This stent-graft is made up of a fully supported surgical polyester-fabric graft (thickness 0.035 mm) on a network of Z-stents (Cook Inc., Bloomington, IN) (Fig. 5–6). The endograft is available as a modular system or as a aortouni-iliac version. The top uncovered suprarenal stent has a length of 26 mm and 10 barbs which are placed at different levels and are 5 mm long (Fig. 5–6B). The introducer size is 20-Fr (ID) for the main system, 16 to 18-Fr (ID) for the contralateral limbs and extension legs, respectively.

Gordon, Lawrence-Brown, et al published their experience in 1996,[64,65] and most recently in 1998[66] with their graft, now commercially available in Europe as the Zenith

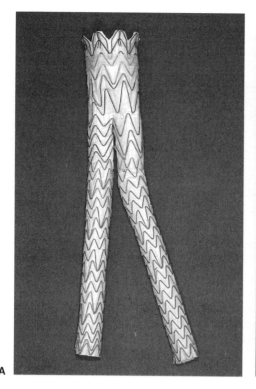
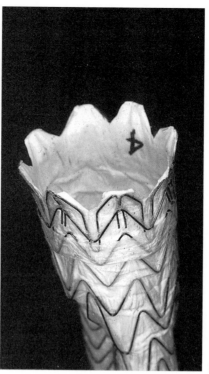

FIGURE 5–5. Excluder endograft (Gore and Assoc., Flagstaff, AZ). The Excluder device is a fully supported graft with a PTFE covering on the inner surface of a nitinol skeleton. (**A**). Prior to deployment of the contralateral limb. (**B**). Close-up of the top of the stent-graft demonstrates small hooks to anchor the leading part.

endograft. The initial report covered 33 patients (5 tube grafts, 22 bifurcated grafts, and 2 aorto-iliac grafts). All were considered high surgical risk patients. The authors reported a perioperative death rate of 5.4% (two patients) from proximal leaks with rupture, with one patient having a disabling stroke caused by angioplasty from a brachial approach. Two procedures were converted to open repair due to delivery system problems. No delayed endoleaks occurred. Three patients with chronic renal insufficiency had progression of their disease.

Their most recent report covered the experience with 108 bifurcated grafts for infrarenal AAAs.[66] They achieved a primary success rate of 87%. They had a total of 15 endoleaks by the 6-week follow-up CT. Seven of these were treated by transcatheter techniques and four sealed spontaneously. There were three patients in whom the graft could not be deployed. Of note is that they experienced four late proximal endoleaks, all due to migration of the device associated with continued expansion of the neck, neck atherosclerotic disease, or flaring of the neck.

■ Complications of Endograft Placement

Endovascular treatment of infrarenal AAAs is associated with certain known complications. There has been noted, however, a shift of their occurrence to more local and vascular complications when compared to open re-

pair. In a nonrandomized comparison of the techniques of open repair versus endovascular repair, Brewster et al noted that the local versus systemic complications were reversed in their rate of occurrence with the two techniques.[44] In their series, endovascular repair had an approximately 50% rate of local/vascular complications in comparison to the 6% rate for open repair. Endovascular repair had an approximately 12% rate of systemic complications in comparison to the 60% rate seen with open surgery. Of note is that most of the local/vascular complications seen with endovascular repair were readily treatable with catheter techniques. We expect the rate of these local and vascular complications to fall dramatically as experience with these devices is gained.

Endoleaks

One of the feared results of endovascular treatment of AAAs is endoleak. The term endoleak, coined by White et al,[67] describes the situation in which there is continued flow of blood into the extragraft portion of the aneurysm sac. They differentiate between 2 types of endoleaks: a type I-endoleak as to be graft-related, and a type II-endoleak as not to be graft-related, such as backbleeding via lumbar arteries or the IMA. This can be seen on the initial completion angiogram, on follow-up CT, or on a follow-up duplex exam. The classification of leaks has been in evolution. Another classification is given by Wain et al.[68] Endoleaks in this classification are described in

59. Machan L, Fry P. Abdominal aortic aneurysm repair using the World Medical Talent prosthesis. Techn Vasc Interv Radiol 1998;1: 25–31.
60. Uflacker R, Robison JG, Brothers TE, Pereira AH, Sanvitto PC. Abdominal aortic aneurysm treatment: preliminary results with the Talent stent-graft system. J Vasc Intervent Radiol 1998;9:51–60.
61. White RA, Donayre CE, Walot I, et al. Modular bifurcation endoprosthesis for treatment of abdominal aortic aneurysms. Ann Surg 1997;226:381–391.
62. Zarins CK, White RA, Schwarten D, et al. AneuRx stent graft versus open surgical repair of abdominal aortic aneurysms: multicenter prospective clinical trial. J Vasc Surg 1999;29:292–308.
63. Blum U, Voshage G, Pfammatter T, et al. Endoluminal treatment of AAA with use of the Excluder device. Personal communication.
64. Gordon MK, Lawrence-Brown MMD, Hartley D, et al. A self-expanding endoluminal graft for treatment of aneurysms: results through the development phase. Aust N Z J Surgery 1996;66: 621–625.
65. Lawrence-Brown MMD, Hartley D, MacSweeney STR, et al. The Perth endoluminal bifurcated graft system-development and early experience. Cardiovasc Surg 1996;4:706–712.
66. Van Schie GP, Sieunarine K, Lawrence-Brown MMD, Hartley D. The Perth bifurcated endovascular graft for infrarenal aortic aneurysms. Sem Interv Radiol 1998;15:63–9.
67. White GH, Yu W, May J. "Endoleak"—a proposed new terminology to describe incomplete aneurysm exclusion by an endoluminal graft. J Endovasc Surg 1996;3:124–125.
68. Wain RA, Marin ML, Ohki T, et al. Endoleaks after endovascular graft treatment of aortic aneurysms: Classification, risk factors, and outcome. J Vasc Surg 1998;27:69–80.
69. Sato DT, Goff CD, Gregory RT, et al. Endoleak after aortic stent graft repair: diagnosis by color duplex ultrasound scan versus computed tomography scan. J Vasc Surg 1998;28:657–663.
70. Malina M, Lanne T, Ivancev K, et al. Reduced pulsatile wall motion of abdominal aortic aneurysms after endovascular repair. J Vasc Surg 1998;27:624–631.
71. Lipski DA, Ernst CB. Natural history of the residual infrarenal aorta after infrarenal abdominal aortic aneurysm repair. J Vasc Surg 1998;27:805–812.
72. Matsumura JS, Chaikof EL. Continued expansion of aortic necks after endovascular repair of abdominal aortic aneurysms. J Vasc Surg 1998;28:422–431.
73. Sonesson B, Resch T, Lanne T, Ivancev K. The fate of the infrarenal aortic neck after open aneurysm surgery. J Vasc Surg 1998;28:889–894.
74. Marin ML, Parsons RE, Hollier LH, et al. Impact of transrenal aortic endograft placement on endovascular graft repair of abdominal aortic aneurysms. J Vasc Surg 1998;28:638–646.
75. Duda SH, Raygrotzki S, Wiskirchen J, et al. Abdominal aortic aneurysms: treatment with juxtarenal placement of covered stent-grafts. Radiology 1998;206:195–198.
76. Matsumura JS, Moore WS. Clinical consequences of periprosthetic leak after endovascular repair of abdominal aortic aneurysm. J Vasc Surg 1998;27:606–613.
77. Resch T, Ivancev K, Lindh M, et al. Persistent collateral perfusion of abdominal aortic aneurysm after endovascular repair does not lead to progressive change in aneurysm diameter. J Vasc Surg 1998;28:242–249.
78. Kato N, Semba CP, Kee ST, et al. Treatment of aortoiliac aneurysms using single-piece tapered stent-grafts. J Vasc Intervent Radiol 1998;9:41–49.
79. Khilnani NM, Sos TA, Trost DW, et al. Embolization of backbleeding lumbar arteries filling an aortic aneurysm sac after endovascular stent-graft placement. J Vasc Intervent Radiol 1996;7: 813–817.
80. Dorffner R, Thurnher S, Holzenbein T, Kretschmer G, Lammer J. Radiologic management of complications encountered with placement of abdominal aortic stent grafts. Sem Interv Radiol 1998;15:47–54.
81. Golzarian J, Struyven J, Abada HT, et al. Endovascular aortic stent-grafts: transcatheter embolization of persistent perigraft leaks. Radiology 1997;202:731–734.

16. Mirich D, Wright KC, Wallace S, et al. Percutaneously placed endovascular grafts for aortic aneurysms: feasibility study. Radiology 1989;170:1033–1037.

17. Boudghene FS, Anidjar S, Allaire E, et al. Endovascular grafting in elastase-induced experimental aortic aneurysms in dogs: feasibility and preliminary results. J Vasc Intervent Radiol 1993;4:497–504.

18. Hagen B, Harnoss BM, Trabbardt S, et al. Self-expandable macroporous nitinol stents for transfemoral exclusion of aortic aneurysms in dogs: preliminary results. Cardiovasc Intervent Radiol 1993;16:339–342.

19. Piquet P, Rolland PH, Bartoli JM, et al. Tantalum-Dacron coknit stent for endovascular treatment of aortic aneurysms: a preliminary experimental study. J Vasc Surg 1994;19:698–706.

20. White R, Kopchok G, Zalewski M, et al. Comparison of the deployment and healing of thin-walled expanded PTFE stented grafts and covered stents. Ann Vasc Surg 1996;10:336–346.

21. Marston WA, Criado E, Baird CA, Keagy BA. Reduction of aneurysm pressure and wall stress after endovascular repair of abdominal aortic aneurysm in a canine model. Ann Vasc Surg 1996;10:166–173.

22. Chuter TA, Viscomi S, Slater JL, et al. Canine model of abdominal aortic aneurysm treated by endovascular graft implantation. Cardiovascular Surgery 1997;5:490–496.

23. Wilson EP, White RA, Kopchok GE, et al. Deployment and healing of an ePTFE encapsulated stent endograft in the canine aorta. Ann Vasc Surg 1997;11:354–358.

24. Eton D, Warner D, Owens C, et al. Results of endoluminal grafting in an experimental aortic aneurysm model. J Vasc Surg 1996;23:819–831.

25. Sanchez LA, Faries PL, Marin ML, et al. Chronic intraaneurysmal pressure measurement: an experimental method for evaluating the effectiveness of endovascular aortic aneurysm exclusion. J Vasc Surg 1997;26:222–230.

26. Quinones-Baldrich WJ, Deaton DH, Mitchell RS, et al. Preliminary experience with the Endovascular Technologies bifurcated endovascular aortic prosthesis in a calf model. J Vasc Surg 1995;22:370–381.

27. Parodi JC. Endovascular repair of abdominal aortic aneurysms and other arterial lesions. J Vasc Surg 1995;21:549–557.

28. Parodi JC, Criado FJ, Barone HD, et al. Endoluminal aortic aneurysm repair using a balloon-expandable stent-graft device: a progress report. Ann Vasc Surg 1994;8:523–529.

29. Parodi JC. Endovascular repair of aortic aneurysms, arteriovenous fistulas, and false aneurysms. World J Surg 1996;20:655–663.

30. Kato N, Semba CP, Dake MD. Use of a self-expanding vascular occluder for embolization during endovascular aortic aneurysm repair. J Vasc Intervent Radiol 1997;8:27–33.

31. Silberzweig JE, Marin ML, Hollier LH, et al. Aortoiliac aneurysms: endoluminal repair—clinical evidence for a fully supported stent-graft. Radiology 1998;209:111–116.

32. Chuter TAM, Green RM, Ouriel K, et al. Transfemoral endovascular aortic graft placement. J Vasc Surg 1993;18:185–197.

33. Scott RAP, Chuter TAM. Clinical endovascular placement of bifurcated graft in abdominal aortic aneurysm without laparotomy. Lancet 1994;343:413.

34. Yusuf SW, Baker DM, Chuter TAM, et al. Transfemoral endoluminal repair of abdominal aortic aneurysm with bifurcated graft. Lancet 1994;344:350–351.

35. Chuter TAM, Wendt G, Hopkinson BR, et al. Transfemoral insertion of a bifurcated endovascular graft for aortic aneurysm repair: the first 22 patients. Cardiovasc Surg 1995;3:121–128.

36. Chuter TAM, Risberg B, Hopkinson BR, et al. Clinical experience with a bifurcated graft for abdominal aortic aneurysm repair. J Vasc Surg 1996;2:655–666.

37. Chuter TAM, Gordon RL, Reilly LM, et al. Abdominal aortic aneurysm in high-risk patients: short- to intermediate-term results of endovascular repair. Radiology 1999;210:361–365.

38. Chuter TAM, Reilly LM, Canto C, et al. Endovascular treatment of aortic aneurysm using the Chuter device. Sem Interv Radiol 1998;15:55–61.

39. Moore WS, Rutherford RB. Transfemoral endovascular repair of abdominal aortic aneurysm: results of the North American EVT phase 1 Trial. EVT Investigators. J Vasc Surg 1996;23:543–553.

40. Edwards WH Jr, Naslund TC, Edwards WH Sr, Jenkins JM, McPherson K. Endovascular grafting of abdominal aortic aneurysms: a preliminary study. Ann Surg 1996;223:568–575.

41. Balm R, Eikelboom BC, May J, et al. Early experience with transfemoral endovascular aneurysm management (TEAM) in the treatment of aortic aneurysms. Eur J Vasc Endovasc Surg 1996;11:214–220.

42. Moore, WS, Vecera CL. Repair of abdominal aortic aneurysm by transfemoral endovascular graft placement. Ann Surg 1994;19:924–933.

43. Colburn MD, Moore WS. Endovascular repair of abdominal aortic aneurysms using the EGS tube and bifurcated graft systems. World J Surg 1996;20:664–672.

44. Brewster DC, Geller SC, Kaufman JA, et al. Initial experience with endovascular aneurysm repair: comparison of early results with outcome of conventional open repair. J Vasc Surg 1998;27: 992–1005.

45. May J, White GH, Saugh R, et al. Treatment of complex abdominal aortic aneurysms by combination of endoluminal and extraluminal aortofemoral grafts. J Vasc Surg 1994;19:924–933.

46. White GH, Yu W, May J, et al. A new nonstented balloon-expandable graft for straight or bifurcated endoluminal bypass. J Endovasc Surg 1994;1:16–24.

47. May J, White GH, Yu W, et al. Endoluminal grafting of abdominal aortic aneurysms: causes of failure and their prevention. J Endovasc Surg 1994;1:44–52.

48. May J, White GH, Yu W, et al. Surgical management of complications following endoluminal grafting of abdominal aortic aneurysms. Eur J Vasc Endovasc Surg 1995;10:51–59.

49. May J, White GH, Yu W, et al. Repair of abdominal aortic aneurysms by the endoluminal method: outcome in the first 100 patients. JAMA 1996;165:549–551.

50. White, GH, Yu W, May J, et al. Three-year experience with the White-Yu endovascular GAD graft for transluminal repair of aortic and iliac aneurysms. J Endovasc Surg 1997;4:124–136.

51. May J, White GH, Yu W, et al. Concurrent comparison of endoluminal versus open repair in the treatment of abdominal aortic aneurysms: analysis of 303 patients by life table method. J Vasc Surg 1998;27:213–221.

52. Blum U, Langer M, Spillner G, et al. Abdominal aortic aneurysms: preliminary technical and clinical results with transfemoral placement of endovascular self-expanding stent-grafts. Radiology 1996;198:25–31.

53. Blum U, Voshage G, Lammer J, et al. Endoluminal stent-grafts for infrarenal abdominal aortic aneurysms. N Engl J Med 1997;336: 13–20.

54. Blum U. Polyester-covered nitinol stents (Stentor/Vanguard Prosthesis) for the treatment of abdominal aortic aneurysms: results and management of complications. Sem Interv Radiol 1998;15: 71–9.

55. Dorffner R, Thurnher S, Polterauer P, et al. Treatment of abdominal aortic aneurysms with transfemoral placement of stent-grafts: complications and secondary radiologic intervention. Radiology 1997;204:79–86.

56. Mialhe C, Amicabile C, Becquemin JP. Endovascular treatment of infrarenal abdominal aneurysms by the Stentor system: preliminary results of 79 cases. J Vasc Surg 1997;26:199–209.

57. Uflacker R, Pereira A, Robison J, et al. Stent grafts in the treatment of abdominal aortic aneurysms: preliminary experience with the Talent system. Cardiovasc Intervent Radiol 1997;20(suppl):S66.

58. Machan L, Morris CD, Doyle L, et al. Experience with Talent endograft as treatment for aortic disease. Cardiovasc Intervent Radiol 1997;20(suppl):S87.

artery or through lumbar collaterals, is another type of leak, one that is usually treated conservatively. We usually employ a strategy of close observation for these endoleaks, given a stable or decreasing sac size. All would agree that intervention would be necessary if the sac size was increasing over time. One report from Sweden indicated that collateral perfusion did not influence aneurysm size.[77] More rare types of endoleaks are those from distal attachment sites, tears in the fabric of the endograft, and from junction sites of modular type endografts. The management of these endoleaks depends on the clinical situation. Any endoleak associated with an increase in sac size warrants intervention. Many endoleaks can be safely watched and in many cases will spontaneously thrombose.

Prophylactic embolization is practiced only in some patients treated endoluminally for AAA. We occasionally embolize a widely patent inferior mesenteric artery before endograft deployment to prevent collateral filling of the aneurysm sac. The internal iliac artery is routinely embolized on one side if the aneurysm process involves the entire common iliac and the limb of the endograft will be placed into the external iliac. Coiling of both internal iliacs is almost never done as there is an increased risk of pelvic ischemic complications.

Management of endoleaks can be either via transcatheter techniques or surgery. Most endoleaks can be treated by endovascular means, as has been the experience of many investigators.[78–81] Proximal leaks can often be treated by repeat balloon angioplasty or by the placement of a proximal tube graft extension component. Most manufacturers can make these individually come as a modular component "off the shelf."

Collateral filling of the aneurysm sac is also easily treated by endovascular means. Access to the offending vessel is via collaterals. The IMA can often be accessed through the arch of Riolan, or less commonly, the marginal artery of Drummond. Lumbar collaterals can often be accessed via branches of the internal iliac artery.[78–81] Coils are recommended for embolization, as gelatin sponge can induce ischemia of distal beds, as described by Golzarian.[81] Leaks between components can often be treated with angioplasty alone.

Distal attachment leaks can sometimes be treated by angioplasty of the distal attachment site or by placing an iliac extension piece. Fabric tears are more problematic, but can be treated with additional endografts of a modular system.

■ Conclusion

A wide variety of devices exist for repair of AAAs. Endograft repair of AAAs is still in its infancy. Many of the devices discussed in this chapter will be antiquated in 2 to 3 years. Continued technologic improvements will lead to new generation devices that will approach many of the ideal characteristics discussed earlier. There is a definite tendency toward development of devices with a low profile, a flexible delivery system, and ease of insertion. The published data support the safety and efficacy of endografts for the treatment of AAAs. Midterm results of these studies indicate that this form of therapy will become a viable alternative to conventional surgical repair. Patient selection, anatomic factors, and indications for endograft treatment will evolve as devices change and as published data support their use.

REFERENCES

1. Ernst CB. Abdominal aortic aneurysm. N Engl J Med 1993;328:1167–1172.
2. Bickerstaff LK, Hollier LH, Van Peenen HJ, Melton LJ III, Pairolero PC, Cherry KJ. Abdominal aortic aneurysms: the changing natural history. J Vasc Surg 1984;1:6–12.
3. Pasch AR, Ricotta JJ, May AG, Green RM, De Weese JE. Abdominal aortic aneurysms: the case for elective resection. Circulation 1984;70(suppl I):I-1–I-4.
4. Estes JE Jr. Abdominal aortic aneurysm: a study of one hundred and two cases. Circulation 1950;2:258–264.
5. Katz DA, Cronenwett JL. The cost-effectiveness of early surgery versus watchful waiting in the management of small abdominal aortic aneurysms. J Vasc Surg 1994;19:980–990.
6. Katz DA, Littenberg BL, Cronenwett JL. Management of small abdominal aortic aneurysms: early surgery vs watchful waiting. JAMA 1992;268:2678–2686.
7. Hollier LH, Taylor LM, Ochsner J. Recommended indications for operative treatment of abdominal aortic aneurysms: report of a subcommittee of the Joint Council of the Society for Vascular Surgery and the International Society for Cardiovascular Surgery. J Vasc Surg 1992;15:1046–1056.
8. Veith FJ, Abbott WM, Yao JST, et al. Guidelines for development and use of transluminally placed endovascular prosthetic grafts in the arterial system. J Vasc Surg 1995;21:670–685.
9. Ahn SS, Reporting standards for infrarenal endovascular abdominal aortic aneurysm repair. Ad hoc committee for standardized reporting practices in vascular surgery of the Society for Vascular Surgery/International Society for Cardiovascular Surgery. J Vasc Surg 1997;25:405–410.
10. Dotter CT. Transluminally placed coilspring endarterial tube grafts: long-term patency in canine popliteal artery. Invest Radiol 1969;4:329–332.
11. Becker GJ, Benenati JF, Zemel G, et al. Percutaneous placement of a balloon-expandable intraluminal graft for life-threatening subclavian arterial hemorrhage. J Vasc Intervent Radiol 1991;2:225–229.
12. Yoshioka T, Wright KC, Wallace S, et al. Self-expanding endovascular graft: an experimental study in dogs. AJR 1988;151:673–676.
13. Lawrence DD, Charnsangavej C, Wright KC, et al. Percutaneous endovascular grafts: experimental evaluation. Radiology 1987;163:357–360.
14. Laborde JC, Parodi JC, Clem MF, et al. Intraluminal bypass of abdominal aortic aneurysm: feasibility study. Radiology 1992;184:185–190.
15. Parodi JC, Palmaz JC, Barone HD. Transfemoral intraluminal graft implantation for abdominal aortic aneurysms. Ann Vasc Surg 1991;5:491–499.

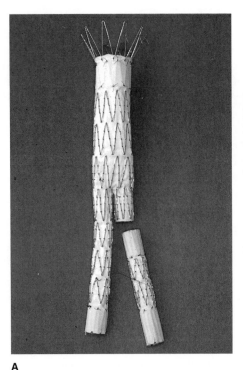

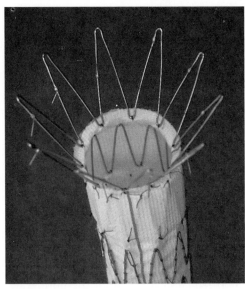

A   B

FIGURE 5–6. Zenith endograft (Cook Inc., Bloomington, IN). (**A**). The stent graft is made up of a fully supported polyester-fabric graft on a network of Z-stents. (**B**). The top of the endoprosthesis is uncovered and allows suprarenal placement (length 26 mm).

terms of their origin, or anatomic characteristics; their chronologic characteristics, or when they appear; or in terms of physiologic characteristics, or how they fill. Detection of endoleaks can be either immediately at postdeployment angiography or at the first or subsequent CT scans. CT is considered to be the most sensitive means of endoleak detection, although this method sometimes fails to define the origin and direction of filling of the leak. Duplex has been confirmed also to be useful for leak detection, but not quite as sensitive as CT.[69] Often one can see persistent pulsatility of the aneurysm on postdeployment angiography as indication of a leak. This phenomenon has been studied with ultrasound investigation of pulsatile wall motion.[70]

Most authors agree that deployment of the endograft as close to the origins of the renal arteries as possible helps reduce proximal endoleaks. Proximal aortic calcification, proximal neck angulation, and atherosclerotic disease increase the rate of endoleaks as well. These trends have been confirmed by several other reports. One other reason for close juxtarenal apposition of the endo-graft has been the observation by authors of the continued expansion of the proximal neck of the aorta after surgical and endovascular repair of aneurysms.[71–73] It is our view that the continued expansion of the infrarenal neck can lead to a proximal endoleak. The

open weave configuration of the Talent device allows deployment of this bare portion of the endograft across the renal arteries. Marin et al used hand made endografts of expanded and tapered PTFE with a Palmaz stent in the proximal portion of the graft. This stent protruded 2 cm proximally from the fabric and was deployed across the renal arteries. The authors noted a significantly lower rate of proximal endoleaks from grafts deployed in this manner when compared to endografts deployed in an infrarenal location (11% vs 38%, respectively).[74] This configuration allows placement of endografts in patients with shorter infrarenal necks than would otherwise be possible.[75]

The management of endoleaks is controversial and undergoing evolution. Some investigators have watched all leaks and only intervened when aneurysmal sac size has increased. Some have treated most leaks seen on follow-up imaging. Few investigators have advocated treatment of all leaks. Proximal leaks have traditionally been regarded as the most dangerous, and there is general accordance to intervene in the presence of a proximal leak. Many of the proximal leaks in the early EVT tube graft experience were associated with attachment wire fractures, device migration, and aneurysm enlargement, some with rupture.[76] Collateral filling of the aneurysm sac, either through a patent inferior mesenteric

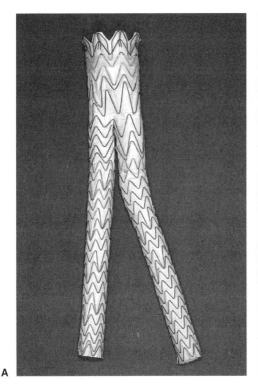
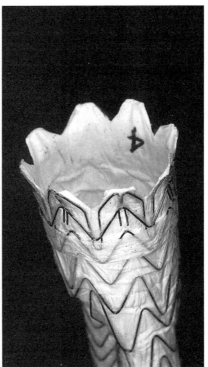

FIGURE 5–5. Excluder endograft (Gore and Assoc., Flagstaff, AZ). The Excluder device is a fully supported graft with a PTFE covering on the inner surface of a nitinol skeleton. (**A**). Prior to deployment of the contralateral limb. (**B**). Close-up of the top of the stent-graft demonstrates small hooks to anchor the leading part.

endograft. The initial report covered 33 patients (5 tube grafts, 22 bifurcated grafts, and 2 aorto-iliac grafts). All were considered high surgical risk patients. The authors reported a perioperative death rate of 5.4% (two patients) from proximal leaks with rupture, with one patient having a disabling stroke caused by angioplasty from a brachial approach. Two procedures were converted to open repair due to delivery system problems. No delayed endoleaks occurred. Three patients with chronic renal insufficiency had progression of their disease.

Their most recent report covered the experience with 108 bifurcated grafts for infrarenal AAAs.[66] They achieved a primary success rate of 87%. They had a total of 15 endoleaks by the 6-week follow-up CT. Seven of these were treated by transcatheter techniques and four sealed spontaneously. There were three patients in whom the graft could not be deployed. Of note is that they experienced four late proximal endoleaks, all due to migration of the device associated with continued expansion of the neck, neck atherosclerotic disease, or flaring of the neck.

■ Complications of Endograft Placement

Endovascular treatment of infrarenal AAAs is associated with certain known complications. There has been noted, however, a shift of their occurrence to more local and vascular complications when compared to open re-

pair. In a nonrandomized comparison of the techniques of open repair versus endovascular repair, Brewster et al noted that the local versus systemic complications were reversed in their rate of occurrence with the two techniques.[44] In their series, endovascular repair had an approximately 50% rate of local/vascular complications in comparison to the 6% rate for open repair. Endovascular repair had an approximately 12% rate of systemic complications in comparison to the 60% rate seen with open surgery. Of note is that most of the local/vascular complications seen with endovascular repair were readily treatable with catheter techniques. We expect the rate of these local and vascular complications to fall dramatically as experience with these devices is gained.

Endoleaks

One of the feared results of endovascular treatment of AAAs is endoleak. The term endoleak, coined by White et al,[67] describes the situation in which there is continued flow of blood into the extragraft portion of the aneurysm sac. They differentiate between 2 types of endoleaks: a type I-endoleak as to be graft-related, and a type II-endoleak as not to be graft-related, such as backbleeding via lumbar arteries or the IMA. This can be seen on the initial completion angiogram, on follow-up CT, or on a follow-up duplex exam. The classification of leaks has been in evolution. Another classification is given by Wain et al.[68] Endoleaks in this classification are described in

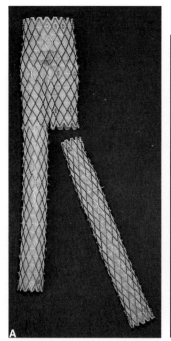
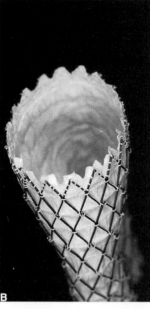

FIGURE 5–4. AneuRx device (Medtronic, Sunnyvale, CA). (**A**). This device is a bifurcated, modular nitinol frame lined by a thin-walled Dacron prosthesis at the inside. (**B**). No fixation system at the top of the endoprosthesis.

thought that this offers more precise measurements than angiography or CT.

These results were followed up with a report by Zarins et al in 1999.[62] They reported on the AneuRx experience in 190 patients in comparison to 60 nonrandomized surgical controls. This covered their FDA phase I and II trials with 40 and 150 patients, respectively. Each center enrolled a small number of surgical controls before they were allowed to perform the endograft deployments. They reported a primary success rate of 78% in the endograft group, defined as a patient alive, with no endoleak, and no reoperation, repeat procedure, or major complication. The rate of endoleaks was 21% at time of discharge, 9% at 6 months, and 6% at 12 months. There were 39 leaks detected at the initial CT scan broken down as follows: seven at the proximal attachment site, 12 from collateral refilling, 10 at the distal attachment site, and 10 at "transgraft" flow. Six (50%) of the collateral leaks sealed spontaneously. Ten endovascular procedures were used to seal endoleaks. Only one patient with a persistent endoleak had enlargement of the aneurysm. There was a significant difference in the need for major reoperation in the two groups (10% in the surgical group versus 1% in the endograft group). There was, interestingly, no difference in the need for local groin exploration in the 2 groups. The rate of medical complications was higher in the surgical group (12% vs 3%). The 30-day mortality rate was 2.6% in the

endograft group and 0% in the surgical group. Two deaths were associated with chronic obstructive pulmonary disease (COPD), one from cholecystitis as described above, one from myocardial infarction (MI) during coronary intervention 3 weeks after successful endograft placement, and one from colon ischemia from covering a patent IMA and internal iliac artery.

Excluder Device

The Excluder endograft (Gore and Assoc., Flagstaff, AZ) is a fully supported graft with a PTFE covering on the inner surface of a nitinol skeleton (Fig. 5–5). The endograft has a low profile and is modular, with both aortic and iliac extenders available. The iliac diameters are available in 12 and 14.5 mm to accommodate iliac arteries 10 to 13.5 mm in diameter. The main trunk and ipsilateral limb comes in 16- and 18-cm lengths. The aortic end of the endograft in 23-, 26-, and 28.5-mm diameters to accommodate aortic diameters of 19 to 26 mm.

The ipsilateral groin sheath is 18-Fr (ID), with the contralateral sheath being 12-Fr (ID). The 18-Fr sheath is placed through a surgical arteriotomy, with the contralateral sheath being placed percutaneously. The graft is unique in its deployment. The device is deployed by pulling off a rip-cord arrangement to unjacket the device and deploy it quickly (identical to the Hemobahn endograft). Appropriately sized balloons are then used to model fully the proximal graft attachment of the main body of the graft and the ipsilateral iliac limb.

Blum et al recently communicated a series of 62 patients treated with the Excluder device.[63] The primary technical success rate was 90%, the rate of type II-endoleaks with lumbar refilling 10%. Apart from one local problem at the access site (laceration of the femoral artery, requiring a patch repair) no further complications occurred. A phase II FDA trial is ongoing in Europe and the USA. Enrollment in this phase of FDA testing should be completed in the fall of 1999.

Zenith Endograft

This stent-graft is made up of a fully supported surgical polyester-fabric graft (thickness 0.035 mm) on a network of Z-stents (Cook Inc., Bloomington, IN) (Fig. 5–6). The endograft is available as a modular system or as a aortouni-iliac version. The top uncovered suprarenal stent has a length of 26 mm and 10 barbs which are placed at different levels and are 5 mm long (Fig. 5–6B). The introducer size is 20-Fr (ID) for the main system, 16 to 18-Fr (ID) for the contralateral limbs and extension legs, respectively.

Gordon, Lawrence-Brown, et al published their experience in 1996,[64,65] and most recently in 1998[66] with their graft, now commercially available in Europe as the Zenith

6

Anesthesia for Endovascular Aortic Aneurysm Stent-Graft Repair

PETER K. SCHOENWALD AND JURAJ SPRUNG

The placement of endovascular stents has traditionally been performed through puncture sites or incisions small enough that they necessitate no more than the injection of a local anesthetic, accompanied perhaps by a small amount of intravenously administered sedative and/or narcotic. The evolution of endovascular stent technology to allow for the repair of select aortic aneurysms has led to the insertion of more complex and concomitantly larger devices. These devices require larger incisions and confer more physiological trespass as they are placed more centrally in the circulation. This may exceed the patient's ability to tolerate the procedure with just local anesthetic injection and sedation. The procedure may require the services of an anesthesiologist to administer general or regional anesthesia. The anesthesiologist may also provide hemodynamic control to allow the successful placement of the graft as well as management of the patient's medical problems.

The administration of anesthesia involves preoperative considerations and preparation, not only of the patient, but also of the physical site at which the procedure is performed. These considerations are discussed in this chapter.

■ Preparatory Considerations

Minimally invasive surgeries and procedures are being promoted for reasons that include decreased physiological insult to the patient, decreased hospital stay, potential cost savings, faster resumption of activities of daily living, decreased pain, and the ability to perform procedures on patients historically deemed too old or ill to tolerate anesthesia and surgery. One fact often lost on nonanesthesia practitioners is that there is no simple, risk-free anesthesia; no such thing as "a little whiff of gas" or a "little bit of anesthesia." Minimally invasive procedures do not necessarily coincide with minimally invasive anesthesia.

Anesthesiologists are perioperative physicians who specialize in the management of pain. Owing to technological advances, this care now extends beyond the operating theater into radiology suites, endoscopy suites, catheterization laboratories, and remote freestanding centers such as those specializing in lithotripsy. Anesthesiologists provide more than just analgesia for surgery. They also provide the quiescent conditions necessary for the performance of a procedure and manage the patient for maintenance of homeostasis. The anesthesiologist's ability to safely administer an anesthetic depends on a properly set up anesthetizing location. The evolution of endovascular suites from other areas may not optimally address these concerns. Preprocedure communication with the anesthesiologist regarding the anesthetic conditions required is essential to maximize patient safety.

Physical Site

Endovascular aortic repair may be done in the operating room or at sites remote to the operating pavilion. These sites may include the radiology department, catheterization lab, and specially designed endovascular surgical suites within or adjacent to the operating pavilion. The specific location is determined, at least initially, by the specialty introducing the procedure. As

Stent-Grafts: Current Clinical Practice. Edited by Dolmatch and Blum. Thieme Medical Publishers, Inc., New York © 2000.

hospitals recognize that multiple specialties may utilize endovascular techniques and there is a need to provide such services, dedicated endovascular suites may be set up to avoid the cost of duplicate equipment and to maximize the efficiency of shared resources.

Unfortunately, incorporating the requirements for a proper anesthetizing location into construction plans at remote sites is an afterthought in many instances, leading to extra expense for retrofitting the site. Regulations, standards, and guidelines, both national and local, varying from locale to locale, may need to be addressed and followed prior to approval as an anesthetizing location. In the United States, the National Fire Protection Association (NFPA) has established standards for health care facilities regarding fire, electrical, and gas system safety in anesthetizing locations.[1] Clearly, the administration of general anesthesia falls into the realm of licensed practitioners, but owing to the proliferation of procedures outside of the operating theater involving only conscious sedation, sedatives may be administered by nonanesthesia personnel who may be unfamiliar or inexperienced with proper airway management or other aspects of sedative administration. The American Society of Anesthesiologists (ASA) has adopted practice guidelines for sedation and analgesia by nonanesthesiologists to address patient safety.[2] To expound on these points further is not the intent of this chapter. Rather, the purpose of mentioning these issues is to advise the nonanesthesia provider that anesthesia services cannot be provided at any location without meeting certain standards, and plans should be made accordingly. If anesthesia services are required, the facility itself must allow for the safe administration of an anesthetic. One must also keep in mind that even if anesthesia services are not planned, a request for their services in emergencies or unforeseen complications requires prior consideration of their involvement.

From an anesthesiologist's perspective, working outside of the operating room environment is not ideal for a number of reasons. The space allocated to them is typically tight for their equipment, and tight space is an uncomfortable environment for rapid management of acute situations in the event of an unforeseen complication. Adequate "elbow room" is needed for the insertion of arterial, central venous and intravenous lines, performance of regional anesthesia and potentially, cardiopulmonary resuscitation. Catheterization laboratories and radiology procedure rooms frequently have large "C-arm" fluoroscopy machines that usurp large amounts of space. The fluoroscopy devices may incorporate the patient's table, which allows movement in three planes but not off-axis moves. The Trendelenburg position for central line insertion may be impossible. Lighting may be poor. A dark environment inhibits optimal assessment of the patient's color (oxygenation and ventilation), man-

agement (drug mixing and administration), and charting (anesthesia record). A distant location may prevent utilization of anesthesia aides for transport of necessary items such as drugs, blood, blood gases, and equipment. Clearly, a well-planned, dedicated area for the performance of endovascular procedures with anesthetizing requirements in mind for air flow, electrical safety, adequate space, adequate lighting, and proximity to ancillary help is not only ideal for the anesthesiologist but also enhances patient safety.

Anesthetic Considerations with Regard to the Type of Endovascular Prosthesis

A variety of endovascular prostheses are undergoing various stages of trials in the United States. The specific types, names, manufacturers, and designs are not reviewed here. However, a review of certain features of these endovascular grafts is necessary because their means of deployment, attachment, and requirement for hemodynamic conditions have important implications for anesthetic management. Briefly, the endovascular grafts must have some way to prevent distal movement once they are properly positioned. Two basic methods are employed to hold the graft in its proper position. One method utilizes hooks incorporated at the proximal and distal ends of the graft, which are embedded into the aortic wall with an intraluminal balloon inflation at the level of the hooks.[3,4] During the period of balloon inflation, the aorta is occluded as if cross-clamped. Alternatively, the graft material may cover a metallic framework where the lateral pressure of the endovascular graft on the aortic wall is sufficient to prevent any distal migration. During deployment of a self-expandable stent-graft, a balloon may or may not be transiently inflated.

Hemodynamic Stability

The use of a balloon has relevance to the anesthesiologist because it is equivalent to a brief period of aortic cross-clamping. The majority of aortic stent-grafts presently utilized are intended for repair of infrarenal aortic aneurysms, so the hemodynamic consequences and stress are minimal when compared to suprarenal or supraceliac aortic cross-clamping. Nevertheless, the increase in afterload for infrarenal stent-graft placement may be of consequence to the sick and elderly vascular patient. Patients with heart disease (inoperable coronary disease or poor myocardial function) are frequently offered an endovascular repair that, because of their comorbidities, may not be considered a reasonable operative risk by conventional open surgical technique.[5,6] The EVT (Endovascular Technologies Inc., Menlo Park, CA) requires the inflation of a balloon to engage securing hooks into the aorta, whereas the AneuRx graft (Medtronic AneuRx Inc., Sunnyvale, CA) may not require intraluminal balloon inflation, but if it does, the impact is brief and minimal in comparison.

In general, patients undergoing endovascular stent-graft repair of infrarenal aortic aneurysms appear to have greater hemodynamic stability compared to those who undergo traditional open repair. This is in spite of the fact that the endovascular group, by selection, contains a sicker group of patients. Baxendale et al[7] demonstrated this when they compared 10 patients receiving a stent-graft via an endovascular technique with a control group receiving surgical repair. All patients received a standard general anesthetic. Systemic pressures, cardiac output, systemic vascular resistance, and lactate levels determined before and after critical events such as aortic occlusion indicated more stability and less stress in the endovascular group. Similarly, Kahn et al,[8] in a retrospective analysis of computerized records, analyzed physiological parameters every 15 seconds in 17 patients undergoing endovascular repair, using a comparison group of 72 patients undergoing open repair. In this series, all of the patients for open repair had a general anesthetic, some of whom also had an epidural catheter for intraoperative analgesia. The endovascular group had regional neuraxial anesthesia except for one patient who had a general anesthetic. This study similarly demonstrated greater hemodynamic stability in the endovascular group.

Conversely, Norgren et al,[9] in a series of six patients under general anesthesia for endovascular aortic stent placement requiring balloon inflation for deployment, had two patients who had sudden and dramatic drops in blood pressure requiring treatment. One patient was somewhat resistant to therapy and responded slowly. The authors did not believe that the hypotension was related to the maneuvers of aortic balloon occlusion. Rather, they surmised that the hypotension might be due to some bleeding into the aneurysm sac after graft implantation or release of factors from the aneurysm sac. Regardless of the mechanism of hypotension, they were impressed enough by the acute hypotension to inform the endovascular community of this potential side effect. Our group similarly reported the occurrence of acute and severe hemodynamic changes from our early experience in a selected group of endovascular patients.[10] In a series of 12 patients undergoing endovascular repair of infrarenal aortic aneurysm with an EVT graft, it was noted that 3 of 12 patients had severe and acute bradycardia with accompanying hypotension, necessitating immediate therapy. All patients were under neuraxial (epidural or continuous spinal) anesthesia, and the events appeared to be related to inflation of the intraluminal balloon during engagement of the proximal hooks into the aorta. Heart rates decreased to 30, 38, and 48 beats per minute. The bradycardia was out of proportion to what one might expect as a result of an in-

crease in peripheral vascular resistance from occlusion of flow during balloon inflation and did not resolve with deflation of the balloon as one might expect. The bradycardia was accompanied by a significant decrease in systemic pressure and rapid treatment with an anticholinergic with vasopressor was necessary. Subsequent work with a self-expanding stent-graft (AneuRx graft) has not resulted in similarly serious bradycardic events. Interestingly, our endovascular surgeon had informed us of the possibility of the occurrence of bradycardia with balloon inflation or distention of large arteries with intraluminal balloons, but we were unable to verify the existence of the phenomenon in the literature.

In a retrospective review of 100 patients for endovascular aortic stent repair, where a combination of general and regional techniques was used, Baker et al[11] alert the reader to considerations of endovascular aortic repair from an anesthetic perspective. The need for a quiet surgical field, anticoagulation, and invasive monitoring, and the possibility of induced hypotension, sudden large blood loss, impaired renal function, and hypothermia are mentioned. However, at no time is there any mention of unanticipated changes in hemodynamic profile (either heart rate or blood pressure).

To reconcile the discrepancies in these reports regarding the hemodynamic stability during the endovascular aortic work, one must choose from a number of possibilities, none of which can at present be verified: (1) the dramatic hemodynamic changes noted in two series were completely serendipitous; (2) the relative stability in the other studies did not have enough power to identify the occurrence of a rare event; or (3) there may be sudden hemodynamic changes during endovascular placement only under certain conditions, possibly related to type of anesthesia, specific graft type, or maneuvers graft deployment.

Induced Hypotension or Decreased Flow for Device Deployment

Some of the grafts require blood pressure and flow alterations during deployment to avoid a "windsock" effect. This refers to the proximal expansion of the compressed graft from within the sheath by the blood initially flowing into it. This expansive filling may generate a significant force, enough to push the device distal to its intended placement site. Should this occur, open correction might be needed. This windsock effect can apparently be largely overcome by decreasing the blood pressure to a mean of approximately 60 mm Hg. One must remember, however, that pressure does not equal flow, and it is the decrease of the forward flow of blood into the graft that one must try to achieve. Attempts to decrease systemic pressure usually utilize methods to decrease the peripheral vascular resistance. Judicious use of vasodilators, β-antagonists, and the sympathectomy from neuraxial regional anesthesia may achieve the desired effect and lessen the windsock effect. Purposefully decreasing the cardiac output primarily by depressing myocardial function is probably not a good method to achieve this end because many of these patients already have impaired myocardial function.

Many of these patients may not tolerate drops in blood pressure from their usual hypertensive state to a mean blood pressure of 60 mm Hg. Their coronary, cerebral, and visceral beds may have pressure-dependent flow through stenosed and compromised beds. Choosing a type of stent-graft that requires dropping the systemic pressure to the degree necessary for device deployment may preclude some patients from being candidates for that type of graft.

An extreme case of decreasing the windsock effect has been demonstrated by the use of adenosine to cause a transient asystole and hypotension during deployment of an endovascular stent for repair of a descending thoracic aortic aneurysm. Two reports describe the technique. Tanito et al[12] describe four patients in whom adenosine 20 to 30 mg was used to cause a transient heart block for less than 1 minute, during which time the stent-graft was expanded. Baker et al[13] report three patients in whom doses of adenosine ranged from 12 to 45 mg to achieve the desired effect of 20 to 30 seconds of asystole for stent-graft deployment. One hazard of this technique, however, is the unpredictability of the exact duration of the adenosine effect. A sudden unexpected ventricular contraction during a slower than expected graft deployment could end up in improper positioning of the graft. Thoracic endovascular grafts have also been deployed without the use of adenosine.

Worst-Case Scenario Preparation

Although most cases of endovascular aortic stent repair proceed without problems, one must always be prepared for the worst-case scenario. During these cases there is the possibility of massive blood loss with the need to convert to an open technique.

Massive blood loss may occur because of aneurysm rupture or leak, but it may also occur at the endovascular access points, usually at the iliac or femoral arteries. The blood loss from this site may be large yet quite insidious because it leaks continuously around the sheaths and catheters and pools in the drapes underneath the patient. Little attention may be given to the amount of blood lost because of a dark room, its occurrence outside of the visual field of the anesthesiologist, and attention drawn away from the surgical site and placed on the fluoroscopy screen. Accordingly, blood must be typed and crossed, at a minimum, and preferably some units stored in close proximity to the procedure site and thus readily available. Also, any unexplained changes in blood pressure or filling pressures should be treated with a high degree of suspicion and investigated. Although usually not needed, adequate, large, intravenous access must be placed prior to the procedure. A dark, crowded room is not optimal for starting this access in an emergency situation. Monitoring should likewise be appropriate for the possibility of large volume shifts (see below).

Consideration must be given to the fact that a finite number of cases will be converted to an open repair. The percentage ranges from 2 to 20% from various groups with an average of approximately 9% from data pooled from several series.[5,10,14–17] The open conversion rate is presently lower than this average rate would indicate because the rates have decreased with experience and with newer versions of the stent-graft systems. A conversion rate of 2% in experienced hands may be a more reasonable estimate. Nevertheless, one should consider that many of these patients are selected for endovascular aneurysm repair, as previously mentioned, owing to their poor state of health. Should there be a massive bleed or a malpositioned graft, one may be obligated to proceed with an open repair in the usual fashion emergently in a high-risk patient. Therefore, the patient must have given informed consent for this scenario in advance, the risks must be fully explained and accepted, and lines and monitoring must be placed in advance commensurate with this possibility.

Even if the procedure proceeds as expected, these patients may experience myocardial ischemia serendipitously, and one must be prepared to treat it and possibly abort the procedure. The patient's cardiac status needs to have been optimized prior to the procedure, and drugs such as nitroglycerin and β-antagonists must be readily available for use.

■ Preoperative Evaluation and Preparation of the Patient

Vascular patients frequently have associated diseases such as hypertension, coronary artery disease (CAD), generalized atherosclerosis of other vascular beds (cerebral, renal, visceral, extremity), pulmonary disease (from smoking), and diabetes. Evaluation of the present state of the diseases and their optimization prior to the planned procedure are necessary to minimize the perioperative morbidity and mortality. Of particular importance is the optimization of the cardiac status in this group of patients because perioperative cardiac morbidity is a major risk. Many resources are available in the literature that address the evaluation and preparation of cardiac patients for noncardiac surgery. The framework and recommendations for this section closely follow guidelines proposed by the American College of Cardiology (ACC) and the American Heart Association (AHA).[18]

Perioperative assessment and optimization of cardiac patients who are to undergo noncardiac surgery necessitates cooperation and communication between all involved medical specialties. Coronary revascularization prior to noncardiac surgery is necessary only for a small subset of very high risk patients. Preoperative testing should be limited to patients in whom the results will affect management and outcome. The ACC and AHA presently recommend a conservative approach to the use of expensive tests and treatments.[18]

Patients with CAD who undergo noncardiac operations have been shown to be at increased risk of perioperative myocardial infarction (PMI) and death.[18–21] The risk is highest among those undergoing vascular surgeries[22,23] because the incidence of CAD is substantially higher in patients requiring vascular surgery than in the general surgical population.[24] Hertzer et al[24] found that only 8% of those undergoing elective vascular surgery had normal coronary arteries and that 15% of patients without clinical evidence of CAD had angiographically proven CAD that needed revascularization or was already inoperable. In addition, they found that half of the patients undergoing elective vascular surgery had 70% stenosis of at least one coronary vessel. In patients with CAD undergoing noncardiac surgery, the overall incidence of PMI is between 1.1[25]–5.6%.[19,25] Two studies, by Tarhan et al[26] and Steen et al,[27] reported an incidence of myocardial reinfarction as high as 37% when surgery was performed within 6 months of the initial myocardial infarction (MI). More recent studies reported a lower incidence of myocardial reinfarction (2–6%)[28,29] after noncardiac surgery performed within 6 months after a MI. Mangano[30] reported a 6.2% average rate (pooled data from multiple studies including 3,306 patients) of perioperative MI and cardiac death after vascular surgery (rate ranged from 2.2 to 19%). This better outcome was speculated to be attributable to improvements in anesthetic techniques, aggressive treatment of CAD, or both.

Main Objectives of Clinical Evaluation

The history, physical examination, and electrocardiographic assessment should focus on the identification of potentially serious cardiac disorders. Signs, symptoms, or history of CAD, congestive heart failure, and abnormal cardiac rhythms should be sought. The severity and stability of the cardiac disease, as well as its treatment history, must be clearly delineated. New guidelines for perioperative cardiovascular evaluation also take into account the patient's functional capacity, age, other disease states (e.g., diabetes mellitus, peripheral vascular disease, renal dysfunction, chronic pulmonary disease)

and type of operation. Surgery-specific cardiac risk classifies operations into three categories: high-risk operations with a reported cardiac risk ≥5% (aortic, thoracic emergency major surgeries, etc.), intermediate-risk operations with cardiac risk between 1 and 5% (carotid endarterectomy, head and neck operations, etc.), and low-risk operations with cardiac risk ≤1% (i.e., cataract, breast operations, etc.). For endovascular stent repair of aortic aneurysms, the risk is probably intermediate, unless open conversion occurs. This would then shift the cardiac risk of the procedure into the high-risk category, warranting extensive evaluation. The preprocedure evaluation of these patients must assess the risk/benefit ratio on an individual basis, yet keep in mind the possibility that the procedure may end up as a high cardiac risk.

Perioperative Management of Specific Cardiovascular Risk Conditions

Hypertension

Surgical candidates who have adequate pharmacological control of their hypertension should be maintained on their regimen throughout the perioperative period. Severe hypertension (i.e., diastolic blood pressure >110 mm Hg) should be electively treated before an operation. The decision to delay an operation because of increased blood pressure should consider the urgency of the surgical procedure. To avoid rebound hypertension, it is especially important to continue antihypertensive treatments perioperatively. Diuretics are the exception and should be held preoperatively to avoid electrolyte disturbances. Patients with hypertension whose blood pressure has been well controlled with medication usually maintain better intraoperative hemodynamic stability than do those whose pressures are poorly controlled.

Valvular Heart Disease

Symptomatic stenotic lesions such as mitral and aortic stenosis are associated with a risk of perioperative congestive heart failure or shock. To lower cardiac risk, surgical treatment may be necessary prior to noncardiac surgery. Severe aortic stenosis is a relative contraindication for neuraxial (spinal or epidural) anesthesia, which is our technique of choice for endovascular aortic aneurysm stent repair. Extensive sympathectomy with neuraxial blockade can cause precipitous hypotension, which, in patients with aortic stenosis, may result in coronary underperfusion. Conversely, symptomatic regurgitant valvular disease is usually better tolerated and may be stabilized preoperatively with intensive medical therapy. These guidelines must be followed regardless of the fact that endovascular aortic repair could be considered a lower stress surgery, again keeping in mind that this procedure in a small percentage of patients may be converted into open, high-stress, aortic repair.

Myocardial Heart Disease

Patients with cardiomyopathy are more prone to perioperative myocardial infarctions, congestive heart failure, and cardiac death. Anesthesiologists should exercise special care in minimizing myocardial stress (hypertension and tachycardia) and fluid overload. In addition, optimal preoperative management as well as intensive postoperative medical therapy and surveillance may improve outcome in these patients.

Dysrhythmias

If a dysrhythmia or cardiac conduction disturbance is present, the clinician should perform a thorough assessment for underlying cardiopulmonary disease, drug toxicity, or metabolic abnormality. Optimally all underlying conditions (electrolyte disturbances, hyperthyroidism, etc.) have to be corrected before surgery. Therapy should be initiated for all symptomatic or hemodynamically significant dysrhythmias. Indications for antiarrhythmic therapy and cardiac pacing are identical to those in the nonoperative setting. If the patient has a pacemaker, its function needs to be evaluated pre- and postoperatively. In addition, the anesthesiologist must recognize the underlying cardiac pathology that required pacemaker insertion. Pacemaker dependency and underlying rhythm should be delineated in case pacing is lost intraoperatively. The anesthesiologist should be familiar with the type of pacemaker and its default pacing mode with a magnet applied over the pulse generator. A magnet must be readily available for conversion to a fixed pacing mode. All automatic implantable cardiac defibrillators (AICDs) in patients with severe malignant recurrent dysrhythmias must be deactivated during surgery, as they can inappropriately discharge because of extraneous signals (electrocautery, succinylcholine induced fasciculations, etc.). While deactivated, an external defibrillator must be available in the operating room at all times until the end of surgery and the AICD should be reactivated prior to leaving the operating room.

Preoperative Coronary Revascularization

Coronary Artery Bypass Grafting (CABG)

A number of studies have shown that patients who have had a previously successful CABG had low rates of MI and death after major surgical procedures.[31,32] However, the argument against more frequent use of prophylactic CABG before vascular surgery is based on a higher combined morbidity and mortality rate for CABG and subsequent vascular surgery as compared to those of vascular surgery alone.[31] For the patient with an unstable coronary syndrome, CABG may lead to improved long-term survival. When the stress of elective noncardiac surgery is likely to exceed that encountered in daily life, consideration of CABG before noncardiac surgery may be reasonable.

Percutaneous Transluminal Coronary Angioplasty (PTCA)

Coronary revascularization by using PTCA is safer,[33] less invasive, less expensive, and requires a shorter recovery period and hospital stay than CABG.[34,35] Gottlieb et al[36] recently demonstrated the cardioprotective role of PTCA in patients undergoing vascular surgery. Allen et al[35] analyzed 148 patients who had PTCA before noncardiac surgery and found a low incidence of PMI and cardiac mortality (both 0.67%). The long-term cardioprotective role of PTCA is still unclear because coronary restenosis occurs in 25 to 40% of patients within 8 months of PTCA.[37]

Medical Therapy for Coronary Artery Disease

Perioperative use of β-antagonists reduces the incidence of PMI,[38] frequency of postoperative ischemia, and the risk of death at 2 years postoperatively.[39] Preoperative therapy with calcium antagonists, however, has not been shown to reduce the incidence of perioperative ischemia,[40] and may even increase the risk of major adverse clinical events and mortality.[41] Presently, data are still not sufficient to determine whether prophylactic intraoperative use of nitroglycerin is helpful or harmful. Current practice is that if a patient is taking β-antagonists, calcium antagonist, or nitrates preoperatively, the drug regimen is continued into the perioperative period. The same is true for the therapies used to control symptoms of congestive heart failure.

Management of Other Associated Comorbidities

Minimization of risk for cerebral and renal insults needs to be addressed and corrected if possible. If the patient is in chronic renal failure, dialysis the day before surgery should be considered with follow-up electrolytes checked. In the patient with diabetes mellitus, blood sugars should be well controlled and checked on the morning of surgery. Usually, one-half the morning insulin dose is given concomitant with a well-functioning intravenous line containing dextrose. Smoking should be discouraged and if possible stopped well before the procedure. Pulmonary function testing may guide optimization of pulmonary function with the use of bronchodilators. Any lung infection should be treated accordingly.

■ Monitoring

Standard anesthesia monitoring of patients undergoing any major vascular surgical procedure includes a five-lead electrocardiogram (ECG) (with lead II and V_5), pulse oximetry, invasive blood pressure monitoring, and at least the capability of temperature monitoring. Direct systemic pressure monitoring via an arterial line provides for instantaneous and accurate data collection in patients who may be labile, not only because of their underlying vascular disease, but also due to changes that may occur during graft placement. The site of arterial line insertion should be carefully considered. Radial artery cannulation is generally adequate, although a brachial line will work as well. Central line access is an additional choice for intravenous volume and medication, in addition to its hemodynamic monitoring capabilities.

The monitoring of filling pressures is an appropriate consideration and should be dictated on an individual basis depending on the cardiac status of the patient. At the very least, central venous pressure (CVP) monitoring should be performed. One might consider the placement of an introducer sheath (8.5 or 9 French) with side port into the jugular vein, which can accommodate either a central line or a pulmonary artery (PA) catheter. If CVP monitoring is deemed adequate, it can be introduced through the sheath, and the side port makes an excellent volume line. However, if the situation changes rapidly, such as during aneurysm rupture or leak, conversion to an open surgical technique, or the onset of signs of cardiac ischemia, the central venous line can be quickly and relatively easily changed to a PA catheter as deemed necessary. This avoids changing lines over a guidewire in a dark and constrained environment.

A CVP line is also beneficial for assessment of occult blood loss, which can easily occur in these cases. A continuous slow bleed occurs from the point where the guidewires enter the devices and around the device sheaths themselves. The blood pools insidiously in the dependent drapes and usually in a darkened environment. A CVP that slowly drifts lower may be one of the earlier signs of occult bleeding outside of the anesthesia provider's visual field.

Continuous ST-segment monitoring is recommended because intraoperative and postoperative ST-segment changes indicating myocardial ischemia have been found to be strong predictors of perioperative MI in patients at high clinical risk who undergo noncardiac surgery.[42] Similarly, postoperative ischemia is a significant predictor of long-term MI and cardiac death.[25] Often, this is not associated with regional wall motion abnormalities; thus, whether this is ischemia or a nonspecific finding is unknown. Currently, few data are available on the cost-effectiveness of ST-segment monitoring for the purpose of reducing perioperative morbidity in any patient population. Accumulating evidence suggests that correct use of computerized ST-segment analysis in appropriately selected high-risk patients may improve sensitivity for detection of myocardial ischemia, which

could lead to improved perioperative and long-term risk assessment and treatment.

Surveillance for postoperative myocardial infarction or ischemia (ECG and myocardial enzymes) should be performed in this patient population. Clinical symptoms, postoperative ECG changes, and elevation of the MB fraction of creatine phosphokinase (CPK) have been most extensively studied. Utilization of the elevation in newer myocardial-specific enzyme markers, such as troponin, may also have value. In patients without known CAD, surveillance should probably be restricted to those who have signs of cardiovascular dysfunction. In patients with known or suspected CAD undergoing high-risk procedures, obtaining an ECG at baseline, immediately after the procedure, and for the first 2 postoperative days is cost-effective. Use of cardiac enzymes is best reserved for patients with clinical, ECG, or hemodynamic evidence of cardiovascular dysfunction.

■ Anesthesia Techniques

Anesthesia for endovascular aortic aneurysm repair may be either general or regional. All anesthetic techniques and drugs are associated with known cardiac effects that should be considered in the anesthetic plan. One of the things frequently stated to convince a patient to accept a regional technique over a general anesthetic technique is its superior safety profile. The issue is controversial, but literature to support this view in the vascular patient exists.[43] There are also other benefits to considering regional anesthesia as the anesthetic of choice, such as its potential to maintain short-term graft patency in peripheral bypass procedures owing to its effects upon the coagulation system.[44,45] A general anesthetic technique is more frequently reported in the earlier literature as having being utilized during endovascular aortic aneurysm repair. This was done owing to the concern regarding preparedness for conversion to open surgical repair. However, one should keep in mind that under most circumstances the only painful site for the patient is the surgical exposure in the groins of the femoral arteries. This can easily be anesthetized with regional anesthesia. The preferred choice of anesthetic has since gravitated from a general anesthetic technique to a regional technique for infrarenal aneurysms. Adequate anesthesia can even be achieved via infiltration of local anesthesia at the access sites, accompanied by monitored anesthesia care with the adjunctive use of narcotics and sedatives. Indeed, U. Blum of the Department of Radiology, University Hospital Zurich, Switzerland, has successfully performed over 100 infrarenal aortic stent-graft repairs in this manner (monitored anesthesia care), with judicious use of supplemental intravenous analgesics (remifentanil) and anxiolytics (midazolam) (personal communication).

Failure to produce complete analgesia at the incision site, however, can lead to an increased stress response, which can in turn lead to myocardial ischemia, particularly in the vascular surgical patient. The incision sites may become too large and the manipulation too intense to keep the patient comfortable for an extended period of time. Furthermore, this still would allow the patient the ability to move the legs since muscle tone and strength are still intact and may not provide for an optimal field during critical parts of the endovascular procedure. Neuraxial regional blockade works quite well for endovascular repair of the abdominal aorta. It provides for a quiet, still field, given appropriate use of local anesthetic agents, and provides for excellent pain relief continued into the postoperative period. Furthermore, the dermatomal level necessary for endovascular aortic repair is usually accompanied by minimal hemodynamic changes. Should it become necessary to extend the incision site or to enter the lower abdominal cavity, this can still be easily accomplished with patient comfort through the use of a neuraxial regional technique.

Monitored Anesthesia Care (Local Standby)

As mentioned above, infrarenal aortic stent placement could be performed under local anesthetic injection at the site of the groin incisions accompanied by intravenous administration of a narcotic analgesic with or without a sedative anxiolytic agent. Prior to proceeding in this manner, however, it must be understood by the patient and personnel performing the procedure that choosing this technique necessitates the acceptance of certain shortcomings and limitations. The physician(s) performing the stent-graft placement must be willing to accept some degree of movement of the patient's legs in the surgical field. Furthermore, once the incisions have been made, should the technique be inadequate for placement of the stent, regional neuraxial blockade is no longer a reasonable option and one may be obligated to proceed to a general anesthetic.

Subcutaneous infiltration of local anesthetic at the incision site in a fan-like manner should provide adequate analgesia for skin incision. A low concentration of anesthetic such as 0.5% lidocaine, 0.25% bupivacaine, or similar agent would be appropriate. Use of retractors and electrocautery may necessitate further infiltration of deeper tissues. Discomfort from electrocautery at high settings may be very difficult to control with local injection, especially when the current spreads to stimulate adjacent nerves and adjustment of the current may be necessary. The femoral nerve may be inadvertently blocked, and its effects may extend into the postoperative period. A running total of the amount of local anesthetic used must be kept to avoid overdosing with a subsequent toxic reaction.

Intravenous narcotics are usually used as adjunctive agents and titrated to the desired analgesic effect. They appear to be anxiolytics or sedatives only because of their central depressant effect and the psychological benefit the patient receives from a decrease in their pain perception. True sedative anxiolytics are usually administered concomitantly. Acceptable choices of narcotics would include low doses of fentanyl (1–2 µg/kg), remifentanil infusion (0.05 µg/kg/min), or other narcotics at low doses.

Midazolam is frequently used as a sedative anxiolytic and titrated to effect with a dose of 1 to 5 mg in a normal-size adult. Titration is important as occasional geriatric patients may be exquisitely sensitive to its effects, and if confusion results, the patient may become uncooperative. A low-dose propofol infusion (1–3 mg/kg/hr or 17–50 µg/kg/min) is also a popular sedative owing to its short duration of action and high clearance. One must be aware that there may be a fine line between conscious sedation and general anesthesia, and the airway must be maintained and protected at all times.

Regional Anesthesia

Regional anesthesia in the form of a continuous epidural or continuous spinal catheter can confer advantages over a general anesthetic approach for endovascular work. The advantages include a decreased incidence of thrombophlebitis, minimization of systemic drugs, decreased afterload, precise control of analgesic level, continuation of pain relief into the postoperative period with the use of an epidural pump, and the ability to converse with the patient regarding symptomatology related to coronary ischemia. One must be careful not to obtain an excessive sympathectomy, otherwise hemodynamic instability and hypotension may result. Continuous neuraxial blockade with a catheter is safe even if the anticoagulant heparin is administered after successful catheter placement. A normal coagulation profile must simply be assured prior to the catheter removal. Thrombolytic agents are a different issue altogether and should not be used in conjunction with neuraxial regional catheters.

The main disadvantage of a neuraxial regional technique involves the degree of sympathetic blockade seen with local anesthetic administration, particularly when the level of blockade exceeds what was planned or predicted. The adverse results of a more extensive sympathectomy than desired are hypotension and, if high enough to block the cardiac accelerators and decrease venous return, bradycardia.

Epidural Anesthesia

Epidural anesthesia is conveniently placed with the patient in the sitting position, although it certainly can be done with the patient in a lateral decubitus position. Verification of a normal clotting profile and absence of a history of anticoagulant use or bleeding disorders is done in advance. Monitoring, both invasive and noninvasive, may also be placed in advance, and should include, at a minimum, ECG and pulse oximetry during insertion of the epidural catheter. Supplemental oxygen, usually by nasal cannula, is administered. A small amount of sedation to alleviate patient anxiety may be helpful, although large doses should be avoided in the sitting position during catheter insertion. The patient's posterior lumbar spinous processes at the appropriate levels are identified. The space between the third and fourth or the fourth and fifth lumbar spinous process is preferred, although spaces above and below may be considered. The reason for the preference stems from the level of analgesia necessary to provide pain relief at the femoral incision while at the same time providing motor blockade of the lower extremities for a motion-free surgical site. Consider that the epidural catheter is preferentially advanced in a cephalad direction such that the catheter is 3 to 4 cm within the epidural space. The local anesthetic is thus delivered at one or two levels higher than the catheter insertion point, approximately at the first or second lumbar dermatome. Only a small amount of local anesthetic dosing is subsequently required for an adequate analgesic level and motor blockade, if desired. The epidural space is identified with an appropriate epidural needle such as an 18-gauge Touhy needle, through which an epidural catheter is inserted. After removal of the epidural needle, the catheter is covered with a sterile dressing and taped into position. A 3-mL test dose of 1.5% lidocaine with 1 : 200,000 epinephrine is administered to identify inadvertent intrathecal or intravenous placement of the catheter. Although arguments have been proposed against the use of epinephrine-containing test solutions in vascular patients, the potential benefits of avoiding inadvertent intravenous or intrathecal administration of significant doses of local anesthetic are felt to outweigh the small and transient risk of the potential administration of 15 μg of intravenous epinephrine in a vascular patient. The dosing of the local anesthetic into the epidural space may be performed with the patient in the sitting position to decrease the onset time of the sensory blockade.[46]

Continuous Spinal Anesthesia

Continuous spinal anesthetics are also appropriate as an anesthetic choice. They may be preferable to an epidural technique under certain circumstances, such as previous lumbar laminectomy where identification of the epidural space may be tenuous at best and may result in a patchy block. Even when a laminectomy at the insertion site is not an issue, arthritic changes in the geriatric person may make identification of the epidural

space and catheter insertion difficult. Conversion from an initial attempt at a continuous epidural to a continuous spinal owing to anatomic difficulties is not unreasonable, but the patient should be advised of this in advance for the proper informed consent. The return of cerebrospinal fluid is a definitive end point. Onset of analgesia is rapid with the intrathecal administration of local anesthetic unless the free flow of cerebrospinal fluid between segments is limited (such as in severe spinal stenosis) or the catheter is not properly placed. If onset of analgesia does not occur with normal intrathecal doses, the technique should probably be abandoned. A typical dose of hyperbaric spinal tetracaine would be a slow injection of 6 to 8 mg. Isobaric bupivacaine 0.5% in a dose of 5 to 10 mg would also be reasonable. Concern about postlumbar puncture headaches is, for the most part, unwarranted in the geriatric population. The incidence of postlumbar puncture headache decreases significantly with age, particularly beyond the fifth decade. Denny et al[47] demonstrated a low incidence (less than 1%) of postdural puncture headache even when an 18-gauge Touhy needle was used to introduce a 20-gauge catheter. An inflammatory reaction owing to the presence of the catheter is postulated to occur at the dural puncture site, resulting in a "fibrin exudate," which effectively seals the dura from cerebrospinal fluid leak and prevents most headaches. Use of a continuous spinal catheter for postoperative pain relief, however, must be carefully considered. Even when clearly marked, the catheter may be mistaken for an epidural catheter, resulting in improper dosing. The older population is also more subject to increased sensitivity to narcotics and subsequently to apnea owing to intrathecal opioids. It is probably safer to avoid postoperative pain control using intrathecal techniques.

General Anesthesia

General anesthesia is most often reported as the anesthetic technique for endovascular stent-grafting. The surgical literature describing initial experiences with aortic stent-graft work is largely responsible for this. Details of the anesthetic are sparse, however, because most reports are authored by nonanesthesiologists. In a recent article by Dake et al[6] on their results in 103 patients receiving stents for descending thoracic aortic aneurysms, the patients had general anesthesia without reference to the specific agents used. It is noted, however, that 60% of the patients were felt not to be candidates for a conventional "open" surgical procedure owing to the severity of their cardiopulmonary or other medical conditions. Most anesthesiologists would prefer a regional anesthetic if possible in a patient with poor ventricular function. This was impossible in this report owing to the patient's right lateral decubitus position, use of a transesophageal echocardiography probe to help in stent placement, and preparation for potential emergency left thoracotomy that included the use of a double-lumen endobronchial tube and cardiopulmonary bypass standby. As previously mentioned, use of adenosine to temporarily induce sinus arrest has been reported during the use of thoracic aortic stent placement. Because no cardiac output occurs during this period, general anesthesia is advisable for patient comfort. Baker et al[11] describe a balanced general anesthetic utilizing nitrous oxide, isoflurane, opioid, and muscle relaxant with intubation and ventilation, a fairly generic technique common for vascular procedures. Baxendale et al[7] report the use of general anesthesia as well and note the use of fentanyl as the narcotic analgesic and etomidate for induction.

For general anesthesia in this sick vascular patient population, induction agents, maintenance agents, and techniques that favor maintenance of ventricular function are preferred. Etomidate or a narcotic with minimal hemodynamic effects such as fentanyl or sufentanil (with or without a low dose of sodium thiopental) should be considered as an induction agent. For maintenance, a balanced technique with the above-mentioned narcotics given intravenously with a low-dose inhalation agent such as isoflurane, with the emphasis on the narcotic as the main agent, could be beneficial in maintaining cardiac output and minimizing myocardial depression.

■ Recovery

The patient undergoing open aortic repair, even when extubated at the end of the procedure in the operating room, is transferred to a surgical intensive care unit because of the risk of postoperative pulmonary problems, fluid shifts, potential electrolyte disturbances, occult bleeding, cardiac rhythm disturbances, and cardiac ischemic events.

If the insertion of an infrarenal aortic stent-graft through the groin is routine, the anesthetic and surgical physiological trespass may indeed be minimal. The greater hemodynamic stability of patients undergoing endovascular aortic repair compared to those undergoing conventional open surgical repair has recently been demonstrated in a comparative study of hemodynamic parameters extracted from computerized anesthesia records.[8] The cardiopulmonary risks mentioned above are minimized and the patient may bypass the surgical intensive care unit completely. Intensive monitoring in the setting of a postanesthesia care unit (PACU), however, is necessary and quite acceptable. Although the total length of stay is arbitrary, a closely monitored stay of 6 to 8 hours is reasonable to establish the stability of the patient and allow any adverse events to occur. In our initial experience of the first dozen patients who underwent endovascular aortic repair at our institution, only one patient who had successful stent placement required a surgical intensive care unit (SICU) stay,[10] owing to an occult retroperitoneal bleed extending from the groin incision but unrelated to the graft placement itself. The safety of a PACU stay rather than SICU care in successful uneventful endovascular aortic repair has subsequently been borne out at our institution in over 100 patients, and our present practice is to bypass SICU care in virtually all patients. Bypassing an SICU stay is considered acceptable at other institutions as well.[11,16]

The overall hospital stay in our institution has also been reduced from approximately 8 days to a median stay of 3 days. Although the cost of the graft appears to be high, averting a 2- or 3-day SICU stay and reducing the overall hospital stay by 5 days or more can realize a considerable cost savings. A decreased hospital stay in turn may reduce the likelihood of nosocomial infection and drug administration error.

Management of postoperative pain is also simplified. The groin incision reportedly is not very painful. Even when regional anesthesia has been used and the opportunity for epidurally administered PCA (patient-controlled analgesia) pump is an option, our surgeons have opted for simpler, alternate forms of postoperative analgesia once the patient is transferred to the nursing floors. This does not rule out a one-time dose of neuraxial delivered narcotic such as epidural morphine with monitoring of respiration or oxyhemoglobin saturation after administration. Obviously, normal clotting parameters must be established prior to the removal of any neuraxial catheter.

■ Comments from an Anesthesiologist's Perspective

Introduction and implementation of new procedures and surgical techniques always provide a challenge to the anesthesiologist. The conditions necessary for the new intervention, the degree of physiological insult, the degree of analgesia necessary, the location, and other new challenges are not always clear until the initial problems are encountered. Communication with other involved services is essential. An appropriate anesthetizing location must be provided. For endovascular aortic repair, patients must be prepared preoperatively as if they were to undergo an open repair to minimize their risk. Although most will successfully undergo endovascular repair, there will always be an occasional change in plans requiring open repair and different approaches, and, in this situation, markedly increased risk to the patient who is probably least likely to tolerate invasive approaches. The worst-case scenario must be prepared for.

Although either regional or general anesthesia can be employed for endovascular aortic stent-graft placement, a regional anesthetic should be considered a very reasonable first choice, at least for infrarenal aneurysms. When properly applied, it has the potential for minimal physiological insult and good pain control, both intraoperatively and in the PACU. If drops in mean blood pressure are required for graft placement, the resulting sympathectomy from a neuraxial block can aid in achieving this goal. Sedation can be minimized, and a relatively alert, comfortable, oriented, and satisfied geriatric patient in the PACU can be the expected result.

From the authors' perspective, the difference in the overall appearance between a patient recovering from an open aortic repair under general anesthesia and a patient immediately postoperatively in the PACU having undergone an endovascular infrarenal aortic stent-graft repair is remarkable. One would not have thought it possible even a decade ago that patients for repair of an aortic aneurysm could be discharged from the hospital within 3 days. It is gratifying to be involved in providing anesthesia care for such a technological advance.

REFERENCES

1. National Fire Protection Association. NFPA 99, Health Care Facilities, 1987 Edition; ANSI/NFPA 99 An American National Standard, February 12, 1987.
2. American Society of Anesthesiologists. Practice guidelines for sedation and analgesia by non-anesthesiologists. Anesthesiology 1996;84:459–471.
3. Balm R, Eikelboom BC, May J, et al. Early experience with transfemoral endovascular aneurysm management (TEAM) in the treatment of aortic aneurysms. Eur J Vasc Endovasc Surg 1996;11:214–220.
4. Katzen BT, Becker GJ, Benenati JF, Zemel G. Treatment of abdominal aortic aneurysms with the Endovascular Technologies tube and bifurcating Endovascular Grafting System: technical aspects. Tech Vasc Intervent Radiol 1998;1:9–18.
5. May J, White GH, Yu W, et al. Surgical management of complications following endoluminal grafting of abdominal aortic aneurysms. Eur J Vasc Surg 1995;10:51–59.
6. Dake MD, Miller DC, Mitchell RS, et al. The "first generation" of endovascular stent-grafts for patients with aneurysms of the descending thoracic aorta. J Thorac Cardiovasc Surg 1998;116:689–704.
7. Baxendale BR, Baker DM, Hutchinson A, et al. Haemodynamic and metabolic response to endovascular repair of infra-renal aortic aneurysms. Br J Anaesth 1996;77:581–585.
8. Kahn RA, Moskowitz DM, Manspeizer HE, et al. Endovascular aortic repair is associated with greater hemodynamic stability compared with open aortic reconstruction. J Cardiothorac Vasc Anesth 1999;13:42–46.
9. Norgren L, Albrechtsson U, Swartbol P. Side-effect of endovascular grafting to treat aortic aneurysm. Br J Surg 1996;83:520–521.
10. Schoenwald PK, Sprung J, Sullivan T. Anesthetic considerations for treatment of abdominal aortic aneurysm (AAA) with an endovascular graft. Anesth Analg 1998;86:S99.
11. Baker AB, Lloyd G, Bookallil MJ Yezerski SD. Retrospective review of 100 cases of endoluminal aortic stent-graft surgery from an anaesthetic perspective. Anaesth Intensive Care 1997;25:378–384.
12. Tanito Y, Endou M, Koide Y, Okumura F. ATP-induced ventricular asystole and hypotension during endovascular stenting surgery. Can J Anaesth 1998;45:491–494.
13. Baker AB, Bookallil MJ, Lloyd G. Intentional asystole during endoluminal thoracic aortic surgery without cardiopulmonary bypass. Br J Anaesth 1997;78:444–448.
14. Blum U, Voshage G, Lammer J, et al. Endoluminal stent-grafts for infrarenal abdominal aortic aneurysms. N Engl J Med 1997; 336:13–20.
15. Machan L, Fry P. Abdominal aortic aneurysm repair using the World Medical Talent Prosthesis. Tech Vasc Intervent Radiol 1998;1:25–31.
16. Moore WS, Rutherford RB. Transfemoral endovascular repair of abdominal aortic aneurysm: results of the North American EVT phase I trial. J Vasc Surg 1996;23:543–553.
17. Nasim A, Thompson MM, Sayers RD, et al. Endovascular repair of abdominal aortic aneurysm: an initial experience. Br J Surg 1996;83:516–519.
18. Ritchie JL, ACC/AHA Task Force. ACC/AHA guidelines for perioperative cardiovascular evaluation for non-cardiac surgery. Circulation 1996;93:1280–1317.
19. Goldman L, Caldera DL, Nussbaum SR, et al. Multifactorial index of cardiac risk in non-cardiac surgical procedures. N Engl J Med 1977;297:845–850.
20. Detsky AS, Abrams HB, McLaughlin JR, et al. Predicting cardiac complications in patients undergoing non-cardiac surgery. J Gen Intern Med 1986;1:211–19.
21. Badner NH, Knill RL, Brown JE, et al. Myocardial infarction after non-cardiac surgery. Anesthesiology 1998;88:572–578.
22. Larsen SF, Olesen KH, Jacobsen E, et al. Prediction of cardiac risk in non-cardiac surgery. Eur Heart J 1987;8:179–185.
23. Eagle KA, Rihal CS, Mickel MC, et al. Cardiac risk of non-cardiac surgery; influence of coronary disease and type of surgery in 3368 operations. CASS Investigators and University of Michigan Heart Care Program. Coronary Artery Surgery Study. Circulation 1997;96:1882–1887.
24. Hertzer NR, Beven EG, Young JR, et al. Coronary artery disease in peripheral vascular patients: a classification of 1000 coronary angiograms and results of surgical management. Ann Surg 1984;199:223–233.
25. Mangano DT. Perioperative cardiac morbidity. Anesthesiology 1987;72:153–184.
26. Tarhan S, Moffitt EA, Taylor WF, Giuliani ER. Myocardial infarction after general anesthesia. JAMA 1972;220:1451–1454.
27. Steen PA, Tinker JH, Tarhan S. Myocardial reinfarction after anesthesia and surgery. JAMA 1978;239:2566–2570.
28. Rao TLK, Jacobs KH, El-Etr AA. Reinfarction following anesthesia in patients with myocardial infarction. Anesthesiology 1983; 59:499–505.
29. Shah KB, Kleinman BS, Sami H, et al. Reevaluation of perioperative myocardial infarction in patients with prior myocardial infarction undergoing non-cardiac operations. Anesth Analg 1990; 71:231–235.
30. Mangano DT. Adverse outcomes after surgery in the year 2001—a continuing odyssey. Anesthesiology 1998;88:561–564.
31. Foster ED, Davis KB, Carpenter JA, et al. Risk of non-cardiac operation in patients with defined coronary disease: the Coronary Artery Surgery Study (CASS) registry experience. Ann Thorac Surg 1986;41:42–49.
32. Mahar LJ, Steen PA, Tinker JH, et al. Perioperative myocardial infarction in patients with coronary artery disease with and without aorta-coronary artery bypass grafts. J Thorac Cardiovasc Surg 1978;76:533–537.
33. Chaitman BR, Rosen AD, Williams DO, et al. Myocardial infarction and cardiac mortality in the bypass angioplasty revascularization investigation (BARI) randomized trial. Circulation 1997; 96:2162–2170.

34. The Bypass Angioplasty Revascularization Investigation (BARI) Investigators. Comparison of coronary bypass surgery and angioplasty in patients with multivessel disease. N Engl J Med 1996;335:217–225.

35. Allen JR, Helling TS, Hartzler GO. Operative procedures not involving the heart after percutaneous transluminal coronary angioplasty. Surg Gynecol Obstet 1991;173:285–288.

36. Gottlieb A, Banoub M, Sprung J, et al. Perioperative cardiovascular morbidity in patients with coronary artery disease undergoing vascular surgery after percutaneous transluminal coronary angioplasty. J Cardiothorac Vasc Anesth 1998;12:501–506.

37. Talley JD, Hurst JW, King SB III, et al. Clinical outcome 5 years after attempted percutaneous transluminal coronary angioplasty in 427 patients. Circulation 1988;77:820–829.

38. Mangano, DT.Layug EL, Wallace A, Tateo I. Effect of atenolol on mortality and cardiovascular morbidity after noncardiac surgery. N Engl J Med 1996;335:1713–1720.

39. Wallace A, Layug B, Tateo I, et al: Prophylactic atenolol reduces postoperative myocardial ischemia. Anesthesiology 1998;88:7–17.

40. Slogoff S, Keats AS. Does chronic treatment with calcium entry blocking drugs reduce perioperative myocardial ischemia? Anesthesiology 1988;68:676–680.

41. Furberg CD, Psaty BM. Calcium antagonists: antagonists or protagonists of mortality in elderly hypertensives? (Editorial). J Am Geriatr Soc 1995;43:1309–1310.

42. Landesberg G, Einav S, Christopherson R, et al. Perioperative ischemia and cardiac complications in major vascular surgery: importance of the preoperative twelve-lead electrocardiogram. J Vasc Surg 1997;26:570–578.

43. Yeager MP, Glass DD, Neff RK, Brinck-Johnsen T. Epidural anesthesia and analgesia in high-risk surgical patients. Anesthesiology 1987;66:729–736.

44. Tuman KJ, McCarthy RJ, March RJ, et al. Effects of epidural anesthesia and analgesia on coagulation and outcome after major vascular surgery. Anesth Analg 1991;73:696–704.

45. Christopherson R, Beattie C, Frank SM, et al. Perioperative morbidity in patients randomized to epidural or general anesthesia for lower extremity vascular surgery. Anesthesiology 1993;79:422–434.

46. Whalley DG, D'Amico JA, Rybicki LA, et al. The effect of posture on the induction of epidural anesthesia for peripheral vascular surgery. Reg Anesth 1995;20:407–411.

47. Denny N, Masters R, Pearson D, et al. Postdural puncture headache after continuous spinal anesthesia. Anesth Analg 1987;66:791–794.

7

Thoracic Aortic Stent-Grafts

CHARLES P. SEMBA AND MICHAEL D. DAKE

Untreated thoracic aortic aneurysms have upward of 50% 5-year and 75% 10-year mortality.[1] Other epidemiological studies show that the 5-year risk is even higher and approaches 75%.[2,3] Aortic rupture is the cause of death in 33 to 50% of these patients, and the remainder die of associated cardiovascular disease. Factors associated with an increased mortality rate include symptomatic aneurysms, advanced age, aneurysms ≥6 cm in diameter, and generalized cardiovascular disease. Although the vast majority of thoracic aortic aneurysms are caused by degenerative atherosclerotic disease aggravated by long-standing hypertension, other etiologies of thoracic aneurysms include congenital weakness in the aortic media owing to Marfan or Ehlers-Danlos syndrome, infective aortitis, traumatic injury, and aortic dissection.

The major reason for treating thoracic aortic aneurysms is to avoid acute rupture, and the only proven method is surgical resection of the aneurysm and placement of a polyester interposition graft.[4] The overall surgical mortality rate with an experienced surgical team is approximately 15%, and long-term follow-up studies support the increased survival in patients undergoing surgery who are at good operative risk. However, the operative mortality increases to nearly 50% in patients requiring emergency treatment or in those with significant comorbidity including advanced age and chronic cardiopulmonary disease.[5,6]

Less invasive endovascular approaches for high-risk patients were developed in the early 1990s—more than two decades after Dotter's[7] first description of the endovascular stent in 1969. The first clinical endovascular repair of an abdominal aortic aneurysm was reported in 1991 when Parodi and colleagues[8] used a Palmaz stent combined with polyester graft material. In 1992, the first successful endovascular thoracic aortic aneurysm repair was performed by the team led by Dake and Miller[9] at Stanford using a polyester covered self-expanding Z-stent. Endovascular stent-graft repair of thoracic aortic aneurysms may provide an attractive, less invasive alternative to thoracotomy and interposition graft placement in high-risk surgical candidates who have isolated aneurysms of the descending thoracic aorta. This chapter outlines the methodology of stent-graft repair of thoracic aneurysms based on the 5-year clinical experience at Stanford University using first-generation technology.[10]

■ Indications

Patients with thoracic aortic aneurysms are evaluated by a cardiovascular surgeon and an interventional radiologist. The stent-graft protocol was approved by the investigational review board at Stanford University Medical Center.

Preoperative Imaging

Prior to any clinical considerations for endovascular repair, the patients are required to meet specific anatomic criteria determined by contrast-enhanced spiral computed tomography (CT) and digital subtraction angiography (DSA) of the thoracoabdominal aorta and pelvis as outlined in Table 7–1.

High-quality spiral CT imaging is essential in any endovascular stent-graft program because it provides the

TABLE 7–1. Anatomic Criteria for Endovascular Repair of Thoracic Aortic Aneurysms Using a First-Generation Stent-Graft

Location of aneurysm	Distal to left subclavian, proximal to celiac arteries
Neck length	≥15 mm
Neck diameter	≤40 mm
Aneurysm length	≤22 cm
Aneurysm diameter	≥40 mm
Abdominal aortic diameter	≥8 mm
Iliac artery diameter[a]	≥8 mm
Common femoral artery diameter[a]	≥8 mm

[a]If the iliofemoral vessels are <8 mm, access into the aorta can be obtained directly using surgical exposure of the left retroperitoneal infrarenal aorta.

crucial information used to determine aortic dimensions, measurements for constructing the stent-graft, and extravascular evaluation of the lung parenchyma, pleural space, and airways. Imaging protocols are derived from the work of Rubin[11–13] using a HiSpeed Advantage scanner (General Electric Imaging systems, Milwaukee, WI) and are utilized for both pre- and post–stent-graft analysis.

After determining the scan delay time, the CT is programmed for the diagnostic study of the thoracic aorta. The scan volume starts 2 to 3 cm above the aortic arch and continues through the lower thoracic aorta using 3-mm collimation and a pitch of 2.0 (120 kV, 280 mA). Total scan duration is approximately 30 seconds (deep breath hold) using 120 to 150 mL of nonionic iodinated contrast (4–5 mL/sec) and a scan delay calculated previously. The length of anatomy covered along the z-axis (table distance) is equal to the total acquisition time multiplied by both the slice thickness and pitch divided by the time required for one 360-degree rotation of the x-ray tube. Axial images are reconstructed at 2-mm increments. Additional images of the aorta are presented in three formats: shaded surface display (SSD), maximum intensity projections (MIPs), and curved planar reformations (CPRs). Three-dimensional reconstructions are used to qualitatively assess the tortuosity of the vascular system and rarely used for quantitative analysis.

Several measurements are documented: (1) the diameter of the proximal and distal aortic neck; (2) the diameter of the outer wall of the aortic aneurysm (maximum diameter); (3) length of proximal and distal necks; (4) distance between the proximal and distal aortic neck; (5) presence of patent intercostal arteries arising from the aneurysm sac; (6) relationship of the subclavian and celiac arteries to the aortic neck; (7) presence of anatomic variations (e.g., aberrant right subclavian artery); (8) presence of significant parenchymal lung disease or unsuspected masses; and (9) presence of extensive mural thrombus or calcifications at

the aortic neck, which may prevent a tight seal following placement of the endoprosthesis. To determine the transverse dimensions of the aortic neck, two perpendicular measurements are made and the diameter is calculated as the mean because many aortas are not round but ovoid in configuration. In certain cases, if the proximal neck is insufficient (≤15 mm), a surgical left subclavian to left common carotid transposition is planned, thereby allowing the proximal portion of the stent-graft to cover the native left subclavian artery.

Clinical Indications

Patients undergoing endovascular repair of a descending thoracic aortic aneurysm must have the appropriate anatomic criteria as outlined above and be considered a high-risk surgical candidate for one or more of the following reasons: severe obstructive pulmonary disease (forced expiratory volume in 1 second <700 mL), coronary artery disease, congestive heart failure, renal insufficiency, advanced age or generalized debility, and multiple previous thoracotomies. Patients must be able to tolerate general anesthesia and endotracheal intubation and should be evaluated preoperatively by an anesthesiologist experienced in the management of patients with significant cardiopulmonary disease.

Contraindications include a positive dobutamine-stress echocardiography exam, generalized sepsis, coagulopathy or other contraindications to intraprocedural systemic anticoagulation, inflammatory aneurysms, aneurysms involving the aorta and great vessels, extremely poor ventilatory reserve and the likely requirement of long-term ventilatory support following the stent-graft procedure, and allergies to iodinated contrast media. Contained aortic rupture and mycotic aneurysms are considered relative contraindications; stent-graft implantation is used when there are no suitable alternatives and the procedure is performed as a lifesaving intervention.

■ Stent-Graft Construction

The stent-graft used at Stanford from 1992 to 1997 was custom built by hand for each patient based on measurements derived from preoperative imaging. The stent-graft is constructed well ahead of time in a clean but nonsterile work space based on measurements acquired from the angiograms and CT. We always have a second, identical stent-graft available as a backup prosthesis. The stent-graft is constructed by combining a Gianturco Z-stent (Cook, Inc., Bloomington, IN) with woven polyester surgical graft material.[14] The Z-stent is a modified tracheobronchial stent (Gianturco-Rosch tracheobronchial Z-stent; Cook, Inc.) with diameters of 15, 20, 25, 30, and 35 mm and a length of 25 mm for each stent body. It is packaged with two stents attached end to end (total length 50 mm) (Fig. 7–1). The stent diameter is usually oversized by 1 to 2 mm to ensure a snug fit at the "landing zone" of the aneurysm neck. The tracheobronchial stents have sharp anchoring hooks that are removed using a wire cutter, and the cut surface is filed smooth prior to placement of the polyester covering. The stent-graft is built in 25-mm length increments; therefore, an aneurysm that has a neck-to-neck length of 60 mm would require four Z-stent bodies to give a total length of 100 mm to sufficiently span the mouth of the aneurysm. To create a sufficiently long stent endoskeleton, the Z-stents are attached to each other using 5–0 polypropylene suture that is threaded through the individual eyelets at the ends of the Z-stent. Changing the diameter of the stent requires that the constraining thread of monofilament be cut and a new loop of 4– or 5–0 polypropylene suture be passed through the eyelets of the stent of the appropriate diameter. This maneuver allows one to create a stent diameter of 36, 38, or 40 mm or any dimension desired.

The graft material used to cover the Z-stent endoskeleton is woven polyester (Cooley Veri-soft, Meadox Medical, Inc., Oakland, NJ). The graft material is available in diameters up to 40 mm. To reduce the profile of the graft, the crimps in the polyester material are removed by smoothing the graft over a cylindrical surface (to avoid creasing the polyester) and pressing with a warm, handheld, standard laundry iron. The graft material is cut to the same length as the Z-stent frame, and the edges of the graft material are sealed using an alcohol flame or cautery probe tip to prevent fraying. The prepared graft material is stretched over the Z-stent frame and should be free of wrinkles or creases. The graft is secured to the Z-stent frame using multiple interrupted 5–0 polypropylene sutures attached to the eyelets on both ends of the graft. To facilitate loading the stent-graft into the loading capsule at the time of deployment, four individual loops of 30-cm-long 2–0 polypropylene suture, referred to as *loading tethers,* are formed by passing the thread through the eyelets at one end of the stent-graft.

■ Delivery System

The delivery of the Z-stent-graft requires five components (Fig. 7–2): a delivery sheath made from 22- or 24-French (Fr) Teflon (Keller-Timmerman sheath; Cook, Inc.) with an external hemostatic valve, tapered dilator, retrieval hook or wire, loading cartridge, and pushing mandrel. Deployment of the stent-graft can be summarized as follows: the stent-graft is constrained and placed in a loading cartridge; the pushing mandrel is used to extrude the stent-graft from the loading cartridge into the delivery sheath; the mandrel pushes the stent-graft through the delivery sheath and is released at the target site.

■ Endovascular Procedure

Stent-graft procedures are performed in the surgical operating suite using a portable C-arm with digital subtraction capabilities (OEC Diasonics; Salt Lake City, UT) or angiography suite with a 16-inch image intensifier (MultiStar TOP; Siemens Medical Imaging Systems, Erlangen, Germany). The angiography suite is

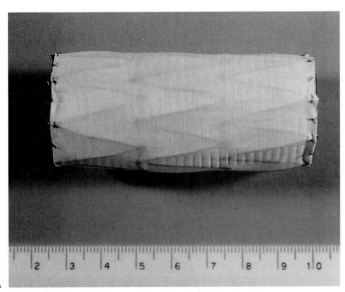
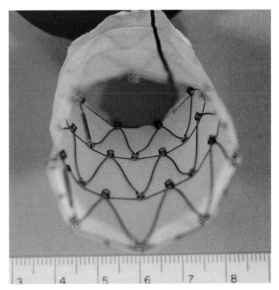

A   **B**

FIGURE 7–1. Outer (**A**) and inner (**B**) view of the Gianturco-Rosch Z-stent covered with woven polyester graft and secured with polypropylene suture.

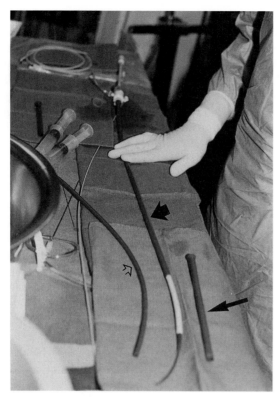

FIGURE 7–2. Delivery system requires a 22- to 24-Fr delivery sheath fitted with a tapered dilator (arrowhead) and a pushing mandrel (open arrow). The stent-graft is loaded into a fluted Teflon cartridge (arrow).

catheter in the steep left anterior oblique projection. The purpose of the predeployment angiogram is to ensure that the patient and image intensifier are positioned optimally to monitor accurate placement of the endoprosthesis.

Following aortography, the patient is systemically anticoagulated with intravenous heparin (150 U/kg) and titrated to maintain the activated clotting time of >250 seconds. The vascular sheath and pigtail catheter are withdrawn over an exchange-length stiff wire (Amplatz Super Stiff; Boston Scientific Vascular, Inc., Watertown, MA). A transverse arteriotomy is performed and the 22- or 24-Fr delivery sheath with inner dilator is introduced over the guidewire and navigated into the thoracic aorta under fluoroscopic guidance. When the delivery system reaches the aorta proximal to the aneurysm, the dilator and guidewire are withdrawn and the Silastic component of the Keller-Timmerman sheath is firmly grasped with the hand to avoid excessive blood loss. The stent-graft is then introduced into the delivery sheath from the loading cartridge with the pushing mandrel. Using fluoroscopic monitoring, the stent-graft is advanced to the target zone with forward motion on the pushing mandrel. The lead edge of the stent-graft is advanced in the delivery sheath until it is flush (tip to tip) with the end of the sheath. The sheath tip is aligned in the proximal neck "landing zone" and is readied for deployment. Prior to release, sodium nitroprusside solution is administered intravenously to transiently decrease the mean arterial blood pressure to a range of 50 to 60 mm Hg to decrease downstream migration of the stent-graft. After final confirmation of position, the stent-graft is deployed by rapidly withdrawing the sheath while the pushing mandrel is maintained in fixed position. The pushing mandrel is removed and a 9-Fr vascular sheath inserted through the Silastic cap of the Rutner adapter. A pigtail catheter is introduced to perform the postdeployment angiogram to detect any perigraft leaks. If the stent-graft does not completely cover the neck of the aneurysm the second backup stent-graft is deployed. If a perigraft leak exists owing to poor sealing and apposition of the stent-graft to the aortic wall, balloon dilatation of the stent-graft is considered using valvuloplasty balloons. Completion angiography should demonstrate exclusion of the aneurysm and no kinks within the prosthesis. At the conclusion of the procedure the arteriotomy is repaired and systemic anticoagulation with heparin is reversed using protamine sulfate.

preferred in cases where high-quality imaging in multiple projections using a large field of view is required. Patients are positioned supine under general anesthesia with endotracheal intubation and fully monitored using pulmonary and radial arterial lines. The patient's thorax is prepped and draped in the routine fashion for a conventional left lateral thoracotomy to facilitate a rapid conversion to an open chest procedure, if necessary. The abdomen, pelvis, and groin are draped for femoral or retroperitoneal iliac/aortic access. Determination of the access site is based on the preoperative angiography. First choice for arterial access is the right common femoral artery. If the common femoral arteries are less than 8 mm in diameter or if there is extensive tortuosity of the iliac vessels, a left retroperitoneal approach is considered for access into the common iliac artery or distal abdominal aorta under direct surgical exposure.

In the majority of cases, the common femoral artery is surgically exposed and a standard 18 G arterial needle is used to puncture the anterior wall of the artery directly and a 0.035" diameter soft guidewire (Bentson; Cook, Inc.) is advanced into the aorta. Following placement of a 5-Fr vascular sheath, aortography of the thoracic aorta is performed using a calibrated pigtail

Alternative access methods are required if the patient has extensive iliofemoral occlusive disease: (1) retroperitoneal access to the distal aorta or common iliac artery; (2) access into existing aortobifemoral bypass graft; and (3) access into a newly placed surgical aortofemoral or aortic tube graft. Direct surgical exposure of the distal aorta or common iliac artery is utilized via a left retroperitoneal approach. The artery is accessed with either typical needle and guidewire technique or, the method we favor, a 20-cm-long, 8-mm-diameter polyester side limb sewn to the aorta or common iliac artery end to side because it is difficult to navigate the long 22- to 24-Fr sheaths into the deep retroperitoneal space. At the conclusion of the procedure, the side limb is oversewn. Femoral access into an existing aortobifemoral graft can be accomplished easily and safely. Because the femoral limbs are commonly 8 mm in diameter and have some radial elasticity, grafts can accommodate the large delivery catheters without difficulty. Thoracic aortic stent-grafting immediately following surgical repair of an abdominal aortic aneurysm has been performed by using the side limb technique.[15]

■ Postprocedure Monitoring

Patients are usually monitored in the intensive care unit for the first 12 to 24 hours after the procedure until they are extubated and hemodynamically stable. On the next day most patients can be transferred to a regular nursing unit. They are discharged from the hospital on the third postoperative day. No postprocedural anticoagulation is administered. Prior to discharge, all the patients undergo a follow-up chest x-ray, arteriogram, and contrast-enhanced spiral CT examination to evaluate the shape and position of the stent-graft, the possibility of perigraft leak, and any residual patency of the aneurysm. A repeat spiral CT is performed 6 months after the stent-graft placement and yearly thereafter.

■ Results

Over a 5-year period at Stanford University, 103 patients underwent thoracic aortic stent-graft repair using the custom fabricated Z-stent device with an average follow-up of 22 months. The preoperative patient profile is summarized in Table 7–2.[10] Complete thrombosis of the aneurysm was achieved in 86 (83%) of patients (Fig. 7–3) and the results are summarized in Table 7–3. The early mortality (<30 days) rate was 9%, and multivariable analysis revealed that myocardial infarction, stroke, or being judged not to be a surgical candidate was associated with a higher likelihood of early death. The overall actuarial survival was 86, 81, and 73% at 6 months, 1 year, and 2 years, respectively.

The most common early postoperative complications included endoleaks (24%), pulmonary insufficiency (12%), early death (9%), acute renal failure (5%), paraplegia/paresis (3%), and myocardial infarction (2%). Twenty-five of 103 patients had evidence of an endoleak documented by angiography or CT scanning. Following further intervention (additional stent-graft or coil embolization), secondary success was accomplished in 11 patients; three patients had spontaneous thrombosis of small endoleaks.

Complications were also analyzed according to whether they were related directly to the stent-graft or

TABLE 7–2. Preoperative Patient Profile of 103 Patients Treated with a First-Generation Endovascular Stent-Graft[10]

Patients	103	(male, 73; female, 30)
Age (years)	76	(range, 34–89)
Operative status		
Emergency	16	(16%)
Nonemergency	87	(84%)
Not surgical candidate	62	(60%)
Etiology (no. of patients)		
Atherosclerosis	64	
Aortic dissection	8	
Trauma	8	
Penetrating ulcer	10	
Other	13	
Size of aneurysm		
Aneurysm length (mm)	86	(range, 10–220)
Aneurysm diameter (mm)	62	(range, 40–110)
Neck diameter (mm)	31.8	(range, 20–45)
Other medical problems (no. of patients)		
Myocardial ischemia	10	(10%)
Congestive heart failure	14	(14%)
Coronary artery disease	31	(30%)
Hypertension	74	(72%)
Diabetes	11	(11%)
Chronic pulmonary disease	32	(31%)
Stroke	11	(11%)
Smoking	63	(62%)
Previous thoracotomy	46	(45%)
NYHA functional class		
I	40	(39%)
II	41	(40%)
III	21	(20%)
IV	1	(1%)

NYHA, New York Heart Association.

TABLE 7–3. Results of 103 Patients Treated with a First-Generation Endovascular Stent-Graft[10]

Aneurysm thrombosis (no. of patients)		
Primary thrombosis (immediate)	75	(73%)
Late thrombosis (≤1 year)	86	(84%)
Early endoleak (<1 year)	25	(24%)
Stent-graft misdeployment	3	(3%)
Early mortality rate (<30 days)	9% ± 3%	(±70% confidence limits)
Paraplegia rate	3% ± 2%	(±1 SE)
Stroke rate	7% ± 3%	(±1 SE)
Actuarial survival		
1 year	81% ± 4%	(±1 SE)
2 year	73% ± 5%	(±1 SE)

SE, standard error.

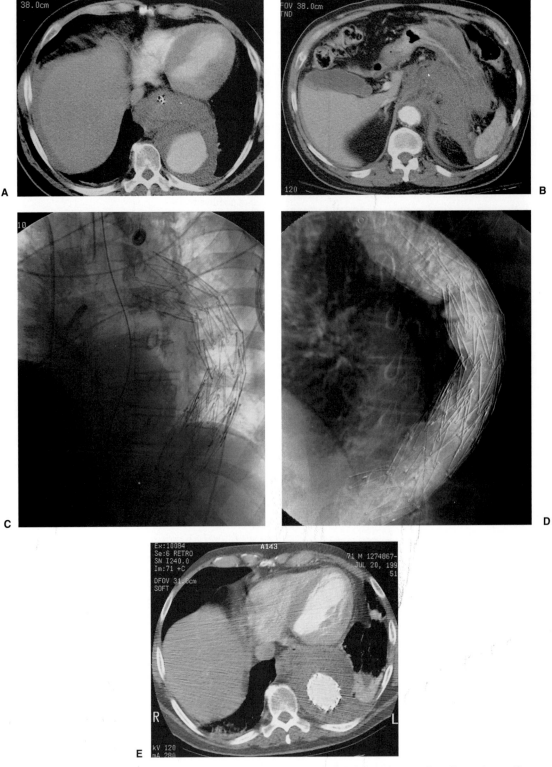

FIGURE 7–3. A 71-year-old patient with an acute rupture of the descending thoracic aortic aneurysm. Preoperative contrast-enhanced spiral computed tomography (CT) reveals (**A**) a contained aortic rupture at the level of the diaphragm and (**B**) extravasation of blood into the retroperitoneal space. (**C**). Two Z-stent-grafts were placed in the descending thoracic aorta and completion angiography shows (**D**) no immediate endoleak, which was confirmed on (**E**) a follow-up CT scan. The patient survived and is alive and well 3 years following the procedure.

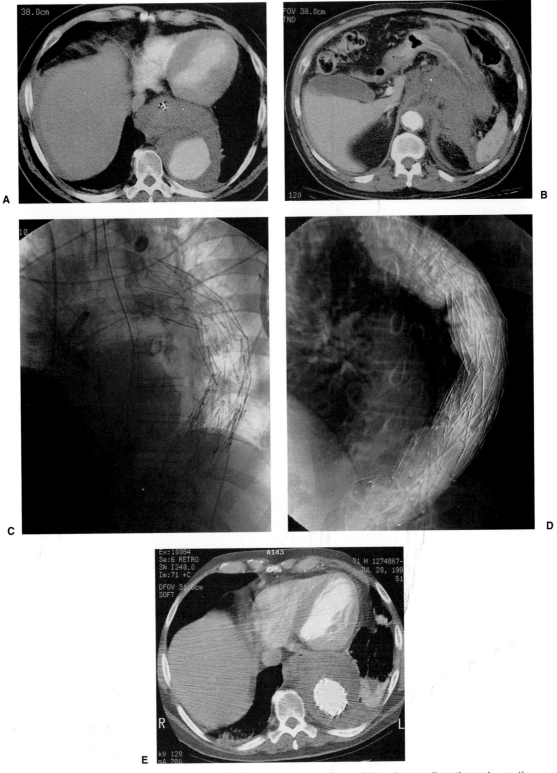

FIGURE 7–3. A 71-year-old patient with an acute rupture of the descending thoracic aortic aneurysm. Preoperative contrast-enhanced spiral computed tomography (CT) reveals (**A**) a contained aortic rupture at the level of the diaphragm and (**B**) extravasation of blood into the retroperitoneal space. (**C**). Two Z-stent-grafts were placed in the descending thoracic aorta and completion angiography shows (**D**) no immediate endoleak, which was confirmed on (**E**) a follow-up CT scan. The patient survived and is alive and well 3 years following the procedure.

aorta or common iliac artery is utilized via a left retroperitoneal approach. The artery is accessed with either typical needle and guidewire technique or, the method we favor, a 20-cm-long, 8-mm-diameter polyester side limb sewn to the aorta or common iliac artery end to side because it is difficult to navigate the long 22- to 24-Fr sheaths into the deep retroperitoneal space. At the conclusion of the procedure, the side limb is oversewn. Femoral access into an existing aortobifemoral graft can be accomplished easily and safely. Because the femoral limbs are commonly 8 mm in diameter and have some radial elasticity, grafts can accommodate the large delivery catheters without difficulty. Thoracic aortic stent-grafting immediately following surgical repair of an abdominal aortic aneurysm has been performed by using the side limb technique.[15]

■ Postprocedure Monitoring

Patients are usually monitored in the intensive care unit for the first 12 to 24 hours after the procedure until they are extubated and hemodynamically stable. On the next day most patients can be transferred to a regular nursing unit. They are discharged from the hospital on the third postoperative day. No postprocedural anticoagulation is administered. Prior to discharge, all the patients undergo a follow-up chest x-ray, arteriogram, and contrast-enhanced spiral CT examination to evaluate the shape and position of the stent-graft, the possibility of perigraft leak, and any residual patency of the aneurysm. A repeat spiral CT is performed 6 months after the stent-graft placement and yearly thereafter.

■ Results

Over a 5-year period at Stanford University, 103 patients underwent thoracic aortic stent-graft repair using the custom fabricated Z-stent device with an average follow-up of 22 months. The preoperative patient profile is summarized in Table 7–2.[10] Complete thrombosis of the aneurysm was achieved in 86 (83%) of patients (Fig. 7–3) and the results are summarized in Table 7–3. The early mortality (<30 days) rate was 9%, and multivariable analysis revealed that myocardial infarction, stroke, or being judged not to be a surgical candidate was associated with a higher likelihood of early death. The overall actuarial survival was 86, 81, and 73% at 6 months, 1 year, and 2 years, respectively.

The most common early postoperative complications included endoleaks (24%), pulmonary insufficiency (12%), early death (9%), acute renal failure (5%), paraplegia/paresis (3%), and myocardial infarction (2%). Twenty-five of 103 patients had evidence of an endoleak documented by angiography or CT scanning. Following further intervention (additional stent-graft or coil embolization), secondary success was accomplished in 11 patients; three patients had spontaneous thrombosis of small endoleaks.

Complications were also analyzed according to whether they were related directly to the stent-graft or

TABLE 7–2. Preoperative Patient Profile of 103 Patients Treated with a First-Generation Endovascular Stent-Graft[10]

Patients	103	(male, 73; female, 30)
Age (years)	76	(range, 34–89)
Operative status		
Emergency	16	(16%)
Nonemergency	87	(84%)
Not surgical candidate	62	(60%)
Etiology (no. of patients)		
Atherosclerosis	64	
Aortic dissection	8	
Trauma	8	
Penetrating ulcer	10	
Other	13	
Size of aneurysm		
Aneurysm length (mm)	86	(range, 10–220)
Aneurysm diameter (mm)	62	(range, 40–110)
Neck diameter (mm)	31.8	(range, 20–45)
Other medical problems (no. of patients)		
Myocardial ischemia	10	(10%)
Congestive heart failure	14	(14%)
Coronary artery disease	31	(30%)
Hypertension	74	(72%)
Diabetes	11	(11%)
Chronic pulmonary disease	32	(31%)
Stroke	11	(11%)
Smoking	63	(62%)
Previous thoracotomy	46	(45%)
NYHA functional class		
I	40	(39%)
II	41	(40%)
III	21	(20%)
IV	1	(1%)

NYHA, New York Heart Association.

TABLE 7–3. Results of 103 Patients Treated with a First-Generation Endovascular Stent-Graft[10]

Aneurysm thrombosis (no. of patients)		
Primary thrombosis (immediate)	75	(73%)
Late thrombosis (≤1 year)	86	(84%)
Early endoleak (<1 year)	25	(24%)
Stent-graft misdeployment	3	(3%)
Early mortality rate (<30 days)	9% ± 3%	(±70% confidence limits)
Paraplegia rate	3% ± 2%	(±1 SE)
Stroke rate	7% ± 3%	(±1 SE)
Actuarial survival		
1 year	81% ± 4%	(±1 SE)
2 year	73% ± 5%	(±1 SE)

SE, standard error.

operative procedure. Five early or late fatal stent-graft complications occurred in four patients, including rupture of the treated aneurysm with the delivery catheter, stent-graft erosion into the esophagus, arterial injury from the delivery catheter requiring graft replacement of the iliac artery, and excessive local bleeding. Overall, 96% ±2% of patients were free from a fatal stent-graft complication at 9 months. Nine patients had a total of 12 early or late postoperative fatal complications including stroke ($n = 3$), pulmonary embolism ($n = 1$), myocardial infarction ($n = 1$), excessive local bleeding ($n = 1$), and pulmonary failure ($n = 4$). In actuarial terms, 90% ±3% of patients were free from fatal postoperative complications at 9 months.

Management of endoleaks can be accomplished by placement of an additional stent-graft and/or selective coil embolization.[16] Based on the initial follow-up spiral CT, the appearance of the leak is confirmed angiographically. For small endoleaks with a small entry channel and no outflow pathway, the channel can be embolized using small metallic coils and microcatheters or managed conservatively by obtaining a follow-up scan in 1 to 2 months. Larger, wide-mouthed leaks owing to incomplete coverage of the proximal or distal neck may require additional placement of a stent-graft device. Prophylactic embolization is reserved only for large vessels communicating directly with the aneurysmal sac.[17]

■ Conclusion

Endovascular stent-graft repair of descending thoracic aortic aneurysms using a first-generation device is technically feasible with acceptable midterm results. The most common complication is incomplete thrombosis of the aneurysm secondary to endoleaks. The described technology is limited by the difficulty in using a Z-stent–based device to accommodate tortuous aortic anatomy, the ability to place the device precisely at the target site, and the relatively large profile of the delivery system. With current development of commercially manufactured dedicated aortic stent-grafts and improved materials and delivery systems, the complication and survival rates for patients will improve significantly.

REFERENCES

1. Joyce JW, Fairbairn JF, Kincaid OW, Juergens JL. Aneurysms of the thoracic aorta: a clinical study with special reference to prognosis. Circulation 1964;29:176–181.
2. Pressler V, McNamara JJ. Thoracic aortic aneurysm: natural history and treatment. J Thorac Cardiovasc Surg 1980;79:489–498.
3. Bickerstaff LK, Pairolero PC, Hollier LW, et al. Thoracic aortic aneurysms—a population based study. Surgery 1982;92:1103–1108.
4. DeBakey ME, McCollum CH, Graham JM. Surgical treatment of aneurysms of the descending thoracic aorta: long-term results in 500 patients. J Cardiovasc Surg 1978;19:571–576.
5. Moreno-Cabral CE, Miller DC, Mitchell RS, et al. Degenerative and atherosclerotic aneurysms of the thoracic aorta. J Thorac Cardiovasc Surg 1984;88:1020–1032.
6. Borst HG, Jurmann M, Buhner B, Laas J. Risk of replacement of the descending aorta with a standardized left heart bypass technique. J Thoracic Cardiovasc Surg 1994;107:126–133.
7. Dotter CT. Transluminally placed coilspring endarterial tube: longterm patency in a canine popliteal artery. Invest Radiol 1969; 4:329–332.
8. Parodi JC, Palmaz JC, Barone HD. Transfemoral intraluminal graft implantation for abdominal aortic aneurysms. Ann Vasc Surg 1991;5:491–499.
9. Dake MD, Miller DC, Semba CP, Mitchell RS, Walker PJ, Liddell RP. Transluminal placement of endovascular stent-grafts for the treatment of descending thoracic aortic aneurysms. N Engl J Med 1994;331:1729–1734.
10. Dake MD, Miller DC, Mitchell RS, Semba CP, Moore KA, Sakai T. The "first generation" of endovascular stent-grafts for patients with aneurysms of the descending thoracic aorta. J Thorac Cardiovasc Surg 1998;116:689–704.
11. Rubin GD. Helical CT of the thoracic aorta. J Thorac Imaging 1997;12:128–149.
12. Rubin GD, Lane MJ, Bloch DA, et al. Optimization of thoracic spiral CT: effects of iodinated contrast medium concentration. Radiology 1996;201:785–791.
13. Semba CP, Razavi MK, Kee ST, Dake MD. Applications of spiral CT in endovascular aortic interventions. Semin Intervent Radiol 1998;15:179–187.
14. Mirich D, Wright KC, Wallace S, et al. Percutaneously placed endovascular grafts for aortic aneurysms: feasibility study. Radiology 1989;170:1033–1037.
15. Moon MR, Mitchell RS, Dake MD, Zarins CK, Fann JI, Miller DC. Simultaneous abdominal aortic replacement and thoracic stent-graft placement for multilevel aortic disease. J Vasc Surg 1997; 25:332–340.
16. Kato N, Semba CP, Dake MD. Embolization of perigraft leaks after endovascular stent-graft treatment of aortic aneurysms. J Vasc Intervent Radiol 1996;7:805–811.
17. Kato N, Semba CP, Dake MD. Use of a self-expanding vascular occluder for embolization during endovascular aortic aneurysm repair. J Vasc Intervent Radiol 1997;8:27–33.

8

Peripheral Aneurysm Stent-Grafts

MICHAEL DEGROOT, DANIEL Y. SZE, AND MAHMOOD K. RAZAVI

The concept of the endovascular use of covered stents was first proposed by Dotter[1] in 1969. After several investigators reported the successful experimental use of these devices in animals in the 1980s, use in human subjects was first described in the subclavian artery by Becker et al,[2] and in the aorta by Parodi et al[3] in 1991. Many reports have since appeared in the literature describing the application of stent-grafts in the treatment of aneurysms, arterial occlusive disease, traumatic vascular injuries, dissections, arteriovenous fistulas, and transjugular portosystemic shunts.

Investigations of stent-graft applications are currently concentrated on the treatment of aortic aneurysms, because of the relatively high incidence and mortality of aortic disease. However, numerous smaller and more flexible devices have also been developed that are designed for applications in vessels other than the aorta. This chapter discusses the use of stent-grafts for the treatment of peripheral arterial aneurysms and compares the treatment to the standard surgical therapy.

■ Devices for Peripheral Applications

Table 8–1 summarizes the devices currently in clinical use in the peripheral vascular system. This is a growing list, with several other manufacturers soon to introduce their products for the peripheral applications. In the United States, some of these devices are in various stages of clinical trials, mainly for the treatment of arterial occlusive disease. The commercial stent-grafts listed are all self-expanding with varying degrees of flexibility, short-

ening, radial strength, and graft porosity. The graft material in these devices is either polytetrafluoroethylene (PTFE) or polyester, fashioned either as an outside covering or as an inside lining of the stent. There are theoretical advantages to each of these configurations. A graft attached to the inside of a stent provides for a smoother luminal surface, which should minimize disturbed flow and in situ thrombus formation. Conversely, with the graft outside of the stent, there is improved apposition of the graft against the vessel wall, and hence minimized risk of perigraft leakage. The Corvita Endograft is an exception to the above design concepts, having graft material integrated over and encapsulating the metallic scaffolding of the stent. Some data are emerging suggesting that these and other design variables affect the outcome of treatment in arterial occlusive disease, but currently there is no evidence supporting this notion in treatment of peripheral aneurysms.

■ Isolated Iliac Artery Aneurysms

Isolated iliac artery aneurysm (IAA) is a relatively rare entity with an estimated prevalence of 0.03% based on large autopsy series.[4] IAAs account for only 2 to 7% of all atherosclerotic aneurysms, and only about 2% of intraabdominal aneurysm repairs are done for isolated IAAs.[5–7] Between 45 and 78% of IAAs are asymptomatic, and many are first detected incidentally on imaging examinations done for other purposes. Owing to the location of these aneurysms deep in the pelvis, detection on routine physical examination is difficult. When patients

Stent-Grafts: Current Clinical Practice. Edited by Dolmatch and Blum. Thieme Medical Publishers, Inc., New York © 2000.

TABLE 8–1. Stent-Graft Devices for Peripheral Applications

Manufacturer	Device Name	Graft Material	Stent	Diameter (mm)	Length (cm)	Introducer Size (French)
Boston Scientific (BSC)	Passager	Polyester	Self-expanding nitinol	6–12	6–10	8–10
W. L. Gore	Hemobahn	PTFE	Self-expanding nitinol	5–12	5–15	8–12
Schneider/BSC	Corvita Endograft	Polycarbourethane	Self-expanding steel alloy	6–12	Adjustable	9–10
Schneider/BSC	Wallgraft	Polyester	Self-expanding steel alloy	6–10	3–9	9–11

PTFE, polytetrafluoroethylene.

become symptomatic, they may present with abdominal or pelvic pain, claudication, congestive heart failure secondary to arteriovenous fistula formation, obstructive urinary symptoms, or neuralgia. Of course, a substantial proportion of patients present with aneurysmal rupture, with sudden abdominal or pelvic pain and hypotension.

Given their relative infrequency, the natural history of IAAs is difficult to document. As with other arterial aneurysms, progressive dilatation and eventual rupture, however, is the expected course. The average rate of increase in the diameter of an IAA is estimated to be similar to that of abdominal aortic aneurysms, at 4 mm per year.[6] Because the natural history of IAAs is incompletely understood, there is no clear consensus on the optimal time and method of management. The smallest ruptured IAA reported measured 3 cm in diameter, and hence many investigators recommend surgical repair for iliac aneurysms larger than 3 cm.[4]

Several large series studying IAAs have been reported. In a series of 50 patients, 78% were asymptomatic at the time of diagnosis, and of the remaining symptomatic patients, 58% presented with a ruptured aneurysm.[6] The most common site of involvement was the common iliac artery (89%). Two-thirds of the patients had a single aneurysm, and one-third had multiple iliac aneurysms. In contradistinction, in another series of 55 patients, multiple iliac aneurysms were seen in 67%,[7] and the most common site of involvement was the internal iliac artery. The mortality rates were 11% and 33% for patients undergoing elective or emergency surgery, respectively. Surgical complications occurred in 34% of the patients, including limb ischemia, sepsis, and excessive hemorrhage. In another series, Sacks et al[5] treated 10 patients with IAAs and reported complications in 50% of the patients, including two with rebleeding owing to incompletely treated aneurysms and one further with uncontrolled bleeding from an arterioenteric fistula.

Although two recent series report significantly fewer complications after surgery,[8,9] it is clear that the risks associated with open surgical repair of IAAs are not trivial. This is especially true in patients with comorbidities such as cardiac or pulmonary disease and advanced age.

Stent-grafts are particularly well suited for this high-risk group of patients, allowing aneurysm repair without the need for general anesthesia. As with stent-graft treatment of aortic aneurysms, hospital stay and recovery periods are significantly shorter.

◼ Results of Endoluminal Treatment of Iliac Artery Aneurysms

Owing to the relatively infrequent occurrence of IAAs, the reports on endovascular treatment of these lesions are limited to small series and case reports (Table 8–2). We first reported our experience in 1995 with the treatment of nine IAAs in eight patients.[10] In that initial report, six of the eight patients were deemed unsuitable candidates for surgical repair. Devices were all custom-made using either Palmaz stents (Cordis/Johnson & Johnson, Inc., Warren, NJ) or Gianturco Z-stents (Cook, Inc., Bloomington, IN) covered with PTFE graft material. To date, we have treated a total of 26 patients with IAAs with a mean follow-up of 29 months (2–62 months). The procedures were all technically successful with placement of the devices across the lesions. There were four small perigraft leaks, three treated by placement of an additional endoprosthesis and one by coil embolization. One patient died within 30 days of the procedure of cardiac causes, resulting in an overall 30-day mortality rate of 4%. There have been no thromboses, clinically evident restenoses, or distal embolizations. Two patients developed deep vein thromboses within a week of the procedure, which were treated by anticoagulation.

Similarly, Marin et al[11] reported a high success and low complication rate treating 11 high-risk patients with a custom-made device consisting of PTFE graft material attached to a balloon-expandable Palmaz stent. There was one complication in their series, consisting of distal embolization to the contralateral limb. Another patient developed a kink in the unsupported portion of the graft, which was corrected by placement of an additional stent. All aneurysms were excluded successfully in this

TABLE 8–2. Reports of Iliac Artery Aneurysm Stent-Graft Repair

Author, Year, Reference	Patients	Device	Initial Technical Success	Restenosis/ Reocclusion	Mean Follow-Up: Months (Range)	Complications (Number of Patients)
Razavi, 1995[10]	9	Palmaz or Z-stent/ PTFE	100%	0	8.5 (1–17)	Contralateral deep venous thrombosis (1)
Marin, 1995[11]	11	Palmaz stent/ PTFE	100%	0	11 (3–21)	Contralateral embolization (1); stent kink—repaired (1); transient colonic ischemia (1)
Cardon, 1996[12]	27	Cragg Endopro	85%	2/24	11.8 (6–19)	Death by hemorrhage from puncture site (1); failed placement (2); graft leak (2)
Dorros, 1997[13]	10	Palmaz stent/ PTFE	100%	1/10	14	Transient renal insufficiency (1); graft thrombosed at 2 weeks, treated successfully (1)
Gasparini, 1997[14]	8	Cragg Endopro	100%	0	6.6 (3–12)	Transient renal insufficiency (1); access site hematoma (1)
Quinn, 1997[15]	7	Palmaz stent/PTFE	86%	0	12	Stent graft leak in tortuous vessel (1)
Dorffner, 1998[16]	6	Dacron-covered nitinol	100%	0	8.8 (3–20)	None
Razavi, 1998[17]	19	Palmaz or Z-stent/ PTFE	100%	0	21 (1–48)	Contralateral deep venous thrombosis (2)
Ruebben, 1998[18]	9	Cragg Endopro	100%	1/9	22	Thrombosis at 2 weeks treated with thrombolysis and additional stent (1)

study, and stent-grafts remained patent after a mean follow-up period of 11 months.

Several published reports have described using the Cragg EndoPro System I and its refined version the Passager (Boston Scientific Vascular, Watertown, MA) to treat iliac aneurysms. In the largest series, Cardon et al[12] reported the results of a multicenter French trial with 27 patients. The periprocedural complication rate was 18.5%. This included one anticoagulated patient who died 2 days after the procedure from bleeding at the site of arterial puncture, two further patients who had a perigraft leak, and two others who failed attempted endovascular therapy and subsequently underwent emergency surgery for aneurysm repair. Overall, 22 of the 24 stent-grafts placed were patent after a mean follow-up period of 11.8 months. Of the two patients with occluded stent-grafts, one underwent subsequent standard surgical repair and the other was treated successfully with angioplasty.

■ Technical Considerations

Devices used in the peripheral circulation, whether custom-made or commercially manufactured, have a variety of performance characteristics that should be taken into consideration before their use. These include radial strength, flexibility of the delivery system and deployed device, profile of the stent-graft prior to deployment, degree of shortening postdeployment, ability for precise deployment, and graft material thrombogenicity and

porosity. Clearly, continued refinement of the design and engineering of these devices will lead to improved performance.

Each custom-made design has its own advantages and shortcomings. In several designs, stent and graft length mismatches may cause persistent leaks, requiring placement of additional devices. During balloon inflation of PTFE-covered Palmaz stents, the PTFE may shrink and leave the ends of the stent uncovered. To minimize this possibility, we use balloons that do not exceed the length of the stent, reducing the degree of "trumpeting" or "dog-boning" during balloon inflation. An alternative strategy is to predilate the PTFE before attachment to the stent. However, larger introducer sheaths may be required to accommodate the predilated graft and to prevent tearing of the material during advancement through the introducer sheath. Another potential problem is the shortening of the stent when dilated to vessel size, which occurs with Palmaz and especially Wallstents. This should be accounted for before tailoring of the graft material. Our preferred custom-made device for iliac applications is the PTFE-covered Z-stent because of the accuracy of deployment and the end-to-end coverage of the stent by graft material. Eventually, the availability of commercially manufactured devices will obviate the need for custom fabrication of stent-grafts in a majority of cases. An exception would be in cases where a tapered device is required (Fig. 8–1). Currently, there are no commercially manufactured tapered devices for peripheral applications.

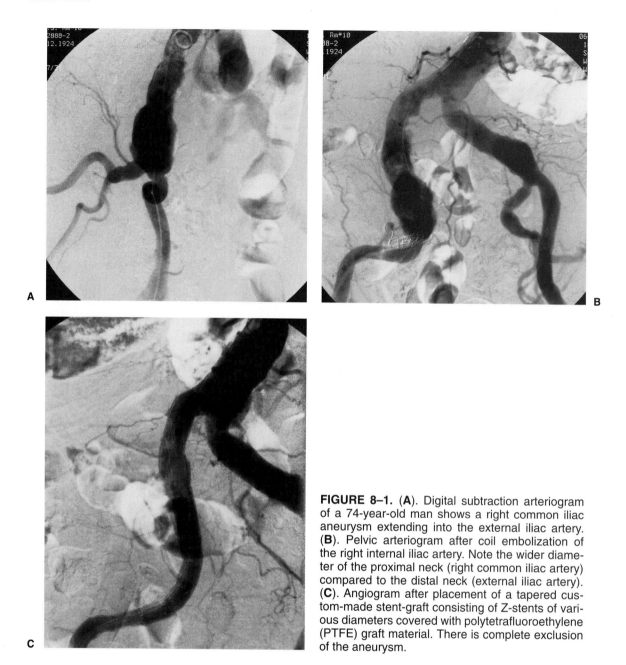

FIGURE 8–1. (**A**). Digital subtraction arteriogram of a 74-year-old man shows a right common iliac aneurysm extending into the external iliac artery. (**B**). Pelvic arteriogram after coil embolization of the right internal iliac artery. Note the wider diameter of the proximal neck (right common iliac artery) compared to the distal neck (external iliac artery). (**C**). Angiogram after placement of a tapered custom-made stent-graft consisting of Z-stents of various diameters covered with polytetrafluoroethylene (PTFE) graft material. There is complete exclusion of the aneurysm.

Regardless of the type of device used, certain anatomic features should be kept in mind when treating an IAA with the use of a stent-graft. The most important consideration is the status of the internal iliac arteries. If the ipsilateral artery is involved, its most proximal normal segment(s) should be coil-embolized prior to stent-graft placement to prevent retrograde flow into the aneurysm (Figs. 8–1B and 8–2B). In our experience, approximately 50% of these patients will develop ipsilateral claudication after embolization, which may last weeks to months. The risk of bowel ischemia does not appear to be significant after internal iliac artery embolization, even in the absence of a patent inferior mesenteric artery. Tortuosity or the presence of significant occlusive disease in the iliac arteries, although complicating factors, are not con-

traindications to endoluminal repair. With use of an appropriate device and pretreatment of stenotic lesions, good technical results may be expected.

■ Subclavian Artery Aneurysms

As with other peripheral locations, subclavian artery aneurysm (SAA) is a rare diagnosis. The etiologies of aneurysms and pseudoaneurysms of the subclavian artery include atherosclerotic disease, thoracic outlet syndrome, and trauma, including iatrogenic causes such as complicated subclavian venous catheter placement.[19–25] Primary SAA is seen more frequently in association with aberrant right subclavian artery, perhaps secondary to its

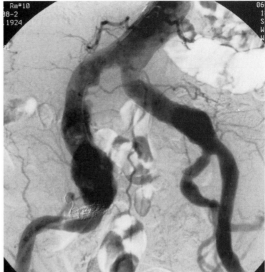

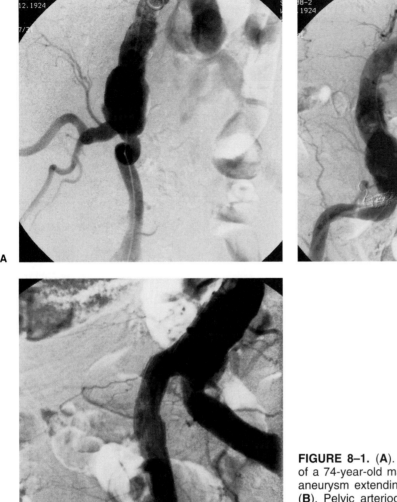

FIGURE 8–1. (A). Digital subtraction arteriogram of a 74-year-old man shows a right common iliac aneurysm extending into the external iliac artery. **(B)**. Pelvic arteriogram after coil embolization of the right internal iliac artery. Note the wider diameter of the proximal neck (right common iliac artery) compared to the distal neck (external iliac artery). **(C)**. Angiogram after placement of a tapered custom-made stent-graft consisting of Z-stents of various diameters covered with polytetrafluoroethylene (PTFE) graft material. There is complete exclusion of the aneurysm.

Regardless of the type of device used, certain anatomic features should be kept in mind when treating an IAA with the use of a stent-graft. The most important consideration is the status of the internal iliac arteries. If the ipsilateral artery is involved, its most proximal normal segment(s) should be coil-embolized prior to stent-graft placement to prevent retrograde flow into the aneurysm (Figs. 8–1B and 8–2B). In our experience, approximately 50% of these patients will develop ipsilateral claudication after embolization, which may last weeks to months. The risk of bowel ischemia does not appear to be significant after internal iliac artery embolization, even in the absence of a patent inferior mesenteric artery. Tortuosity or the presence of significant occlusive disease in the iliac arteries, although complicating factors, are not con-

traindications to endoluminal repair. With use of an appropriate device and pretreatment of stenotic lesions, good technical results may be expected.

■ Subclavian Artery Aneurysms

As with other peripheral locations, subclavian artery aneurysm (SAA) is a rare diagnosis. The etiologies of aneurysms and pseudoaneurysms of the subclavian artery include atherosclerotic disease, thoracic outlet syndrome, and trauma, including iatrogenic causes such as complicated subclavian venous catheter placement.[19–25] Primary SAA is seen more frequently in association with aberrant right subclavian artery, perhaps secondary to its

TABLE 8–2. Reports of Iliac Artery Aneurysm Stent-Graft Repair

Author, Year, Reference	Patients	Device	Initial Technical Success	Restenosis/ Reocclusion	Mean Follow-Up: Months (Range)	Complications (Number of Patients)
Razavi, 1995[10]	9	Palmaz or Z-stent/ PTFE	100%	0	8.5 (1–17)	Contralateral deep venous thrombosis (1)
Marin, 1995[11]	11	Palmaz stent/ PTFE	100%	0	11 (3–21)	Contralateral embolization (1); stent kink—repaired (1); transient colonic ischemia (1)
Cardon, 1996[12]	27	Cragg Endopro	85%	2/24	11.8 (6–19)	Death by hemorrhage from puncture site (1); failed placement (2); graft leak (2)
Dorros, 1997[13]	10	Palmaz stent/ PTFE	100%	1/10	14	Transient renal insufficiency (1); graft thrombosed at 2 weeks, treated successfully (1)
Gasparini, 1997[14]	8	Cragg Endopro	100%	0	6.6 (3–12)	Transient renal insufficiency (1); access site hematoma (1)
Quinn, 1997[15]	7	Palmaz stent/PTFE	86%	0	12	Stent graft leak in tortuous vessel (1)
Dorffner, 1998[16]	6	Dacron-covered nitinol	100%	0	8.8 (3–20)	None
Razavi, 1998[17]	19	Palmaz or Z-stent/ PTFE	100%	0	21 (1–48)	Contralateral deep venous thrombosis (2)
Ruebben, 1998[18]	9	Cragg Endopro	100%	1/9	22	Thrombosis at 2 weeks treated with thrombolysis and additional stent (1)

study, and stent-grafts remained patent after a mean follow-up period of 11 months.

Several published reports have described using the Cragg EndoPro System I and its refined version the Passager (Boston Scientific Vascular, Watertown, MA) to treat iliac aneurysms. In the largest series, Cardon et al[12] reported the results of a multicenter French trial with 27 patients. The periprocedural complication rate was 18.5%. This included one anticoagulated patient who died 2 days after the procedure from bleeding at the site of arterial puncture, two further patients who had a perigraft leak, and two others who failed attempted endovascular therapy and subsequently underwent emergency surgery for aneurysm repair. Overall, 22 of the 24 stent-grafts placed were patent after a mean follow-up period of 11.8 months. Of the two patients with occluded stent-grafts, one underwent subsequent standard surgical repair and the other was treated successfully with angioplasty.

■ Technical Considerations

Devices used in the peripheral circulation, whether custom-made or commercially manufactured, have a variety of performance characteristics that should be taken into consideration before their use. These include radial strength, flexibility of the delivery system and deployed device, profile of the stent-graft prior to deployment, degree of shortening postdeployment, ability for precise deployment, and graft material thrombogenicity and

porosity. Clearly, continued refinement of the design and engineering of these devices will lead to improved performance.

Each custom-made design has its own advantages and shortcomings. In several designs, stent and graft length mismatches may cause persistent leaks, requiring placement of additional devices. During balloon inflation of PTFE-covered Palmaz stents, the PTFE may shrink and leave the ends of the stent uncovered. To minimize this possibility, we use balloons that do not exceed the length of the stent, reducing the degree of "trumpeting" or "dog-boning" during balloon inflation. An alternative strategy is to predilate the PTFE before attachment to the stent. However, larger introducer sheaths may be required to accommodate the predilated graft and to prevent tearing of the material during advancement through the introducer sheath. Another potential problem is the shortening of the stent when dilated to vessel size, which occurs with Palmaz and especially Wallstents. This should be accounted for before tailoring of the graft material. Our preferred custom-made device for iliac applications is the PTFE-covered Z-stent because of the accuracy of deployment and the end-to-end coverage of the stent by graft material. Eventually, the availability of commercially manufactured devices will obviate the need for custom fabrication of stent-grafts in a majority of cases. An exception would be in cases where a tapered device is required (Fig. 8–1). Currently, there are no commercially manufactured tapered devices for peripheral applications.

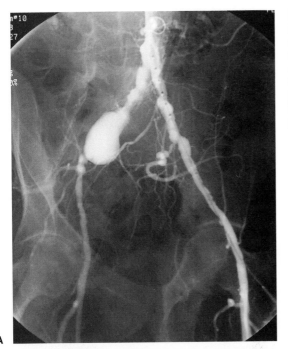

A

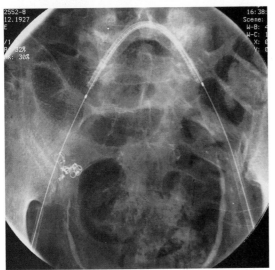

B

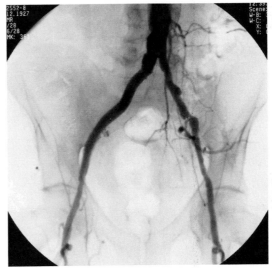

C

FIGURE 8–2. (**A**). Pelvic arteriogram of a 71-year-old man shows a right iliac aneurysm involving the origin of the internal iliac artery. There is also associated occlusive disease of both iliac arteries. (**B**). Advancement of a flexible self-expanding PTFE-covered nitinol stent through a contralateral approach after coil embolization of the right internal iliac artery. (**C**). Pelvic arteriogram after stent-graft placement, confirming exclusion of the aneurysm.

tortuous course, or to compression by the trachea and the esophagus. Finally, although mycotic SAAs were, as a rule, secondary to tuberculosis and syphilis, this entity is now most commonly associated with intravenous drug abuse in Western countries.[26,27]

SAA is frequently asymptomatic. Patients may present with a supraclavicular pulsatile mass, upper extremity thromboembolism and ischemia, central neurologic deficits secondary to retrograde embolization, or compression of the brachial plexus presenting as neuropathy. Other rare presentations include Horner syndrome, dysphagia, and hemoptysis.

The surgical approach to SAA depends on the location of the aneurysm. Intrathoracic right SAA is usually approached through a median sternotomy. For a left SAA, however, a high lateral thoracotomy is preferred.

The less invasive supraclavicular approach on either side is only appropriate for aneurysms of the second and third portions of the subclavian artery. Resection or endoaneurysmorrhaphy is preferred to direct ligation because of the decreased risk of ischemia and recurrence. In aneurysms secondary to thoracic outlet syndrome, partial resection of the clavicle, first rib, or scalenus muscles may also be performed. Despite the highly invasive nature of these surgical approaches, exposure of the affected artery is frequently incomplete. The suboptimal visualization can result in insufficient control of the vessel.[20,22,28] The reported mortality of operative repair of SAA varies from 5 to 39%.[29,30] The mortality is highest in the setting of traumatic pseudoaneurysm secondary to a gunshot wound. Operative morbidity is also substantial and may involve hemor-

TABLE 8–3. Reports of Subclavian Artery Aneurysm Stent-Graft Repair

Author, Year, Reference	Patients	Device	Technical Success	Mean Follow-Up: Months (Range)	Complications
May, 1993[31]	1	Palmaz stent/PTFE	Yes	4	None
MacSweeny, 1996[32]	1	Polyester-covered Z-stents	Yes	8	None
Patel, 1996[33]	5	Palmaz stent/PTFE	100%	19 (7–30)	None
Sullivan, 1996[34]	2	Palmaz stent/PTFE	100%	6 (9–3)	None
Meyer, 1998[35]	1	Cragg EndoPro	Yes	24	None
Szeimies, 1998[36]	2	Cragg EndoPro	100%	18 (14–22)	Both with stent stenosis, one treated successfully with angioplasty
Stanford experience	9	Custom-made	100%	34 (6–54)	Restenosis at 6 months treated with angioplasty (1)

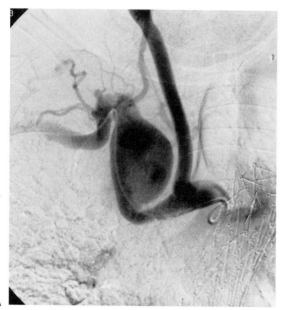

A

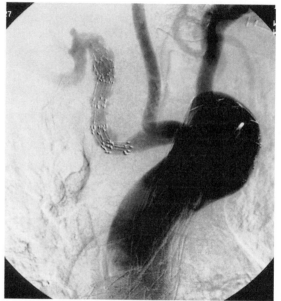

C

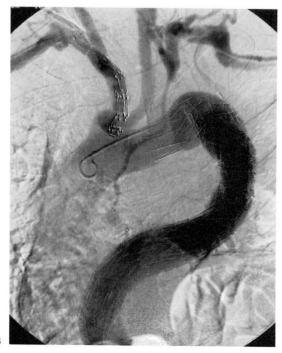

B

FIGURE 8–3. (**A**). Selective right upper extremity arteriogram reveals an aneurysm of the subclavian artery originating a few centimeters beyond the origin of the common carotid artery and extending to the origin of the vertebral artery. A thoracic aortic aneurysm has already been treated in this patient using a stent-graft. (**B** and **C**). Post–stent-graft thoracic aortograms in two different projections demonstrating complete exclusion of the right subclavian artery aneurysm.

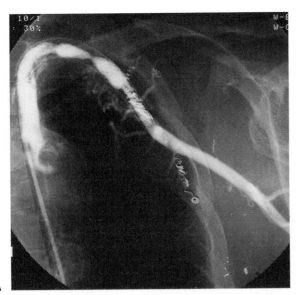
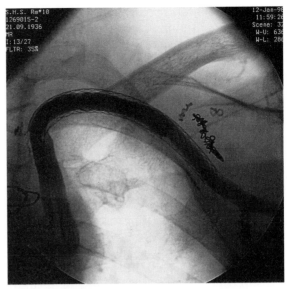

A

B

FIGURE 8–4. (A). Left subclavian arteriogram in a 61-year-old man who was treated with a PTFE-covered Wallstent for an arteriovenous fistula (AVF) and vascular malformation 1 year prior to this study. Restenosis involving the middle and proximal portions of the stent-graft were balloon dilated successfully at the time of this examination. (B). Repeat arteriogram 1 year after angioplasty and 2 years after placement of the initial device shows widely patent stent-graft with neointimal layer covering the inner surface of the entire device.

rhage, brachial plexus injury, distal embolization to the upper extremity or vertebral circulation, or pneumothorax.

■ Results of Endoluminal Treatment of Subclavian Artery Aneurysms

Given the rarity of SAA, there are no large series reported using stent-grafts to treat this disease. Several case reports and small series have been published and are summarized in Table 8–3. The very first published case report of stent-graft use in a human patient was Becker et al's[2] treatment of a traumatic pseudoaneurysm. They used a silicone-covered Palmaz stent to stop the life-threatening hemorrhage. Patel et al[33] treated five patients with endoprostheses assembled from PTFE-covered Palmaz stents with a mean follow-up period of 19 months. There was one late complication owing to stent fracture necessitating placement of a second device. Several other case studies similarly report successful exclusion of SAA with no procedural morbidity or significant postprocedural complications after follow-up periods ranging from 4 to 24 months.[31–39]

At Stanford, we have treated nine patients with subclavian artery lesions including aneurysms, pseudoaneurysms, and fistulas with a mean follow-up of 34 months (6–54 months). All devices used were custom-made from PTFE and Palmaz stents, Z-stents, or Wallstents (Schneider/Boston Scientific, Watertown, MA). There was a 100% initial technical success rate with exclusion of

all lesions (Fig. 8–3). There have been no thromboses or infections after a mean follow-up of 34 months. There was one distal embolization in a patient with a contraindication to anticoagulation. This was treated successfully by thromboaspiration. One further patient developed a stenosis along the entire length of the endoprostheses after 6 months, which was treated by angioplasty alone. The stent-graft in this patient has thus far remained patent for 36 months (Fig. 8–4). Szeimies et al[36] also reported a stent-graft stenosis secondary to thoracic outlet compression, which was in a similar location to the patient in our series reported above. Devices extending across the thoracic outlet may be prone to restenosis or stent fracture owing to the external musculoskeletal compressive forces.

Two patients who were treated for vascular malformations in our series had symptomatic recurrences. The recurrent arteriovenous malformations in both of these patients were treated by particulate and/or alcohol embolization. Because of the aggressive recruitment and parasitization of neovascularity, skeletonization of vascular malformations by stent-graft placement does not appear to be a durable solution. However, in both cases mentioned above, stent-grafts successfully excluded the coexisting fistulas, and symptoms, though persistent, were significantly diminished.

■ Technical Considerations

Owing to the inherent anatomic features, endoluminal treatment of SAA is technically more challenging than treatment of IAA. Subclavian supply to the vertebral artery and the proximity to the carotid arteries introduce the risk of embolic stroke, necessitating meticulous technique and periprocedural anticoagulation. In addition, the target vessels are a long distance from the groin, and the affected patient population frequently have very elongated and tortuous aortic arches. Ipsilateral axillary or brachial access, while allowing a more direct route, increases the risk of hematoma or pseudoaneurysm and resultant neuropathy. To reduce this risk, a cut-down may be required to introduce the device. Our preference is to use the femoral approach. For this purpose we routinely use long introducer sheaths to cross the lesion prior to the delivery of the stent-graft. In cases of extreme arch tortuosity or inability to maneuver the sheath into the subclavian artery, we use a "through and through" wire technique where the end of a guidewire introduced from a brachial approach is snared from below, and the introducer sheath is advanced over it from the groin.

As with IAAs, the presence and potential involvement of subclavian artery branches are important preprocedural considerations. The option of vertebral artery sacrifice, although rarely necessary, should be kept in mind. In patients in whom the vertebral artery arises from or close to the aneurysm and may be covered, complete cerebral angiography should be performed to determine the eligibility of the patient for endovascular treatment. In addition, the past or future use of the internal mammary artery for coronary bypass grafting should be considered, and efforts should be made to preserve it. Finally, in treatment of SAAs extending beyond the thoracic outlet, a flexible self-expanding device should be used to diminish the risk of stent fracture or deformity caused by external impingement. Supplemental surgical decompression of the region may be considered to ensure success.

■ Femoropopliteal Aneurysms

Although the femoral artery is the second most common site of peripheral aneurysms, there is little experience with stent-graft repair in this location. This is mainly because aneurysms usually occur in the common or deep femoral arteries and are easily accessible for surgical repair, which carries a high rate of technical success, very low morbidity, and good long-term patency. Furthermore, use of stent-graft devices in this location is problematic in patients who may require further angiographic and endoluminal procedures. A stent-graft may not accommodate larger introducer sheaths, and pseudoaneurysms may form after each instrumentation. For these reasons, there is currently no good indication for the use of stent-grafts in the treatment of common or deep femoral artery aneurysms.

Distal superficial femoral and popliteal artery aneurysms frequently coexist and are often in continuity with each other. For this reason, we have grouped these two together under popliteal aneurysms. The popliteal artery is the most common site of peripheral aneurysms.[40] The most common etiology is atherosclerosis, with mycotic and traumatic causes being far less prevalent. Unlike aneurysms of the iliac and subclavian arteries, a majority (52–86%) of patients are symptomatic at presentation, usually secondary to thromboembolic ischemia. Rupture and compression of adjacent structures are other rare presentations.[41]

As with other peripheral aneurysms, the natural history of this disease is incompletely understood, and the indications for intervention are thus debatable. In asymptomatic patients with small popliteal aneurysms (<2 cm), the incidence of limb loss and other complications is reported to be low.[42] There is consensus, however, that surgery should be performed on all symptomatic patients because the incidence of limb loss and associated complications are unacceptably high in such patients if treated conservatively. Wychulis et al[43] reported a 31% complication rate in symptomatic patients who were managed without surgery. In the series of 71 popliteal aneurysms in 50 patients reported by Dawson et al,[44] 74% of the patients treated conservatively suffered complications. In contrast, the operative morbidity and mortality in elective popliteal aneurysm repair is as low as 2%. The 10-year cumulative patencies of elective repair range from 66 to 92%.[44,45] Given the available data, it is clear that symptomatic patients should be treated aggressively. In addition, it is now generally accepted that aneurysms larger than 2 cm should also undergo repair.

There is currently insufficient data to allow an evaluation of the role of stent-grafts in the treatment of popliteal artery aneurysms. Based on several theoretical concerns, it appears that the current generation of devices are not a viable alternative to elective surgery. The inherent thrombogenicity of graft materials, combined with the smaller lumen of the popliteal artery, may result in a high occlusion rate. Furthermore, devices would be subject to repetitive trauma owing to traversal of a highly mobile joint and proximity to the skin surface. Despite these disadvantages, some investigators have used stent-grafts to treat popliteal aneurysms with mixed outcomes. Marcade[46] reported the treatment of six popliteal aneurysms using a Cragg Endo-Pro System I. Incomplete distal exclusion led to the recurrence of the aneurysm in one patient. Another patient suffered stent-graft thrombosis 7 months after the initial procedure, requiring placement of an additional stent-graft. The remaining four devices were patent after a mean follow-up period of 5.5 months. Gieskes et al[47] reported on three patients with popliteal aneurysms treated with the use of endoprostheses, which one thrombosed after 15 days. Similarly, one of two patients treated with use

of this polyester-covered nitinol stent occluded after 1 month.[48] There are two other case reports in the literature, both with initial technical success and patencies of up to 6 months.[49,50] A single case of successful treatment of a mycotic femoral artery aneurysm is also reported using a stent covered with autologous vein, with primary patency and no graft infection after 1 year of follow-up.[51]

Given these preliminary results in popliteal artery aneurysms, it is clear that the current generation of stent-grafts should be reserved for unusual circumstances. With continued refinement of endoluminal device design and increasing experience in this location, however, stent-graft repair of popliteal aneurysms may find wider applicability.

■ Conclusion

Review of the collective experience of the investigators cited suggests that the use of stent-grafts in the treatment of certain peripheral aneurysms is safe and effective. In larger-diameter vessels, stent-grafts appear to be a viable alternative to surgery, especially in patients in whom surgery presents an unacceptably high risk. Although endovascular repair of peripheral aneurysms is less invasive and generally safer than surgery, these procedures have their own potential pitfalls and complications. These include perigraft leak, thrombosis, restenosis, distal embolization, kinking, misplacement and migration, branch vessel occlusion, infection, initial technical failure, and unknown long-term durability of stent and graft material. Although this list is long, the reported incidence of complications is very low.

Long-term data on the outcome of patients treated with stent-grafts are needed to clarify the indications for their use before they can be recommended as the treatment of choice in patients with peripheral arterial aneurysms. It is evident, however, that outcome is dependent on the nature of the lesion, the anatomic location, and the type of device used.

REFERENCES

1. Dotter CT. Transluminally-placed coil spring endarterial tube grafts: long term patency in canine popliteal artery. Invest Radiol 1969;4:329–332.
2. Becker GJ, Benenati JF, Zemel G, et al. Percutaneous placement of a balloon-expandable intraluminal graft for life-threatening subclavian arterial hemorrhage. J Vasc Intervent Radiol 1991;2:225–229.
3. Parodi JC, Palmaz JC, Barone HD. Transfemoral intraluminal graft implantation for abdominal aortic aneurysms. Ann Vasc Surg 1991;5:491–499.
4. Brunkwall J, Hauksson H, Bengtsson Bergqvist D, Takolander R, Bergentz SE. Solitary aneurysms of the iliac arterial system: an estimate of their frequency of occurrence. J Vasc Surg 1987;10:381–384.
5. Sacks NP, Huddy SJ, Wegner T, Giddings AE. Management of solitary iliac aneurysms. J Cardiovasc Surg 1992;33:679–683.
6. McCready RA, Pairolero PC, Gilmore JC, Kazmier FJ, Cherry KJ, Hollier LH. Isolated iliac artery aneurysms. Surgery 1983;93:688–693.
7. Richardson JW, Greenfield LJ. Natural history and management of iliac aneurysms. J Vasc Surg 1988;8:165–170.
8. Kasirajan V, Hertzer NR, Beven EG, O'Hara PJ, Krajewski LP, sullivan TM. Management of isolated common iliac artery aneurysms. Cardiovasc Surg 1998;6:171–177.
9. Krupski WC, Selzman CH, Floridia R, Strecker PK, Nehler MR, Whitehill TA. Contemporary management of isolated iliac aneurysms. J Vasc Surg 1998;281:1–13.
10. Razavi MK, Dake MD, Semba CP, Nyman URO, Lidell RP. Percutaneous endoluminal placement of stent-grafts for the treatment of isolated iliac artery aneurysms. Radiology 1995;197:801–804.
11. Marin ML, Veith FJ, Lyon RT, Cynamon J, Sanchez LA. Transfemoral endovascular repair of iliac artery aneurysms. Am J Surg 1995;170:179–182.
12. Cardon JM, Cardon A, Joyeux A, Vical V, Noblet D. Endovascular repair of iliac artery aneurysm with endoprosystem 1: a multicentric French study. J Cardiovasc Surg 1996;37(suppl 1):45–50.
13. Dorros G, Cohn JM, Jaff Mr. Percutaneous endovascular stent graft repair of iliac artery aneurysms. J Endovasc Surg 1997;4:370–375.
14. Gasparini D, Lovaria A, Saccheri S, et al. Percutaneous treatment of iliac aneurysms and pseudoaneurysms with Cragg endopro system 1 stent-grafts. Cardiovasc Intervent Radiol 1997;20:348–352.
15. Quinn SF, Sheley RC, Semonsen KG, Sanchez RB, Hallin RW. Endovascular stents covered with pre-expanded polytetrafluoroethylene for treatment of iliac artery aneurysms and fistulas. J Vasc Intervent Radiol 1997;8:1057–1063.
16. Dorffner R, Thurnher S, Puig S, et al. Treatment of arterial aneurysms of the pelvic leg vessels using Dacron-covered nitinol stents. Fortschr Roentgenstr 1998;168:275–280.
17. Razavi M, Kee S, Slonim S, Semba C, Dake M. Iliac artery aneurysms: stent-grafting techniques. Tech Vasc Intervent Radiol 1998;1:37–41.
18. Ruebben A, Tettoni S, Muratore P, Rossato D, Savio D, Rabbia C. Percutaneous endoluminal bypass of iliac aneurysms with a covered stent. Cardiovasc Intervent Radiol 1998;21:339–342.
19. Nehler MR, Taylor LM, Moneta GL, Porter JM. Upper extremity ischemia from subclavian artery aneurysm caused by bony abnormalities of the thoracic outlet. Arch Surg 1997;132:527–532.
20. Hood DB, Kuehne J, Yellin AE, Weaver FA. Vascular complications of thoracic outlet syndrome. Am Surg 1997;63:913–917.
21. Dougherty MJ, Calligaro KD, Savarese RP, DeLaurentis DA. Atherosclerotic aneurysm of the intrathoracic subclavian artery: a case report and review of the literature. J Vasc Surg 1995;21:521–529.
22. Pairolero PC, Walls JT, Payne S, Hollier LH, Fairbairn JF. Subclavian-axillary artery aneurysms. Surgery 1981;90:757–763.
23. Brzowski BK, Mills JL, Beckett WC. Iatrogenic subclavian artery pseudoaneurysms: case reports. J Trauma 1990;30:616–618.
24. Baldwin RT, Kieta DR, Gallagher MW. Complicated right subclavian artery pseudoaneurysm after central venipuncture. Ann Thorac Surg 1996;62:581–582.
25. Pastores SM, Marin ML, Veith FJ, Bakal CW, Kvetan V. Endovascular stented graft repair of a pseudoaneurysm of the subclavian artery caused by percutaneous internal jugular vein cannulation: case report. Am J Crit Care 1995;4:472–475.
26. Earl GM Jr, Mohr JA, White RH, Stein PD. Subclavian arterial-pulmonary arterial fistula associated with healed cavitary tuberculosis. Am Rev Respir Dis 1972;106:898–903.
27. Egami J, Fujiki T, Sudo K, et al. Aneurysm of a branch of the subclavian artery with multiple arteriovenous fistulae. J Cardiovasc Surg (Torino) 1996;37:355–357.
28. Hyer CE, Cikrit DF, Lalka SG, Sawchuk AP, Dalsing MC. Aggressive management of vascular injuries of the thoracic outlet. J Vasc Surg 1998;27:880–885.

29. George SM, Croce MA, Fabian TC, et al. Cervicothoracic arterial injuries: recommendations for diagnosis and management. World J Surg 1991;15:134–140.

30. Degiannis E, Velmahos G, Krawczykowski D, Levy RD, Souter I, Saadia R. Penetration injuries of the subclavian vessels. Br J Surg 1994;81:524–526.

31. May J, White G, Waugh R, Yu W, Harris J. Transluminal placement of a prosthetic stent-graft device for treatment of subclavian artery aneurysm. J Vasc Surg 1993;18:1056–1059.

32. MacSweeney ST, Holden A, Hartley D, Lawrence-Brown M. Endovascular repair of subclavian artery aneurysm. J Vasc Surg 1996;24:304–305.

33. Patel AV, Marin ML, Vieth FJ, Kerr A, Sanchez LA. Endovascular graft repair of penetration subclavian artery injuries. J Endovasc Surg 1996;3:382–388.

34. Sullivan TM, Bacharach JM, Perl J, Gray B. Endovascular management of unusual aneurysms of the axillary and subclavian arteries. J Endovasc Surg 1996;3:389–395.

35. Meyer T, Merkel S, Lang W. Combined operative and endovascular treatment of a post traumatic embolizing aneurysm of the subclavian artery. J Endovasc Surg 1998;5:52–55.

36. Szeimies U, Kueffer G, Stoeckelhuber B, Steckmeier B. Successful exclusion of subclavian aneurysms with covered nitinol stents. Cardiovasc Intervent Radiol 1998;21:246–249.

37. Ruebben A, Merlo M, Verri A, et al. Combined surgical and endovascular treatment of a traumatic pseudo-aneurysm of the brachiocephalic trunk with anatomical anomaly. J Cardiovasc Surg (Torino) 1997;38:173–176.

38. Babatasi G, Massetti M, Le Page O, Theron J, Khayat A. Endovascular treatment of a traumatic subclavian artery aneurysm. J Trauma 1998;44:545–547.

39. Ackroyd R, Singh S, Beard JD, Gaines PA. Simultaneous brachial embolectomy and endoluminal stenting of a subclavian artery aneurysm. Eur J Vasc Endovasc Surg 1995;10:248–249.

40. Dent TL, Lindenauer SM, Ernst CB, et al. Multiple arteriosclerotic arterial aneurysms. Arch Surg 1972;105:338–341.

41. Vermillion BD, Dimmins SA, Pace WG. A review of one hundred forty-seven popliteal aneurysms with long term follow-up. Surgery 1981;90:1009–1015.

42. Shellack J, Smith RB III, Perdue GD. Nonoperative management of selected popliteal aneurysms. Arch Surg 1987;122:372–378.

43. Wychulis AR, Spittell JA, Wallace RB. Popliteal aneurysms. Surgery 1970;68:942–947.

44. Dawson I, vanBockel JH, Brand R, et al. Popliteal artery aneurysms. Long-term follow-up of aneurysmal disease and results of surgical treatment. J Vasc Surg 1991;13:398–404.

45. Shortell CK, DeWeese JA, Ourial K, et al. Popliteal artery aneurysms: a 25 year surgical experience. J Vasc Surg 1991;14:771–778.

46. Marcade JP. Stent graft for popliteal aneurysms. Six cases with Cragg Endo-Pro System 1 Minitec. J Cardiovasc Surg (Torino) 1996;37(suppl 1):41–44.

47. Gieskes L, Rousseau H, Otal P, et al. Percutaneous treatment of popliteal aneurysms using a covered stent: preliminary clinical experience. J Mal Vasc 1995;20:264–267.

48. Link J, Muller-Hulsbeck S, Brossmann J, Schwarzenberg H, Heller M. The initial results of percutaneous therapy of popliteal aneurysms with stent. Fortschr Roentgenstr 1996;164:244–248.

49. Marin ML, Veith FJ, Panetta TF, et al. Transfemoral endoluminal stented graft repair of a popliteal artery aneurysm. J Vasc Surg 1994;19:754–757.

50. Dorffner R, Winkelbauer F, Kettenbach J, Staudacher M, Lammer J. Successful exclusion of a large femoropopliteal aneurysm with a covered nitinol stent. Cardiovasc Intervent Radiol 1996;19:117–119.

51. Schneider P, Abcarian P, Leduc J, Ogawa D. Stent-graft repair of mycotic superficial femoral artery aneurysm using a Palmaz stent and autologous saphenous vein. Ann Vasc Surg 1998;12:282–285.

9

Stent-Grafts for Peripheral Occlusive Disease

MICHAEL S. ROSENBERG, ABBAS CHAMSUDDIN, AND ANDREW H. CRAGG

Charles Dotter[1] in 1969 proposed placement of tightly wound steel coils to act as endoluminal stents. Since then, the use of endoluminal metallic stents to treat occlusive peripheral vascular disease has become a widespread practice. Stenting achieves a greater lumen diameter than angioplasty and prevents postangioplasty recoil that may contribute to restenosis.

During the evolution of clinical stenting, the occasional need for stents covered with graft material became apparent. In 1984, Cragg et al[2] demonstrated the potential application of a stent-graft–type device using metallic tube grafts (Fig. 9–1). Becker et al[3] placed the first stent-graft in a human in 1991, when they treated a life-threatening injury to the subclavian artery. Stent-grafts were also being developed for aneurysmal disease at this time, and both Volodos et al[4] and Parodi et al[5,6] described in 1991 the application of endoluminal stent-graft technology in the treatment of aortic aneurysms.

In 1993, Marin et al[7] and Cragg and Dake[8] described the use of endovascular stent-grafts in the treatment of arterial occlusive disease in the aortoiliac and femoropopliteal circulation. The first series of patients with life-threatening ischemia caused by multilevel arterial occlusive disease treated with endovascular stent-grafts in combination with standard bypass grafting was published by Marin et al[9] in 1995.

The potential for covered stents became apparent as the limitations of both percutaneous transluminal angioplasty (PTA) and "bare" stents were recognized. For instance, in Becker et al's[10] meta-analysis of 4,304 PTAs for occlusive lesions in the superficial femoral artery (SFA), the 2-year patency rate was 43 to 79%. Adding a stent did little to reduce restenosis in the SFA. Sapoval et al[11] noted a 1-year unassisted patency rate following SFA stenting of 49%. Gray et al[12] reported a 1-year unassisted patency of 22% following stenting of SFA stenoses and occlusions. Covered stents offer the potential to reduce these relatively high rates of restenosis following both stand-alone PTA and PTA-stenting of SFA stenoses and occlusions. Stent-grafts also offer the possibility of improving upon results obtained after PTA in other vascular locations, too.

■ Design of Stent-Grafts for the Treatment of Occlusive Vascular Disease

Different constructions of stents and covering materials have been developed with the intent of preventing neointimal proliferation through the interstices of metal mesh stents. Although many different kinds of stent-graft designs have been described, the majority of devices are distinguished by several principles of design, such as whether the graft material is supported or unsupported by the stent, the type of stent, and the type of graft material.

The basic design concept for an *unsupported* endoluminal stent-graft calls for placement of a stent at one or both ends of a segment of conventional surgical bypass graft conduit that has been delivered into the vascular lumen. The stents can be either balloon-expandable or self-expanding and are typically sutured to the graft, where they act as anchors for the remainder of the graft conduit that is not stent-supported. Stent-grafts for treatment of long segments of occlusive disease can be easily constructed using this design simply by using longer

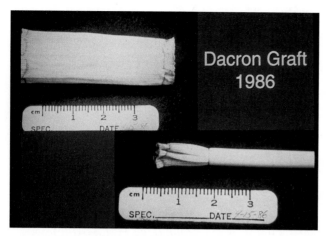

FIGURE 9–1. Early endovascular graft prototype. The basic design of expandable stent-grafts consists of an expandable metallic stent framework covered by conventional polyester graft material.

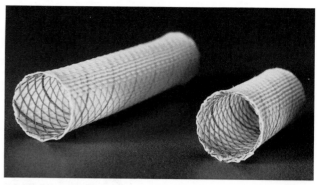

FIGURE 9–2. The Wallgraft endoprosthesis is an example of a fully supported endoskeleton stent-graft. [Courtesy of Schneider (USA) Inc.]

graft conduit segments. Usually, expanded polytetrafluoroethylene (ePTFE) has been used as the graft material for treatment of aortoiliac and femoropopliteal occlusive disease with unsupported endoluminal stent-grafts.[7–9] One limitation of any unsupported stent-graft, however, is the need for a specialized delivery system because the stent-graft has little longitudinal strength ("column strength"). Any attempt to push an unsupported stent-graft in the standard fashion through a delivery sheath will likely kink, collapse, and foreshorten the stent-graft appreciably. If delivery has been successfully achieved, the unsupported segment may be prone to other adverse mechanical forces. Luminal narrowing may be seen immediately after deployment or may develop over time owing to radial compression by the surrounding blood vessel, trapped blood, or subgraft neointima.

Fully supported stent-grafts rely on the presence of a stent throughout the entire length of the graft. This makes the graft less prone to kinking, foreshortening, and external compression. This design also requires a less complicated delivery mechanism because the metallic stent "skeleton" supports the stent-graft as it is delivered into position. The stent framework can be on the inner luminal surface of the graft (endoskeleton) (Fig. 9–2), on the outer surface of the graft (exoskeleton) (Fig. 9–3), or incorporated into the graft material without any exposed stent at all. Advantages of an endoskeleton include a potentially simpler manufacturing process and a more secure fixation of the graft to the stent.[13] A potential disadvantage of designs that place the stent on the inner surface of the graft is that the stent-graft has a significant amount of metal in contact at the flow surface. A metal endoskeleton of this type leads to stent-associated neointimal proliferation within the stent-graft lumen in animal investigation.[14] Designs that utilize an

external stent framework (exoskeleton) or a design that incorporate the stent into the graft material so that no stent is exposed on the inside or outside of the stent-graft can potentially avoid this problem.

Because there were no suitable devices available when stent-grafts were first considered for use in occlusive vascular disease, all of the early experience was obtained with home-made designs. Most of these devices combined commercially available stents with commercially available vascular graft conduit. The Wallstent has been fashioned into a stent-graft for treatment of a variety of conditions.[15] Many authors have described incorporation of the Palmaz stent into a stent-graft. The Palmaz stent has also been used as an anchoring device for unsupported polytetrafluoroethylene tube grafts.[7,9,16] Covered Gianturco-Rosch Z stents (Cook, Inc., Bloomington, IN) have also been reported in the treatment of aneurysmal disease of the iliac artery,[17] but there is little information regarding this type of stent-graft for treatment of peripheral occlusive disease.

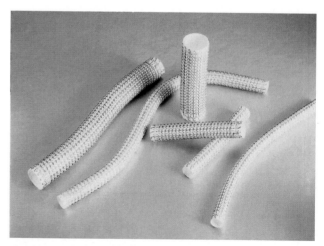

FIGURE 9–3. The Hemobahn endovascular prosthesis is an example of a fully supported exoskeleton stent-graft. (Courtesy of W.L. Gore & Associates, Inc.)

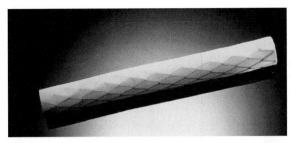

FIGURE 9–4. The Cragg EndoPro System 1 is an example of a fully supported endoskeleton stent-graft. Although not commercially available in the United States, it has widespread use in Europe. It is made of nitinol wire with low-porosity polyester graft.

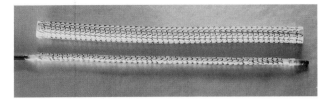

FIGURE 9–6. The Hemobahn endovascular prosthesis in restrained and fully deployed states. (Courtesy of W.L. Gore & Associates, Inc.)

Different graft materials have been used to produce stent-grafts for occlusive disease, including ePTFE, polyethylene terephthalate (PET), and polyurethanes such as Corethane. Although there are no commercially produced stent-grafts currently available in the United States for treatment of peripheral vascular disease, the Cragg EndoPro System 1 (Fig. 9–4) or Passager stent-graft is available outside the United States. This design utilizes a flexible, self-expanding stent-like prosthesis made of nitinol wire to afford the endoskeleton a fully supported stent-graft. Nitinol is a biocompatible nonmagnetic alloy of nickel and titanium that has the property of shape memory (the ability to recover its initial diameter and shape). This stent-graft is covered with woven PET of low porosity.

There are ongoing U.S. clinical trials evaluating the Wallgraft endoprosthesis (Fig. 9–5) (Schneider, Minneapolis, MN) and the Hemobahn (Fig. 9–6) endovascular prosthesis (W.L. Gore and Assoc., Flagstaff, AZ). The Wallgraft endoprosthesis is based on the self-expanding braided wire Wallstent composed of Elgiloy, a supermetal alloy. This stent-graft is fully supported and uses the stent as an endoskeleton that is covered with PET.

The Hemobahn endovascular prosthesis combines a self-expanding nitinol exoskeleton stent with an ultrathin ePTFE graft on the inner surface. It is constrained on a delivery catheter that uses a rip-cord system for releasing the stent-graft.

The Corvita endoluminal graft is another commercially produced stent-graft that initially entered clinical trials in the United States and Europe. This stent-graft consists of a self-expanding exoskeleton wire stent that is treated in a unique process that applies layers of Corethane predominantly on the luminal side of the stent. Corethane, a member of the broad group of polyurethane elastomers, is believed to be more resistant to biological conditions than most other polyurethanes that have been studied in the past.

Other stent-grafts are being designed. An ePTFE stent-graft currently in development by Impra/Bard uses a process of encapsulating a nitinol stent within the graft material. This design reduces the direct influence of the stent upon ultimate healing of the device and may limit neointimal hyperplasia within the stent-graft lumen. The encapsulation process also allows for ePTFEs of different design to be incorporated into the final stent-graft. This, too, may have an effect upon stent-graft healing and incorporation into the arterial wall.

■ Stent-Grafts for Femoropopliteal Arterial Occlusive Disease

PTA, alone, is still a very successful and durable method for percutaneous revascularization of atherosclerotic occlusive disease in the femoropopliteal system. In general, patients with short stenoses or occlusions, particularly in large vessels (≥6-mm diameter) do well. It is established, however, that patency following PTA for long lesions is worse than for short ones. For example, SFA lesions longer than 10 cm have a restenosis/occlusion rate as high as 80% at 5 years.[18,19]

As noted earlier, the use of stents for femoropopliteal occlusive disease does not appear to reduce the restenosis rate. A number of factors may contribute to the failure of stents in this location, such as the long lesion length and the small arterial diameters in the stented SFA segments.

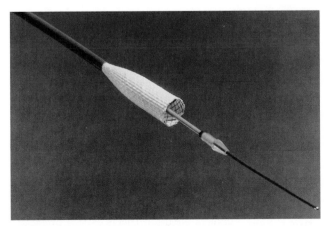

FIGURE 9–5. A partially deployed Wallgraft endoprosthesis. [Courtesy of Schneider (USA) Inc.]

In addition, the superficial location of the SFA may result in exposure of the stented segment to repeated extrinsic compression and stent deformity that may, in turn, lead to a greater tendency for restenosis. For whatever reasons, stenting of the femoropopliteal segment has a very high rate of restenosis related to neointimal ingrowth through the interstices of the stent.

Early investigation into SFA stent-graft placement for occlusive disease was provocative. In 1994, Cragg[20] presented a cohort of 12 patients treated with ePTFE stent-graft for femoropopliteal occlusive disease. The device was constructed as an unsupported stent-graft with anchoring stents attached to both ends of a segment of ePTFE conduit. Favorable clinical response was seen in 10 patients. With a mean follow up of 1 year, nine stent-grafts were patent.

Henry et al[22] reported a series of patients with symptomatic peripheral vascular disease treated with the Cragg EndoPro System 1 stent-graft implanted in the iliac, femoral, and popliteal artery[21,22] (Fig. 9–7). With a follow-up of 18 months, primary patency at the femoral level was 59% and secondary patency was 81%. At the 1999 Eleventh Annual International Symposium on Endovascular Therapy, Henry and Amor[23] presented 5-year follow-up data. The primary patency rate was 64% at the femoral level with a secondary patency of 73%. It was noted that primary patency at the femoral level was not significantly different for lesions shorter or longer than

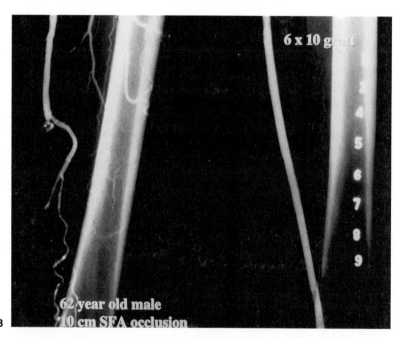

A, B

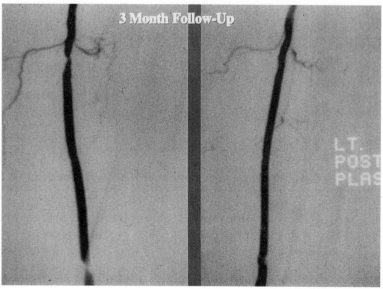

C, D

FIGURE 9–7. Treatment of a superficial femoral artery occlusion using the Cragg EndoPro System 1. (**A** and **B**). A 10-cm occlusion of the superficial femoral artery (SFA) treated by placement of a stent-graft. (**C**). At 3 months, the patient returned with focal stenoses at the proximal and distal ends of the graft. This is usually owing to intimal hyperplasia at the stent-graft margins. (**D**). Angioplasty was used to assist patency.

15 cm; however, secondary patency rates were better for shorter lesions than for longer ones (93% vs. 73%). Popliteal patency rates were low, with primary patency of 33% and secondary patency of 50%.

Henry and Amor[23] also reported data from the Corvita endoluminal graft iliac and femoropopliteal trial. A total of 75 stent-grafts were implanted in 64 patients for aneurysmal and occlusive disease; 20 occlusions and 27 stenoses were treated with 100% immediate technical success but with six early thromboses, three at the femoral level (all were long lesions) and one at the popliteal level (following treatment of an aneurysm). In addition, three late thromboses were encountered, of which two were at the femoral level. At a maximum 30-month follow-up for all patients (mean 18.6 ± 6.7 months) there were four restenoses—two iliac, one femoral, and one popliteal.

Henry and Amor[23] also reported results of a multicenter feasibility study investigating the Hemobahn endovascular prosthesis for occlusive disease (Fig. 9–8). This study was performed at three sites in the United States and at 12 European centers. A total of 100 lesions were treated in 93 patients, including 58 iliac and 42 femoral sites. There was a 99% primary technical success for all 100 lesions. Primary femoral patency rates were 100, 91, and 80% at 1, 3, and 6 months, respectively. The Hemobahn endovascular prosthesis is currently in the midst of phase II clinical trials in the United States. This trial involves a maximum of 25 centers, which have per-

formed approximately 400 implants in lesions up to 13 cm in length. It will be interesting to see whether the primary patency rates will mirror those that have been reported in the preliminary European and U.S. trials. If so, the Hemobahn endovascular prosthesis may usher in a new era for percutaneous treatment of occlusive atherosclerotic disease in the SFA.

■ Stent-Grafts for Iliac Artery Occlusive Disease

Application of stent-grafts for iliac artery occlusive disease is a controversial topic. In Becker et al's[10] meta-analysis of 2,697 iliac artery angioplasties, PTA, alone, had a technical success of 92% and a mean 5-year patency of 72% (range 50–87%). Although this suggests that angioplasty may suffice for most iliac artery lesions, the reality is that many of these iliac angioplasties were performed for focal stenosis or limited occlusion, where PTA works well. Current use of stents has encouraged treatment of more complex iliac stenoses and occlusions, where PTA has a higher technical failure rate and lower patency. Bosch and Hunink's[24] meta-analysis of iliac artery PTA and stenting confirmed that stents improved upon the technical success of iliac PTA and offers better long-term patency than PTA alone. In their analysis of over 2,000 patients who had undergone either PTA without or with stent placement, technical suc-

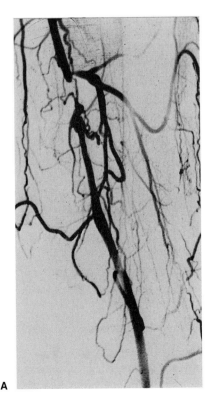
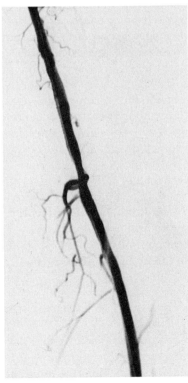

FIGURE 9–8. Treatment of an SFA occlusion using the Hemobahn endovascular prosthesis. (**A**). Initial angiogram reveals complete occlusion of the distal SFA with collateral formation. (**B**). Result after placement of a Hemobahn endovascular prosthesis. (Courtesy of W.L. Gore & Associates, Inc.)

A   B

cess for PTA was 91%; for PTA with stenting the technical success increased to 96% (p <.05). The risk of long-term failure at 4 years was reduced by 43% following stent placement.

Given these data, some may argue that stents have improved upon iliac PTA so that there is no need for further advance. Others view Bosch and Hunink's work differently and believe that stents are just another step along the way to more durable adjuncts for iliac artery PTA. There are data in Bosch and Hunink's meta-analysis that suggest that long-term durability can be improved. The 4-year primary patency for stents on an "intent-to-treat" basis was 72%, which was only 15% better than the 4-year result for PTA. Whether the solution for long-term patency is a stent-graft, however, is an issue that is currently being explored.

In 1995, Pernes et al[25] published a series of 10 patients treated for long iliac artery stenosis using the Cragg EndoPro System 1, a PET-covered nitinol stent-graft. There was no residual postprocedure stenosis, even when the stenotic arterial lesions were densely calcified. Although primary patency of 80% at 6 months was similar to patency for uncovered stents placed in short iliac stenoses (91% patency),[24] this study substantiated the feasibility of stent-graft placement for iliac artery occlusive disease.

Henry et al[21,22] also used the Cragg EndoPro System 1 to treat occlusive iliac artery disease. There was virtually no residual stenosis (0.5% ±3%) after stent-graft implantation (pooled iliac and femoral arterial lesions). At 18 months, primary patency in the iliac artery was 97% and secondary patency was 100%. Five-year follow-up data, presented at the 1999 Eleventh Annual International Symposium on Endovascular Therapy, cited primary iliac artery patency of 92% and secondary patency of 100%.[23] Unfortunately, the Cragg EndoPro System 1 is not available in the United States.

The Hemobahn endovascular prosthesis has been studied in the iliac artery in both the United States and European phase I clinical trials.[23] A total of 58 iliac arteries were treated, with primary and secondary iliac patency rates of 96% at 6 months. Although these data are encouraging, the current U.S. clinical trial of the Hemobahn is focused on the SFA, and we may not see further data regarding iliac artery use for a while.

Krajcer et al[26] presented 3-month follow-up data from a multicenter randomized study comparing the Wallgraft endoprosthesis and the Wallstent for treatment of complex iliac artery lesions. These lesions were defined as those that are greater than 3 cm in length, calcified, eccentric, or totally occluded. A total of 161 iliac lesions were treated in 196 patients over a 16-month period with 83 Wallgrafts and 78 Wallstents. Results demonstrated no significant difference between the two treatment groups with regard to immediate and secondary success (98 and 99%, respectively), rate of major complications,

percent claudication-free, or percent increase in ankle-brachial index. It was concluded that there was equivalent safety and efficacy; however, more patients and longer follow-up are required to make a full statistical comparison of the restenosis rates for the Wallgraft compared with the Wallstent. The Wallgraft endoprosthesis is currently in a phase II clinical trial that involves 20 centers. More than two-thirds of the 300 patients have been enrolled.

Complications of peripheral stent-graft placement include hematoma, pseudoaneurysm, puncture site thrombosis, early graft thrombosis, graft misplacement, distal embolization, pain, and fever.[13,22] The development of pain and fever postdeployment of stent-grafts represents an interesting finding that has been described by many authors in both animal studies and clinical trials, and is typically seen with PET-covered stent-grafts.[13,14,21,22,27] Typically, patients develop fever, leukocytosis, and elevation of C-reactive protein levels. Pain is usually present in the region of the implant and can last for 2 to 3 weeks. This postimplantation syndrome has been studied using ultrasound, magnetic resonance imaging, and computed tomography, in addition to laboratory analyses of blood. In all reported cases, the process appears to be inflammation, not infection. Although the cause of this phenomenon remains unclear, treatment, for the most part, has been administration of nonsteroidal antiinflammatory medications.

In animal models, one of the most severe inflammatory stent-graft–related responses has been caused by heparin-coated PET-covered stent-grafts. Magnetic resonance images demonstrated contrast enhancement and edema of the implanted arterial segment. Macroscopic examination showed marked vascular wall thickening and adventitial adhesions. Microscopic examination showed a pronounced giant cell foreign-body inflammatory response. In comparison, there was a moderate inflammatory response to the plain PET-covered stent-grafts (no heparin coating) and almost no response to noncovered stents.[27]

While the postimplantation syndrome associated with PET stent-grafts is of some concern, it is limited in duration to several weeks and does not seem to recur. Furthermore, there have not been any permanent sequelae associated with this syndrome in the peripheral arterial system. Aside from the fear of infection and the cost of any tests associated with this syndrome, it seems to be of little consequence in the long term.

■ Future Directions

The Cragg EndoPro System 1 is being used at many centers in Europe. In the United States, two stent-graft designs for use in occlusive peripheral vascular disease are on the horizon: the Wallgraft endoprosthesis and the Hemobahn endovascular prosthesis. Both stent-grafts are well under way in clinical trials in the United States, the Wallgraft for iliac artery disease and the Hemobahn for SFA lesions.

Although stent-grafts represent potentially important advances in the treatment of occlusive peripheral vascular disease, it is important to remember that these devices represent first-generation technology. Our current concept of stent-grafts for occlusive disease will likely be challenged by newer designs with smaller delivery systems. Along the way, some devices will not meet the clinical challenge. For instance, the Corvita endoluminal graft has been withdrawn from clinical trial owing to the discovery of an unacceptably high thrombosis rate. Although preliminary results from clinical trials of other stent-grafts are encouraging, the ultimate performance of the Wallgraft, the Hemobahn, or any other stent-graft designed for treating peripheral occlusive disease must await completion of controlled clinical trials, with ultimate confirmation of efficacy through continued clinical use.

REFERENCES

1. Dotter C. Transluminally-placed coilspring endarterial tube grafts: long term patency in canine popliteal artery. Invest Radiol 1969;4: 329–332.
2. Cragg A, Lund G, Rysavy J, Salomonowitz E, Castaneda-Zuniga W, Amplatz K. Percutaneous arterial grafting. Radiology 1984;150: 45–49.
3. Becker GJ, Benenati JF, Zemel G, et al. Percutaneous placement of a balloon-expandable intraluminal graft for life threatening subclavian arterial hemorrhage. J Vasc Intervent Radiol 1991;2:225–229.
4. Volodos NL, Karpovich IP, Troyan VI, et al. Clinical experience of the use of self-fixing synthetic prostheses for remote endoprosthetics of the thoracic and the abdominal aorta and iliac arteries through the femoral artery and as intraoperative endoprosthesis for aorta reconstruction. Vasa Suppl 1991;33:93–95.
5. Parodi JC, Palmaz JC, Barone HD. Transfemoral intraluminal graft implantation for abdominal aortic aneurysms. Ann Vasc Surg 1991;5:494–499.
6. Parodi JC. Endovascular repair of abdominal aortic aneurysms and other arterial lesions. J Vasc Surg 1995;21:549–557.
7. Marin ML, Veith FJ, Panetta TF, et al. Transfemoral stented graft treatment of occlusive arterial disease for limb salvage: a preliminary report. Circulation 1993;88:1–11.
8. Cragg AH, Dake MD. Percutaneous femoropopliteal graft placement. J Vasc Intervent Radiol 1993;4:455–463.
9. Marin ML, Veith FJ, Sancehz LA, et al. Endovascular aortoiliac grafts in combination with standard infrainguinal arterial bypasses in the management of limb-threatening ischemia: preliminary report. J Vasc Surg 1995;22:316–325.
10. Becker GJ, Katzen BT, Dake MD. Noncoronary angioplasty. Radiology 1989;170:921–940.
11. Sapoval MR, Long AL, Raynaud AC, Beyssen BM, Fiessinger J-N, Gaux J-C. Femoropopliteal stent placement: long-term results. Radiology 1992;184:833–839.
12. Gray BH, Sullivan TM, Childs MB, Young JR, Olin JW. High incidence of restenosis/reocclusion of stents in the percutaneous treatment of long-segment superfirial femoral artery disease after suboptimal angioplasty. J Vasc Surg 1997;25:74–83.
13. Cragg A, Dake M. Treatment of peripheral vascular disease with stent-grafts. Radiology 1997; 205:307–314.
14. Dolmatch BL, Dong YH, Trerotola SO, Hunter DW, Brennecke LH, Labounty R. Tissue response to covered Wallstents. J Vasc Intervent Radiol 1998;9(3):471–478.
15. Kato N, Sze DY, Semba CP, Razavi MK, Kee ST, Dake MD. Custommade stent-graft of polytetrafluoroethylene-covered Wallstents: technique and applications. J Vasc Intervent Radiol 1999;10:9–16.
16. Sanchez LA, Marin ML, Veith FJ, et al. Placement of endovascular stented grafts via remote acces sites: a new approach to the treatment of failed aortoiliofemoral reconstructions. Ann Vasc Surg 1995;9:1–8.
17. Razavi MK, Kee ST, Slonim SM, Semba CP, Dake MD. Iliac artery aneurysms: stent-grafting techniques. Tech Vasc Intervent Radiol 1998;1(1):37–41.
18. Murray RR, Hewes RC, White RL, et al. Long segment femoropopliteal disease: is angioplasty a boon or bust? Radiology 1987; 162:473–476.
19. Capek P, Mclean GK, Berkowitz HD. Femoropopliteal angioplasty: factors influencing long-term results. Circulation 1991;83(suppl 2):170–180.
20. Cragg AH. Percutaneous femoropopliteal graft placement. Paper presented at the 19th Annual Meeting of the Society of Cardiovascular and Interventional Radiology, San Diego, March 1994.
21. Henry M, Amor M, Ethevenot G, et al. Initial experience with the Cragg EndoPro System 1 for intraluminal treatment of peripheral vascular disease. J Endovasc Surg 1994;1:31–43.
22. Henry M, Amor M, Cragg A, et al. Occlusive and aneurysmal peripheral arterial disease: assessment of a stent-graft system. Radiology 1996;201(3):717–724.
23. Henry M, Amor M. Covered stents. Paper presented at the Eleventh Annual International Symposium on Endovascular Therapy, January 1999, Miami, FL.
24. Bosch JL, Hunink MGM. Meta-analysis of the results of percutaneous transluminal angioplasty and stent placement for aortoiliac occlusive disease. Radiology 1997;204:87–96.
25. Pernes JM Auguste M, Hovasse D, Gignier P, Lasry B, Lasry JL. Long iliac stenosis: initial clinical experience with the Cragg endoluminal graft. Radiology 1995;196:67–71.
26. Krajcer Z, Zaqqa M, Diethrich E, Ansel G, Lipman J, Murphy T. Wallgraft versus Wallstent endoprosthesis for treatment of complex stenotic arterial lesions: three months follow-up of a multicenter, randomized study. Paper presented at the 48th Annual American College of Cardiology, March 1999, New Orleans, LA.
27. Schurmann K, Vorwerk D, Bucker A, et al. Perigraft inflammation due to Dacron-covered stent-grafts in sheep iliac arteries: correlation of MR imaging and histopathologic findings. Radiology 1997;204(3):757–763.

10

Stent-Grafts for Coronary Occlusive Disease

ROBERT S. SCHWARTZ

The intracoronary stent is an indispensable part of the interventional coronary practice. Stents have proven value for two important clinical applications: as bailout for failed angioplasty, and for long-term effects on decreasing restenosis.[1-5] Restenosis rates, using current third-generation devices in straightforward lesions, are now less than 10%. Advances in stenting have had a remarkable effect on the safety and efficacy of clinical practice. Now that stents are easily deployed, and have shown substantive clinical impact, what does the future hold for stenting? Answers to this question center on several remaining problems with current stent technology and interaction with the biology of coronary arteries.

■ Stent Efficacy Is Purely Mechanical

The efficacy of modern stents arises solely from their mechanical scaffolding abilities. The artery at risk of acute closure typically promotes thrombosis for mechanical reasons, including flow disturbances from plaque disruption or intimal dissection. The stent mechanically seals this region, compressing residual plaque and flaps, and creating a smoother surface for improved rheology. The stent creates large initial lumina and limits recoil.[6-10] These long-term effects on restenosis are mediated by the larger postangioplasty lumen, permitting more neointimal ingrowth long-term and a larger long-term lumen. The stent also limits vascular remodeling by its scaffolding effects. This late lumen efficacy is generally smaller than widely thought. In the STRESS and BENESTENT trials, angiographic binary restenosis rates were lowered from 32 to 22% and 41 to 32%, respec-

tively.[11,12] However, the absolute differences in lumen size between stent and balloon angioplasty groups were minuscule, respectively only 0.18 and 0.09 mm. These numbers are put into perspective by considering that a human hair is about 0.08 mm in diameter. The minute differences between stented and control groups indicate that the effects may have been due to factors other than lumen size alone.

Importantly, patients and lesions were highly selected in these trials; in non-STRESS/non-BENESTENT lesions (small vessels, vein grafts, ostial lesions, and those with thrombus) the binary restenosis rates remain at 40% or more even when stented.[2,13] To summarize, the stent reduces restenosis by mechanical means only and possesses no inherent biological activity. It does not inhibit neointimal thickening, and indeed it actually enhances neointimal hyperplasia[14-16] compared to balloon angioplasty.

■ Stent Thrombosis Remains a Problem

Recent application of newer pharmacological regimens has dramatically reduced the incidence of stent thrombosis. Using standard coumadin and aspirin anticoagulation, the BENESTENT trial found a subacute closure rate of 3.5% for the stent group and 2.7% in the percutaneous transluminal coronary angioplasty (PTCA) group.[12] The need for anticoagulation required an 8.5-day stay in hospital for the stented group. Similarly, the STRESS study found subacute stent closure in 3.4% of stented group compared to 1.5% of the PTCA group.[11] These studies were reported prior to the demonstration that high pressure inflation to attain full stent deployment could limit stent thrombosis.[17] However, stent thrombosis remains a concern in diabetes, in small arteries, and in bailout after failed angioplasty. There is also concern about stent thrombosis in cases of preexisting coronary artery thrombus as occurs in acute myocardial infarction or unstable angina.[18,19] Ticlopidine has recently emerged as an antiplatelet adjunct to aspirin for limiting subacute stent thrombosis. Schomig et al[20] reported an important, randomized trial of aspirin/ticlopidine compared to aspirin/coumadin in 517 patients undergoing coronary stenting. These authors found stent occlusion in 5.4% of the coumadin/aspirin group compared to 0.8% in the ticlopidine/aspirin group. Yet even an acute closure rate of 0.8% may be too high, since placement of 800,000 stents annually in the world would still result in over 6,000 acute closures. This number remains too high considering that stent closure is a catastrophic event for all patients in whom it occurs.

■ Potential Solution: The Stent-Graft

The typical metallic coronary stent covers between 13 and 20% of the coronary artery surface. If a stent were made of a biocompatible material, and this material made to cover the stent fully, a stent-graft would result. A typical such configuration is shown in Fig. 10–1. The purposes of such devices are several. The underlying atherosclerotic coronary artery disease can be completely covered by such a device. If placed over a site of ruptured vulnerable plaque, it is easy to see that such a thrombogenic surface could be covered completely by a solid stent-graft. The material of such a graft should be antithrombogenic and simultaneously antineointimal. This likely will require biological activity of the stent, either the form of pharmacological or genetic modification of the local stent environment.

Pharmacological means to effectively limit neointima remain unknown, although several candidates are being considered.[21,22] Restenosis from neointima is intimately related to mural thrombus and to cell accumulation at the injury site by migration and proliferation.[23–26] Anticoagulant strategies to limit acute closure may thus have efficacy against neointimal hyperplasia as well, if such agents can be released over time to limit chronic thrombotic deposition.

Other strategies will involve antiproliferative effects to limit neointimal growth. Several strategies are under active investigation. Clinical trials have begun with a beta-emitting radioactive stents using the isotope [32]P.[27] The short (14-day) half-life of this agent, and its excellent safety profile make it clinically practical. Efficacy studies are pending.

Additional strategies are pharmacologically based, and include the use of physiological molecules such as nitric oxide.[28–32] This strategy seeks to restore arterial homeostasis to limit neointima. Other pharmacological treatments involve limiting neointimal growth by steroids or toxins. Gene therapy is also rapidly advancing in vascular biology.[33–35] Deoxyribonucleic acid (DNA) delivery for gene therapy by stent is under active investigation by a number of groups. These strategies are similarly antiproliferative, aimed at cycle specific events in actively proliferating cells.

■ Solutions to Stent Thrombosis: Anticoagulant Coatings

Stents must also have potent anticoagulant properties and be able to deliver this therapy locally. It is highly inefficient and potentially dangerous to anticoagulate the entire 5-L blood volume of a patient when only 15 mm of coronary artery is at immediate thrombosis risk. A logical solution is to add local anticoagulant to the stent surface. This has been implemented in the form of heparin coatings, but others are under consideration such as glycoprotein (Gp) IIb/IIIa receptor blockade.[36–38] The stent should be more than nonthrombogenic; because it will be placed in regions of active thrombotic potential, it should be antithrombogenic. This feature, in conjunction with local activity, would permit conversion of a highly thrombotic coronary artery segment into a smooth, anticoagulant surface, with obvious clinical benefit. Heparin in its current use is a poor antiplatelet agent, and will likely be surpassed by other, more potent antiplatelet agents.

■ Stent-Graft Material: Polymers

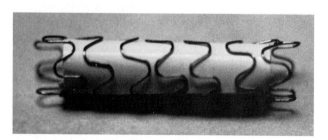

FIGURE 10–1. Configuration of a prototype stent-graft. The device consists of a metallic backbone and a polymer covering. In this prototype, the polymer is polypropylene, and has been placed inside the stent. Other configurations have the metal structure embedded within the polymer to conserve profile.

In consideration of coronary stent-grafts, it is important to understand several issues regarding materials. Intracoronary stents in current use include both balloon expandable and self-expanding designs, all of which are metal. These metals are generally spring-tempered stainless steel, nitinol, or elemental tantalum. The physical and mechanical properties of metals make these stents easily deployable using common PTCA techniques. Excellent radial strength results from both designs in their expanded configuration. The documented ease of deployment, coupled with acceptable tissue biocompatibility, represents the initial engineering solution to stent design. Indeed, such designs originated with Dotter's early work in 1969, and current devices have not changed conceptually in the 30 years since this early work.

Recent advances in biomaterials technology permit consideration of alternative, nonmetallic intracoronary stents. Such devices may allow improved physiological and clinical results. Because device design typically proceeds through many iterations, it is likely that current metal designs will be considerably modified to overcome current limitations, and additional applications may develop. Current designs likely represent an early phase in an evolutionary course of improved stent designs.

Polymers for Coronary Stent-Grafts

Other chapters of this book discuss materials related to arterial stenting in the periphery. Since polymers are a likely material of the stent-graft, and it is unclear whether the same considerations apply to the coronary arteries, a brief discussion of polymers in the coronary arteries is worthwhile.

Polymers by definition contain many repeating structural subunits.[39,40] They have many medical, industrial, and commercial applications. The chemical industry has synthesized thousands of polymers. Selection of potentially useful polymers for an intracoronary stent draws upon much industrial research and development. Most polymers were initially developed for industrial purposes, owing to the large costs associated with new polymer research and development, and were later found to be useful in biomedical applications.

The biological behavior of a polymer depends on the repeating subunit configurations, the conformations of the polymerized molecule, and the inter- and intramolecular bonding forces. Polymers frequently exist in forms in which polymerized chains of many different lengths make up the macroscopic material. Its properties can be influenced by the range and shape of the molecular weight distribution. Low molecular weight portions arise from short chains and usually are waxy or liquid. Additives and reaction residues also contribute to the low molecular weight content of polymers. The higher molecular weight portions arise from long chains, and usually are harder and less flexible.

Polymeric blood compatibility is dominated by the outermost molecular layers in blood contact. The polymer surface is thus critical for blood contact applications. In some polymers, surface characteristics are quite different from those of the bulk polymer just a few molecular layers deeper. Agents used to synthesize the polymer or give it desirable physical features such as flexibility (plasticizing agents) frequently migrate to the polymer surface, resulting in altered biocompatibility. Much study is thus concentrating on polymer surface properties and their modification. Certain additives incorporated during polymer synthesis result in novel, potentially beneficial biological surface properties. These additives are called surface modifying additive (SMA) substances. SMA substances migrate to the polymer surface after synthesis, and may provide a useful compromise between desirable surface and bulk polymer properties. The polymeric intracoronary stent will need suitable bulk properties for practical intracoronary delivery. It will also require excellent surface properties to prevent thrombosis and to avoid stimulation of neointimal hyperplasia. Surface modifying technology may be helpful in satisfying both of these needs.

Typical polymers used for biomedical devices today exhibit good tissue compatibility (Table 10–1). They also provide adequate mechanical strength. These polymers are biostable, and do not degrade significantly over time within the body. They also cannot deliver drugs easily. While they are termed biocompatible, they are somewhat thrombogenic.

Thrombosis and coagulation are powerful survival mechanisms in all higher animal species. Blood normally clots only at sites of vascular injury, yet remains fluid elsewhere in the body. Endothelial cells, continuous throughout the vascular tree, are critical for regulating the delicate balance between fluid and clotted blood. The endothelium as described by Virchow was historically considered an inert cell layer. He postulated that endothelial violation exposed thrombogenic subintima, activating protective clotting mechanisms. He viewed the endothelium as a passive protective lining. Recent evidence reveals the endothelial cell is far from inert. It synthesizes a variety of antithrombotic substances including von Willebrand factor, tissue-type plasminogen activator (t-PA), urokinase, prostacyclin, and thrombomodulin, which collectively enable low local thrombogenic potential. The normal homeostatic coagulation milieu may thus be a highly active equilibrium process modulated by endothelium. Endothelial surfaces continually neutralize thrombin and lyse fibrin.

TABLE 10–1. Polymers with Potential Use in Stent Grafts

Polyethylene
Polytetrafluoroethylene (PTFE; Teflon, Goretex)
Polypropylene (Prolene)
Polyethylene terephthalate (Dacron, Mylar)
Polyurethane (Tecothane, Tecoflex)

This finding has significant impact for polymeric stents within arteries. Foreign surfaces may be recognized as such by blood if key substances are not actively elaborated. A nonthrombogenic man-made material may not be possible, at least in passive form. Some investigators have considered seeding foreign arterial implants with endothelial cells to help overcome problems of passive material surfaces.

An understanding of coagulation is critical to polymeric intracoronary stent design. Studies of foreign surface/blood interfaces indicate the importance of surface electric charge, thermodynamic surface energy and chemistry, and surface texture. These studies may have oversimplified the interactions. For example, it was thought that materials with net negative surface charge (negative electrochemical potentials) are highly blood compatible. After rigorous testing, however, this hypothesis may be an erroneous simplification. There are no simple rules governing interactions between blood and foreign materials.

The interaction between blood and polymers is initiated by the attachment of plasma proteins. Such proteins are usually fibrinogen and fibrin, constituting a *conditioning film*. This film initiates a second phase of biological interaction, platelet adhesion, and aggregation. Complement activation by C3 and C5 also occurs early in foreign material–blood interactions. Following platelet adhesion and aggregation, activation of the extrinsic clotting system by damaged tissue completes the clotting process.[41,42]

Polymeric blood compatibility relates to which specific plasma proteins deposit on the implanted material. Many passive foreign surfaces become albumin coated (as in some artificial organs), which may be beneficial. Fibrin may attach to those foreign bodies that are less blood compatible. Currently, many problems remain; there is no truly blood compatible foreign material.

An important distinction should be made between materials that are *blood compatible* and those that are *biocompatible* (soft tissue compatible). Materials that are blood compatible are biocompatible, but the converse is not always true since blood compatibility requirements are much more stringent. Little is known about blood compatibility of many polymers, and no universally accepted evaluation standards exist.

Useful Polymer Characteristics— Bioabsorbability and Drug Elution

The coronary stent-graft may be made from biostable polymers such as polypropylene. Vascular sutures made of polypropylene remain intact for many years. Theoretical advantages of an intracoronary stent made from such biostable materials are uncertain; one improvement might be lower thrombogenicity. An alternative approach to biostable materials is a bioabsorbable stent-graft, remaining intact for a predetermined time and gradually dissolving. The bioabsorbable polymers generally disintegrate by chemical hydrolysis. Three hydrolytic mechanisms are known. First, long-chain polymers connected by hydrolyzable cross-linkages separate when the cross-links are hydrolyzed. Second, other polymers are water insoluble, but easily hydrolyze to soluble products, which may be carried away by body fluids. These solubilization products are frequently large molecules, not easily eliminated via the kidney or liver. Polymers used systemically that erode via this mechanism are problematic. They are thus used principally in topical applications. Third, insoluble polymers with labile backbones split through hydrolysis of that backbone. The resulting products are low molecular weight and water soluble, making these polymers most suitable for systemic uses. many polymers erode through combinations of hydrolytic mechanisms.

Polymer degradation has two types of macroscopic behavior, homogeneous and heterogeneous. Heterogeneous degradation occurs at the polymer surface only. Gross structural integrity of the polymer remains, much like ice melting in a glass of warm water. Homogeneous degradation, by comparison, occurs evenly throughout the structure. This causes fragmentation and structural integrity loss soon after implantation, much like the piecemeal breakup of an iceberg. Most bioabsorbable polymers degrade via both mechanisms. More hydrophobic polymers tend toward heterogeneous mechanisms, and hydrophilic polymers tend toward homogeneous dissolution through hydration. Fragmentation of an absorbable polymeric stent could have adverse effects if gross embolization occurred. If the polymer maintains its structural integrity for more than a few weeks, concerns for embolization may be unnecessary because thrombus and neointima would likely cover the device.

Degradation times can be as short as a few hours, or as long as many years, even for the same polymer. Degradation times depend on bulk polymer configuration, additives, and fabrication methods. Through changes in synthetic methods, polymers can be programmed for different degradation rates. This property is a definite advantage to their potential use in intracoronary stenting. It is thus important to establish how long a coronary stent must remain in place.

Biodegradability provides a means for controlled release of incorporated drugs.[41,43–46] This scheme permits continuous, concentrated, local elution of desired bioactive agents. High local concentrations could translate into low systemic doses that would be well tolerated. All polymer and drug would disappear at the end of the programmed degradation time. This concept provides potential solutions to the two major problems in PTCA today: acute vessel closure and long-term restenosis. First, the macroscopic configuration of the polymeric covered stent-graft could maintain the dilated state of the vessel, and also support intimal dissections. Second, as yet undefined pharmacological agents that limit intimal hyperplasia could be incorporated directly into such a stent. Antithrombotic agents might also be incorporated into the polymer matrix to reduce local thrombosis at the dilated site.

A few bioabsorbable polymers are well suited for drug impregnation and delivery during polymer degradation. Polymers degrading through the backbone hydrolysis mechanism will likely be most useful for the intracoronary stent. Some of these polymers are in use for intramuscular, intraperitoneal, and subcutaneous drug delivery systems. Table 10–2 lists some candidate bioabsorbable polymers for coronary stent-graft applications. The most promising of these are the following:

1. *Polylactic acid (PLA), polyglycolic (PGA) acid copolymers* are polyesters. They have been studied most comprehensively of all degradable and drug-eluting polymers. Their first use was in absorbable sutures during the early 1970s. PLA/PGA erodes relatively homogeneously to lactic acid, glycolic acid, water, and carbon dioxide. These degradation products have little toxicity, but do generate an inflammatory response. These polymers have been considered for implantable, long-acting contraceptives. One problem our group encountered in using thin, extruded PLA/PGA fibers was brittleness resulting in the inability to make tight bends without fracture. Such fibers must be formed into a stent and mounted in a delivery system, later to expand into a supportive stent form. Plasticizers or other synthetic methods may result in better PLA/PGA physical properties. Little has been published regarding blood compatibility of PLA/PGA. Vessel inflammation at the implant site remains a theoretical concern. Drug loading of this polymer is also more difficult.

2. *Polyanhydrides* were discovered early in this century. These polymers underwent extensive study in the late 1950s when they were under consideration as replacements for polyester fibers. They were discarded due to their hydrolyzability. The polyanhydrides erode heterogeneously, typically through surface erosion. They exhibit good tissue biocompatibility and minimal degradation product toxicity. Rare inflammation and mild fibrosis resulted when implanted subcutaneously in rats. Exposure of these polymers to ultrasonic energy may be a means of modulating drug release. Current clinical applications include local delivery of chemotherapeutic agents active against central nervous system malignancies. These polymers will require blood compatibility studies prior to use in stents.

3. *Polyorthoesters* are another biodegradable polymer that hydrolyze rapidly in acid but are more slowly hydrolyzed in alkaline media. These compounds are in clinical tests for releasing contraceptive steroids within subcutaneous implants. They undergo heterogeneous degradation. Incorporated drugs may form small "bubbles" within the polymer during manufacture. During hydration, the polymer swells, and adjacent bubbles are connected. Eventually the bubbles become confluent with the polymer surface, causing drug release. A skeleton of absorbable bulk polymer remains after all drug is gone. The polymer skeleton usually erodes more slowly than the time required for drug release. Through compositional and fabrication manipulations, constant drug release can be obtained.

4. *Polyiminocarbonates* are also potential polymers for the biodegradable, drug-eluting, intracoronary stent. These compounds have not been used in medical or industrial applications. The polyiminocarbonates are hydrolyzed either by acid or basic media. They degrade to carbon dioxide, ammonia, and alcohols or phenols related to the original polymer makeup. Little toxicity has been found from initial work with these substances. Subcutaneous mouse implants revealed little inflammatory reaction. Their mechanical properties may permit use as an intracoronary stent.

5. *Polyphosphate esters* are an interesting, new group of polymers that show promise for formability into mechanically useful stent configurations. They are bioabsorbable and capable of eluting drugs. Such drugs can reportedly be proteins. Another advantage to this family of polymers is that their degradation time can be readily changed by varying the composition.

Experimentation on pharmacological agents that may be incorporated into bioabsorbable polymers is expanding. Previously, only drugs of molecular weight 600 or less were usable, but more recently these limitations have been overcome. Small proteins can now be incor-

TABLE 10–2. Bioabsorbable Polymers with Possible Coronary Stent-Graft Applications

Polylactic acid/polyglycolic acid
Polyanhydrides
Polyorthoesters
Polyphosphate esters
Polyiminocarbonates
Polyurethanes (absorbable)
Polyhydroxy butyrate
Polycaprolactone
Polytrimethylene carbonate

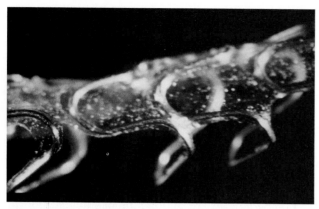
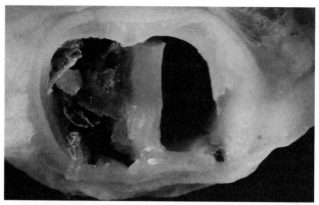

FIGURE 10–2. (A). Preimplant hybrid stent/stent-graft. In this configuration, a polymer is coated on one side of the metallic stent. The stent configuration here is a balloon-expandable wire stent. The devices were implanted in pig coronary arteries to test for polymer biocompatibility. This configuration permits a control in the form of bare stent wires to be located quite close to the polymer, on the opposing side of the artery. **(B).** Cross section through explanted pig coronary artery. At 28 days, marked inflammation and thrombus were seen on the side of the polymer. The tissue is organizing into a large amount of neointimal hyperplasia. Portions of the polymer are evident at the right side of the image.

porated for slow release in some classes of polymers. Polymers capable of delivering proteins may be quite useful, as many growth factors and other vasoactive substances are proteins.

Little has been published about development of bioabsorbable, drug-eluting intracoronary stents, likely because of the newness of this concept.[47–49] Polymer implantation at angioplasty sites has been proposed in the form of "polymeric endoluminal paving."[50–52] In this method, a polymer is heat formed at the arterial delivery site. Few in vivo results have been published about this method.

Research into biodegradable stents is proceeding in parallel with research into the pathophysiology of restenosis.[42,44,53–57] When the etiology of restenosis is better defined, more effective pharmacological targeting should be possible. Local, chronic, high concentrations of one or more drugs delivered by polymer may better approach this difficult clinical problem.

Studies using synthetic biopolymer stents in animal models have met with mixed results. Polyglycolic acid stents tested in canine coronaries showed thrombus formation beginning 3 hours after the procedure. Stent degradation was associated with a foreign body reaction although endothelialization did occur without subacute vessel closure. Poly-L-lactide stents deployed in canine femoral arteries resulted in reliable vessel patency, with a minimal inflammatory response, and no vessel closure at 18 months. The porcine model of coronary restenosis, unlike other models in common use, more closely reflects the process observed in human atherectomy and autopsy specimens. Initial results with polymeric stenting using the porcine model were disappointing. A polyethylene terephthalate meshwork stent caused an extensive inflammatory, proliferative response with coronary occlusion in all stented segments.

In a recent multicenter study, five biodegradable and three nonbiodegradable polymers incorporated in wire coil stents were implanted in the porcine coronary model.[58] Five to ten stents were placed in four to six animals in each of the eight polymer groups. The arterial patency at 4 weeks ranged from 70 to 100%. Five polymer groups demonstrated an eccentric coronary lumen reduction angiographically at the site of the stent implant. All eight polymers evoked a marked vessel wall inflammatory reaction. This powerful induction of neointimal thickening by polymeric stenting would have to be controlled before its potential could be investigated in humans. These results were discouraging for the use of synthetic polymers in a stent-graft configuration, but work continues to determine whether the reaction to the polymer can be moderated. A typical example of marked incompatibility from this study is shown in Figure 10–2.

■ Biomaterials and the Coronary Stent-Graft: Fibrin Films

One key issue regarding the poor results obtained with synthetic polymers is whether the material itself is the reason for the apparent problems of biocompatibility. It is clear that injury to the artery is responsible for neointimal thickening. Studies using the porcine coronary restenosis model indicate that the structural integrity of the internal elastic lamina (IEL) is essential to minimize neointimal thickening. Exposure of the injured IEL to the blood within the coronary lumen initiates the first, thrombotic phase of the restenosis process.

Using this model, we hypothesized that a fibrin film stent might be able to completely cover an artery, and

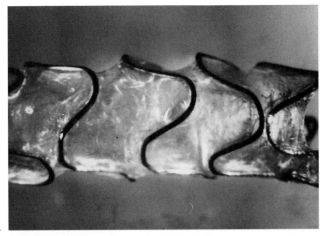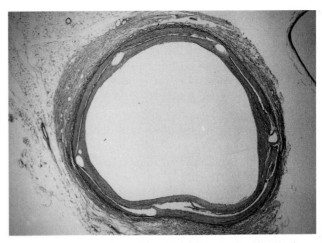

A   B

FIGURE 10–3. (A). Fibrin film stent. This is a thin (0.005″) coating of fibrin over a tantalum Wiktor stent. The excellent viscoelastic properties of the fibrin make it easily able to compress and expand with the stent during crimping and deployment. **(B).** Histopathological results of the fibrin film stent in a porcine coronary artery after 28 days of implant. The fibrin is nearly completely resorbed, and there is little inflammation or negative tissue reaction. (Hematoxylin/eosin stain, 50 ×.)

yield little long-term reaction.[56,59] Stents were fabricated with fibrin film, and implanted for long-term observation. Figure 10–3 shows this stent and early preclinical results. The results with these fibrin-coated stents were more encouraging than with the polymer coatings. Specifically, the neointima was thin and inflammation minimal. Most of the fibrin had dissolved by 1 month. The study showed safety of fibrin film stents compared to a bare metal stent in that there were no differences among the fibrin film group and the bare stent groups. The short-term to midterm data demonstrate no significant neointimal obstruction or late mortality up to 1 year after stenting. The fibrin film stent did not inhibit neointimal thickening compared to the bare metal stent. However, this result in itself is important when compared to previous synthetic polymer stent studies. In contrast to these studies, the fibrin film stent did not stimulate neointimal thickening despite achieving total arterial coverage at the treatment site. A similar stent-graft could be made from other materials such as collagen. The advantages of bioabsorbability are uncertain, except that drug elution may be facilitated by this option.

■ The Vein-Covered Stent: A Living Graft

Autologous vein grafts covering stents have been used recently.[60–67] The purpose of this connection is to achieve total natural stent coverage. Encouraging initial experimental results are emerging from this concept. In the porcine model, 27 autologous vein graft stents (AVGSs) were deployed within iliac arteries with uncoated stents acting as controls. Follow-up ranged from 7 days to 6 months. All AVGSs remained patent and became incorporated into the arterial wall after 2 months. Also, no exaggerated neointimal response was observed. The same group has deployed AVGSs in seven patients without complications to a mean follow-up of 4 months.

■ The Stent-Graft as a Concept

The most immediate applications of a coronary stent-graft are for covering perforations and coronary aneurysms, similar to those in peripheral vessels. The ability to seal such lesions is key, yet the prevalence of these problems in the coronary practice is quite low. Another application includes potential use in saphenous vein graft disease. While unproven, it is possible that embolization could be limited by a stent-graft that covers entirely the inner surface of a saphenous vein. The vein graft could theoretically be given a new endothelial/neointimal lining as the stent-graft healed into the old vein graft. Another advantage would be in completely covering an injured arterial site with a biocompatible, nonthrombogenic material.

To be clinically applicable, the stent-graft must incorporate sufficient mechanical support to maintain luminal gain and vessel patency. The device should allow for endothelialization of the diseased arterial segment after the procedure. In addition, the stent should be biocompatible and not initiate local thrombus formation or foreign body reaction. Such stents could also act as vehicles for local drug delivery during the period associated with neointimal thickening. Whether this concept has application in the native coronary circulation is unclear but will undoubtedly be tried for efficacy at some point in the near future. The major disadvantages include covering side branches and enhanced thrombosis.

■ The Ideal Stent-Graft

What would constitute the ideal intracoronary stent-graft? Such a device should be easily deployed, and have good fluoroscopic visibility. It should be nonthrombogenic (and possibly antithrombogenic), and be temporary, remaining in place only as long as needed to permit adequate arterial healing. It should abolish restenosis, creating instead a thin, smooth, reendothelialized, fibrocellular conduit of sufficient diameter to permit unimpeded blood flow. Ideally, the natural tissue conduit left by the stent would remain unchanged for the remainder of the patient's life. An ideal stent may not be realizable in practice; the design requirements are quite stringent. Biocompatible polymers have some properties that may provide alternatives to purely metallic devices.

Luminal obstruction by neointimal hyperplasia and/or thrombosis remains likely to be the most severe clinical problem for both the native circulation and synthetic vascular stent-grafts. Routine success has not been achieved in synthetic grafts of less than 6 mm, since smaller grafts develop occlusive proliferative neointima. This neointima typically emanates from anastomotic sites, eventually causing prosthetic thrombosis. Similarly, late restenosis after coronary angioplasty is caused by neointimal proliferation. Histopathologically, the neointima in each of these situations has many common properties. Smooth muscle cell–derived myofibroplasia is frequently seen in conjunction with intercellular ground substance. It thus appears quite likely that the problems of restenosis and prosthetic graft failure are closely related problems. The histopathological similarities between these processes suggest that arteries respond both to injury and foreign bodies in similar ways, although the mechanisms are not well understood.

The ideal stent-graft should promote organized neointimal growth to a point, and then cease. This would result in a patent, endothelialized biological lumen for flowing blood. Toward this end, the elucidation of neointimal pathophysiology and control will be an achievement of major clinical proportions. Resolution of restenosis, longer synthetic vascular graft lifetimes, and successful smaller-diameter synthetic grafts would result. Coronary bypass with synthetic grafts would be possible.

■ Summary

Technological advances in interventional cardiology have markedly increased the range of lesions amenable to dilation. The major remaining limitation of percutaneous revascularization is restenosis, a problem of neointimal hyperplasia that has successfully resisted all mechanical and systemic pharmacological approaches. A mechanism for controlling this hyperplasia may be local, targeted drug delivery via dissolving polymer matrix, simultaneously providing mechanical support to the freshly dilated coronary artery. The implications, if such a solution can be found, will be far-reaching and likely have application in areas as diverse as small-diameter synthetic vascular grafts for coronary bypass. Practical realization of this idealized concept will remain hampered until the mechanisms of restenosis and neointimal proliferation are better understood and effective pharmacological therapy is devised.

REFERENCES

1. Antoniucci D, Valenti R, Santoro GM, et al. Bailout coronary stenting without anticoagulation or intravascular ultrasound guidance: acute and six-month angiographic results in a series of 120 consecutive patients. Cathet Cardiovasc Diagn 1997;41:14–19.
2. Colombo A, Di Mario C, Reimers B, et al. Coronary stenting in 1000 consecutive patients. Long-term clinical and angiographic results. G Ital Cardiol 1997;27:19–31.
3. Gambhir DS, Sudha R, Singh S, et al. Elective coronary stenting after recanalization for chronic total occlusion: clinical and angiographic follow-up results. Indian Heart J 1997;49:163–168.
4. Goldberg SL, Di Mario C, Hall P, Colombo A. Comparison of aggressive versus nonaggressive balloon dilatation for stent deployment on late loss and restenosis in native coronary arteries. Am J Cardiol 1998;81:708–712.
5. Kastrati A, Schuhlen H, Hausleiter J, et al. Restenosis after coronary stent placement and randomization to a 4-week combined antiplatelet or anticoagulant therapy: six-month angiographic follow-up of the Intracoronary Stenting and Antithrombotic Regimen (ISAR) Trial [see comments]. Circulation 1997;96:462–467.
6. Dussaillant GR, Mintz GS, Pichard AD, et al. Small stent size and intimal hyperplasia contribute to restenosis: a volumetric intravascular ultrasound analysis. J Am Coll Cardiol 1995;26:720–724.
7. Ikari Y, Hara K, Tamura T, Saeki F, Yamaguchi T. Luminal loss and site of restenosis after Palmaz-Schatz coronary stent implantation. Am J Cardiol 1995;76:117–120.
8. Kuntz RE, Hinohara T, Robertson GC, Safian RD, Simpson JB, Baim DS. Influence of vessel selection on the observed restenosis rate after endoluminal stenting or directional atherectomy. Am J Cardiol 1992;70:1101–1108.
9. Mintz G, Pichard A, Kent K, et al. Endovascular stents reduce restenosis by eliminating geometric arterial remodeling: a serial intravacular ultrasound study. J Am Coll Cardiol 1995;26:36A.
10. Post M, de Smet B, van der Helm Y, Kuntz R, Borst C. Arterial remodeling contributes to restenosis after angioplasty, but is prevented by stenting in the atherosclerotic micropig. J Am Coll Cardiol 1995;26:303A.
11. Fischman DL, Leon MB, Baim DS, et al, for the Stent Restenosis Study Investigators. A randomized comparison of coronary-stent placement and balloon angioplasty in the treatment of coronary artery disease. N Engl J Med 1994;331:496–501.
12. Serruys PW, de Jaegere P, Kiemeneij F, et al. A comparison of balloon-expandable stent implantation with balloon angioplasty in patients with coronary artery disease. N Engl J Med 1994;331:489–495.
13. Colombo A, Ferraro M, Itoh A, Martini G, Blengino S, Finci L. Results of coronary stenting for restenosis. J Am Coll Cardiol 1996;28:830–836.
14. von Birgelen C, Mintz G, de Vrey EA, et al. Atherosclerotic coronary lesions with inadequate compensatory enlargement have smaller

plaque and vessel volumes: observations with three dimensional intravascular ultrasound in vivo. Heart 1998;79:137–142.

15. Mintz GS, Kent KM, Pichard AD, Satler LF, Popma JJ, Leon MB. Contribution of inadequate arterial remodeling to the development of focal coronary artery stenoses. An intravascular ultrasound study. Circulation 1997;95:1791–1798.

16. Mintz GS, Kent KM, Pichard AD, Popma JJ, Satler LF, Leon MB. Intravascular ultrasound insights into mechanisms of stenosis formation and restenosis. Cardiol Clin 1997;15:17–29.

17. Columbo A, Hall P, Nakamura S. Intracoronary stenting without anti-coagulation accomplished with intravascular ultrasound guidance. Circulation 1995;91:1676–1688.

18. de-Jaegere PP, de-Feyter PJ, van-der-Giessen WJ, Serruys PW. Endovascular stents: preliminary clinical results and future developments. Clin Cardiol 1993;16:369–378.

19. Foley JB, Brown RI, Penn IM. Thrombosis and restenosis after stenting in failed angioplasty: comparison with elective stenting. Am Heart J 1994;128:12–20.

20. Schomig A, Neumann F, Kastrati A, et al. A randomized comparison of antiplatelet and anticoagulant therapy after the placement of coronary-artery stents. N Engl J Med 1996;334:1084–1089.

21. Kikuchi S, Umemura K, Kondo K, Nakashima M. Tranilast suppresses intimal hyperplasia after photochemically induced endothelial injury in the rat. Eur J Pharmacol 1996;295:221–227.

22. Stephan D, Nabel EG. Gene and other biological therapies for vascular diseases. Fundamen Clin Pharmacol 1997;11:97–110.

23. Schwartz CJ, Sprague EA, Valente AJ, Kelley JL, Edwards EH. Cellular mechanisms in the response of the arterial wall to injury and repair. Toxicol Pathol 1989;17:66–71.

24. Schwart RS, Murphy JG, Edwards WD, Camrud AR, Vlietstra RE, Holmes DR Jr. Restenosis occurs with internal elastic lamina laceration and is proportional to severity of vessel injury in a porcine coronary artery model. Circulation 1990;4:III-656.

25. Schwartz RS, Edwards WD, Murphy JG, Camrud AR, Holmes DR Jr. Restenosis develops in four stages: serial histologic studies in a coronary injury model. J Am Coll Card 1991;17:52A.

26. Schwartz RS, Murphy JG, Edwards WD, Camrud AR, Vlietstra RE. Restenosis occurs with internal elastic lamina laceration and is proportional to severity of vessel injury in a porcine coronary artery model (abstr). Circulation 1990;82:III-656.

27. Fischell T, Carter A, Laird J. The beta-particle-emitting radioisotope stent (isostent): animal studies and planned clinical trials. Am J Cardiol 1996;78:45–50.

28. Pipili-Synetos E, Papageorgiou A, Sakkoula E, et al. Inhibition of angiogenesis, tumour growth and metastasis by the NO-releasing vasodilators, isosorbide mononitrate and dinitrate. Br J Pharmacol 1995;116:1829–1834.

29. Struck AT, Hogg N, Thomas JP, Kalyanaraman B. Nitric oxide donor compounds inhibit the toxicity of oxidized low-density lipoprotein to endothelial cells. FEBS Lett 1995;361:291–294.

30. Tronc F, Wassef M, Esposito B, Tedgui A. Role of nitric oxide in blood flow-induced vascular remodeling. Circulation 1995;92:2680.

31. Welch G, Loscalzo J. Nitric oxide and the cardiovascular system. J Cardiac Surg 1994;9:361–371.

32. Marks DS, Vita JA, Folts JD, Keaney JF Jr, Welch GN, Loscalzo J. Inhibition of neointimal proliferation in rabbits after vascular injury by a single treatment with a protein adduct of nitric oxide. J Clin Invest 1995;96:2630–2683.

33. Fujiik S, Vinogradsky B, Sawa H, Guala A, Lundgren C. Seeding of stents with genetically modified endothelial cells: overexpression of urokinase receptor results in increased seeded cell retention. Circulation 1996;94:I-261.

34. Rajasubramanian G, Meidell RS, Landau C, et al. Fabrication of resorbable microporous intravascular stents for gene therapy applications. ASAIO J 1994;40:M584–589.

35. Tanguay JF, Zidar JP, Phillips HR, Stack RS. Current status of biodegradable stents. Cardiol Clin 1994;12:699–713.

36. Schafer AI. Antiplatelet therapy with glycoprotein IIb/IIIa receptor inhibitors and other novel agents. Tex Heart Inst 1997;24:90–96.

37. Schulman SP, Goldschmidt-Clermont PJ, Topol EJ, et al. Effects of integrelin, a platelet glycoprotein IIb/IIIa receptor antagonist, in unstable angina. A randomized multicenter trial. Circulation 1996;94:2083–2089.

38. Lincoff AM, Califf RM, Anderson KM, et al. Evidence for prevention of death and myocardial infarction with platelet membrane glycoprotein IIb/IIIa receptor blockade by abciximab (c7E3 Fab) among patients with unstable angina undergoing percutaneous coronary revascularization. EPIC Investigators. Evaluation of 7E3 in Preventing Ischemic Complications. J Am Coll Cardiol 1997;30:149–156.

39. van der Giessen W, Lincoff A, Schwartz R, et al. Marked inflammatory sequelae to implantation of biodegradable and non-biodegradable polymers in porcine coronary arteries. Circulation 1996;94:1690–1697.

40. Greisler HP, Dennis JW, Schwarcz TH, Klosak JJ, Ellinger J, Kim DU. Plasma polymerized tetrafluoroethylene/polyethylene terephthalate vascular prostheses [published erratum appears in Arch Surg 1990;125(1):96]. Arch Surg 1989;124:967–972.

41. Ozaki Y, Violaris AG, Serruys PW. New stent technologies. Prog Cardiovasc Dis 1996;39:129–140.

42. Palmaz JC. Review of polymeric graft materials for endovascular applications. J Vasc Intervent Radiol 1998;9:7–13.

43. Ye YW, Landau C, Willard JE, et al. Bioresorbable microporous stents deliver recombinant adenovirus gene transfer vectors to the arterial wall. Ann Biomed Eng 1998;26:398–408.

44. Lincoff AM, Furst JG, Ellis SG, Tuch RJ, Topol EJ. Sustained local delivery of dexamethasone by a novel intravascular eluting stent to prevent restenosis in the porcine coronary injury model. J Am Coll Cardiol 1997;29:808–816.

45. Aggarwal RK, Ireland DC, Azrin MA, Ezekowitz MD, de Bono DP, Gershlick AH. Antithrombotic potential of polymer-coated stents eluting platelet glycoprotein IIb/IIIa receptor antibody. Circulation 1996;94:3311–3317.

46. Ye YW, Landau C, Meidell RS, et al. Improved bioresorbable microporous intravascular stents for gene therapy. ASAIO J 1996;42:M823–827.

47. Zidar J, Mohammad S, Culp S, Brott B, Phillips H, Stack R. In vitro thrombogenicity analysis of a new bioabsorbable, balloon-expandable, endovascular stent. J Am Coll Cardiol 1993;21:483A.

48. Zidar J, Gammon R, Chapman G, et al. Short and long-term tissue response to the Duke bioabsorbable stent. J Am Coll Cardiol 1993;21:439A.

49. Tanguay JF, Zidar JP, Phillips HR 3rd, Stack RS. Current status of biodegradable stents. Cardiol Clin 1994;12:699–713.

50. Slepian MJ. Polymeric endoluminal gel paving: therapeutic hydrogel barriers and sustained drug delivery depots for local arterial wall biomanipulation. Semin Intervent Cardiol 1996;1:103–116.

51. Slepian MJ, Massia SP, Whitesell L. Pre-conditioning of smooth muscle cells via induction of the heat shock response limits proliferation following mechanical injury. Biochem Biophys Res Commun 1996;225:600–607.

52. Slepian MJ. Polymeric endoluminal paving. A family of evolving methods for extending endoluminal therapeutics beyond stenting. Cardiol Clin 1994;12:715–737.

53. Salzmann DL, Yee DC, Roach DJ, Berman SS, Williams SK. Healing response associated with balloon-dilated ePTFE. J Biomed Mater Res 1998;41:364–370.

54. Bertrand OF, Sipehia R, Mongrain R, et al. Biocompatibility aspects of new stent technology. J Am Coll Cardiol 1998;32:562–571.

55. Murphy JG, Schwartz RS, Edwards WD, Camrud AR, Vlietstra RE, Holmes DR Jr. Percutaneous polymeric stents in porcine coronary arteries. Initial experience with polyethylene terephthalate stents. Circulation 1992;86:1596–1604.

56. Holmes DRJ, Camrud A, Jorgenson M, Edwards W, Schwart R. Polymeric stenting in the porcine coronary artery model: differential outcome of exogenous fibrin sleeves versus polyurethane-coated stents. J Am Coll Cardiol 1994;24:525–531.

57. Fontaine AB, Koelling K, Passos SD, Cearlock J, Hoffman R, Spigos DG. Polymeric surface modifications of tantalum stents. J Endovasc Surg 1996;3:276–283.

58. van der Giessen WJ, Lincoff AM, Schwartz RS, et al. Marked inflammatory sequelae to implantation of biodegradable and non-biodegradable polymers in porcine coronary arteries [see comments]. Circulation 1996;94:1690–1697.

59. McKenna CJ, Camrud AR, Sangiorgi G, et al. Fibrin-film stenting in a porcine coronary injury model: efficacy and safety compared with uncoated stents. J Am Coll Cardiol 1998;31:1434–1438.

60. Byer A, Ussia G, Galleti G. Autologous vein lined and vein covered stents in swine arteries. An experimental study to assess and compare patency and intimal hyperplastic response [in process citation]. J Cardiovasc Surg (Torino) 1998;39:393–398.

61. Clark DA. Reconstructing diseased vein grafts—great potential raises old issues [editorial; comment]. Cathet Cardiovasc Diagn 1998;43:322.

62. Gruberg L, Roguin A, Beyar R. Percutaneous closure of a coronary aneurysm with a vein-coated stent. Cathet Cardiovasc Diagn 1998;43:308–310.

63. Schellhammer F, Haberstroh J, Wakhloo AK, Gottschalk E, Schumacher M. Vein graft-coated vascular stents: a feasibility study in a canine model. Cardiovasc Intervent Radiol 1998;21:158–164.

64. Stefanadis C, Tsiamis E, Vlachopoulos C, et al. Arterial autologous graft-stent for treatment of coronary artery disease: a new technique. Cathet Cardiovasc Diagn 1997;40:302–307.

65. Stefanadis C, Tsiamis E, Vlachopoulos C, et al. Autologous vein graft-coated stents for the treatment of thrombus-containing coronary artery lesions. Cathet Cardiovasc Diagn 1997;40:217–222.

66. Stefanadis C, Toutouzas K, Vlachopoulos C, et al. Stents wrapped in autologous vein: an experimental study. J Am Coll Cardiol 1996;28:1039–1046.

67. Stefanadis C, Toutouzas K, Vlachopoulos C, et al. Autologous vein graft-coated stent for treatment of coronary artery disease. Cathet Cardiovasc Diagn 1996;38:159–170.

11

Stent-Grafts in Hemodialysis Shunts

MARC R. SAPOVAL, LUC TURMEL-RODRIGUES, ALAIN C. RAYNAUD,
BERNARD M. BEYSSEN, AND JEAN-CLAUDE GAUX

Covered stents were originally conceived as an endovascular therapy for treatment of aneurysms and arterial stenoses. They have more recently been proposed in the treatment of conditions associated with angioaccess where they may prove useful for acute angioplasty-induced rupture, shunt pseudoaneurysms, and possibly in the treatment of restenosis after venous angioplasty. This chapter briefly presents the devices and materials that are likely to be used to treat hemodialysis shunts, and reviews the theoretical background and clinical results that have been obtained so far.

■ Different Stent-Grafts

Five devices are theoretically suitable for use in hemodialysis angioaccess:

The Passager (Boston Scientific Corp., Natick, MA)
The covered Jostent (Jomed Implantate, Rangendingen, Germany)
The Wallgraft (Boston Scientific Corp., Natick, MA)
The Hemobahn (W. L. Gore and Assoc., Scottsdale, AZ)
The Impra/Bard encapsulated stent-graft (Impra Inc., Tempe, AZ)

To our knowledge, only the first two have been clinically used for hemodialysis access intervention. Published data are available only for the Passager.

The Passager stent-graft was initially manufactured by Mintec (Cragg Endopro, La Ciotat, France) and has been slightly modified by the Boston Scientific Corp. It is made of a monofilament nitinol wire with thermal shape memory alloy, with wire that is 0.27 mm in diameter. This wire is shaped into a tube configuration with a series of longitudinal zigzags. Every zigzag is attached to the next row with 7–0 polypropylene suture. The nitinol-polypropylene skeleton is covered with low-porosity woven polyethylene terephthalate (PET) graft material 0.1 mm thick. This stent-graft is self-expanding and can be delivered through a 9-French (Fr) sheath. Beside hemodialysis shunts, this stent-graft has been used for a variety of indications including the treatment of iliac artery stenoses and occlusions, popliteal aneurysms, and abdominal and thoracic aortic aneurysms.[1–3]

Another device that has recently been released in Europe is the covered Jostent. It is a stainless steel balloon-expandable expanded polytetrafluoroethylene (ePTFE)-covered stent delivered through a 7- or 8-Fr sheath. This stent-graft can be dilated from 4 to 12 mm in diameter. Owing to its lack of elasticity, however, it is not recommended for use in superficial vessels because there is a risk that extrinsic force may cause irreversible deformity of this device. Nevertheless, the ePTFE-covered Jostent may potentially be used in deeper venous outflow stenoses or possibly in central venous obstructions.

The Wallgraft is a PET-covered Wallstent that is currently in clinical trial for treatment of iliac artery occlusive and aneurysmal diseases. For sizes that are most suited to dialysis shunt use, it can be delivered through a 9-Fr sheath. Similarly to a Wallstent, it is difficult to determine its final implanted length because of the complex relationship between length and diameter. Potential advantages include its flexibility and self-expanding properties. There are no data regarding the use of this device in arteriovenous shunts or venous stenoses.

The Gore Hemobahn is a self-expanding ePTFE-covered nitinol stent with its graft material on the inner aspect of the stent. It is delivered through a 10-Fr sheath. To our knowledge, this device has been used only in peripheral arteries through European and U.S. multicenter clinical trials.

The final device is the Impra/Bard encapsulated ePTFE stent-graft. It consists of a Memotherm nitinol stent that is encapsulated within ePTFE. The ePTFE is carbon loaded, with the goal of reducing thrombogenicity by increasing the negative charge of ePTFE. This modification has been shown to reduce interaction of this graft material with platelets while increasing the adsorption of passivating proteins like albumin that may reduce the thrombogenic potential of ePTFE.[4,5] This device has been tested in pig iliac arteries[6] and will soon enter canine arteriovenous shunt testing followed by multicenter European and U.S. dialysis access studies.

■ Stent-Grafts for the Prevention of Anastomotic and Venous Outflow Stenoses

Neointimal growth at the venous anastomosis of a synthetic arteriovenous (AV) shunt (Fig. 11–1A) and in the venous outflow of both synthetic and native AV shunts (Fig. 11–1B) is a natural process. It occurs for a number of reasons including compliance mismatch, shear stress on the vein wall related to blood flow, vibratory effects, upstream and downstream cellular and molecular mechanisms, and vein wall injury at the time of surgical shunt formation.[7] The final result is a stenosis at the distal end of the shunt that reduces blood flow. Untreated, this leads to shunt thrombosis. Primary patency for a newly placed synthetic dialysis shunt ranges from 1 to 3 years, and the average hemodialysis patient can expect an episode of shunt thrombosis every 12 to 15 months.[8,9] The rationale for using stent-grafts to treat shunt-related stenoses is based on the assumption that cellular proliferation and intercellular matrix secretion will be decreased by the presence of a cellular barrier of polymeric graft, as proposed by Cragg and Dake.[10] They suggested that tissue ingrowth can be prevented by the tightness of the graft material.

One of the main interests for use of stent-grafts in hemodialysis access intervention is the potential for reducing the rate of postangioplasty restenosis. This is a clinically important problem because patency following angioplasty of a stenosed shunt is relatively poor. The recent National Kidney Foundation document regarding dialysis outcomes (Dialysis Outcomes Quality Initiative; DOQI) states that the anticipated primary patency rate following venous angioplasty of a synthetic dialysis shunt

should be at least 40% at 6 months.[11] The DOQI document sets the standard even lower for thrombosed grafts following successful declotting, where venous angioplasty is expected to yield primary patency of only 40% at 3 months. These low expectations following angioplasty indicate that there is clearly room for improvement.

The mechanism for recurrent postangioplasty angioaccess stenosis is predominantly related to luminal narrowing caused by growth of neointimal hyperplasia with some contribution from postangioplasty elastic recoil.[12] Although elastic recoil may play a role as supported by an intravascular US study in AV shunts and other arteries, it does not explain all of the restenotic process, as patency rates following placement of a stent, however, are no better than results achieved with angioplasty alone.[13–15] When one looks at angiograms of stenosed stents in hemodialysis shunts, it is obvious that neointimal tissue, propagating through the interstices of the stent, is the dominant cause (Fig. 11–2).

As noted earlier, there are two types of graft materials that can be incorporated into a stent-graft for use in angioaccess: PET, a medical-grade textile that has been reviewed elsewhere in this text; and ePTFE. Soon after PET has been placed into the vascular system as a bypass conduit, a luminal fibrin layer forms. An external fibrous capsule begins to form as well. There is gradual ingrowth of fibroblasts through the interstices of the graft material.[16] The healing response for *endovascular* stent-graft implantation of PET graft material is different from that for surgically placed PET bypass grafts. This may be, in part, because endoluminal PET is placed in apposition to the biochemically active endothelial surface rather than within interstitial tissues where the PET conduit is often located.[17] Inflammatory and myointimal cells may pass directly into the interstices of the endoluminal PET from the vascular intima that is in contact with the outer graft surface.

From various animal models, it appears that PET stent-grafts are infiltrated and lined by a fibrocellular neointimal layer similar to that seen for surgical grafts. However, endothelialization occurs to a greater degree than for surgical grafts. In dogs[18] and minipigs,[19] neointimal tissue was found throughout PET stent-grafts with a complete endothelial surface by 6 weeks. Criado et al[20,21] studied stented PET grafts in dogs and demonstrated complete incorporation at 3 months. These implants developed a fibrocellular neointima that was approximately 250 μm thick, with endothelial coverage at 6 months. Eton et al,[22] in a dog model, noted incorporation with fibrocellular growth up to 0.9 mm thick after 6 months.[22] A greater degree of neointimal proliferation has been reported in a sheep model by Schurmann et al,[23] who noted more neointimal hyperplasia related to PET-covered stents when compared to bare stents.

visible means only that it is thrombosed but not necessarily sealed. One must always keep in mind that development of a pseudoaneurysm may be delayed, occurring many weeks or months after rupture. Therefore, patients who have sustained any degree of rupture must be followed closely. It is of interest to note that in surgical series, repair of false aneurysms represent 1 to 7% of all secondary procedures performed on dialysis shunts.[42] Although many of these are not directly related to angioplasty ruptures, it is nevertheless prudent to confirm durability of treatment when rupture occurs. We recommend a control fistulogram at least once at 6 months for any case of angioplasty-related rupture.

In cases where prolonged balloon inflation does not correct a rupture, or when the rupture is severe, Wall-stent placement is a proven method of treatment. Although the Wallstent is admittedly not covered, it seems to correct most ruptures by lowering the pressure within the shunt. It accomplishes this by relieving the extrinsic compression caused by an expanding hematoma. A Wallstent may also tack back part of the ruptured vein that obstructs blood flow through the shunt. In our experience in a series of 40 ruptures, Wallstent implantation alone was effective in 39.[43] In the report from Funaki et al,[44] 23 ruptures were treated successfully with Wallstents with only one pseudoaneurysm seen in the midterm follow-up.

When a Wallstent fails to stop bleeding, a covered stent is of value (Fig. 11–5). In our series of 14 patients treated with the Cragg Endopro, three patients were

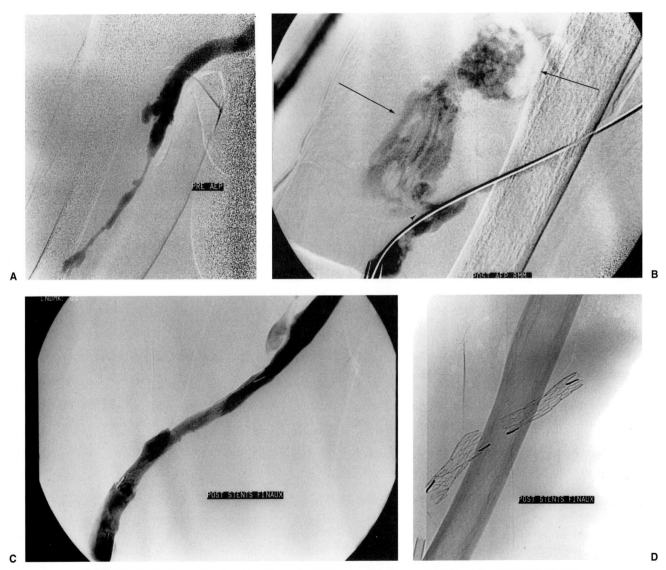

FIGURE 11–5. Superficialized basilic vein AV fistula. (**A**). Preangioplasty. (**B**). Postangioplasty: massive rupture (arrowhead) with active extravasation of contrast (arrows). (**C**). Control angiogram after placement of two 4-cm-long Passager stent-grafts. (**D**). Passager stent-grafts are easily seen on a nonsubtracted image.

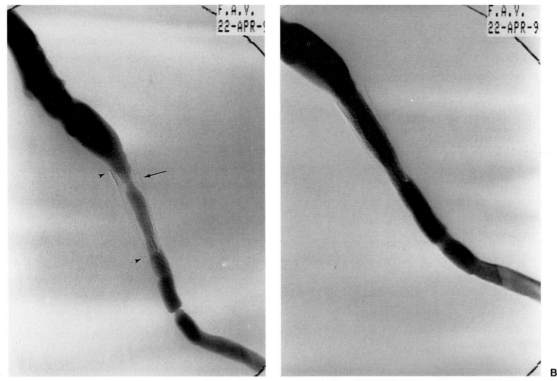

FIGURE 11–4. This expanded polytetrafluoroethylene (ePTFE) brachioaxillary shunt developed clinical restenosis 4 months after it was placed. Angioplasty resulted in a severe rupture that was treated with implantation of a covered Cragg stent. (**A**).This angiogram at 1 year was performed because of increased venous pressure during dialysis. There is restenosis within the stent-graft (arrow). Arrowheads delineate the margin of the stent-graft. (**B**). Successful angioplasty of neointimal tissue within the lumen of the stent-graft.

year after placement of a Cragg Endopro stent-graft initially implanted for angioplasty-related rupture.

We concluded from this study that this stent-graft could not prevent restenosis when used to treat dialysis shunt stenoses. Furthermore, in some cases we observed the development of a new stenosis immediately upstream or downstream of the stent-graft. This may be related to compliance mismatch between the stent-graft and the native vein, to creation of a neoanastomosis, or perhaps to technical factors during implantation. We have made similar observation following placement of Passager stent-grafts inside restenotic Wallstents (unpublished data). This raises the possibility that placement of a stent-graft may incite stenosis in an adjacent segment of vein. If this is true, the benefits of a dialysis shunt stent-graft may be outweighed by the accelerated loss of vein that could otherwise have been used to create another angioaccess.

A recently published report (38) tends to contradict our results, however. In a series of 20 patients treated with the Cragg Endopro (native vein, $n = 10$; venous anastomosis of synthetic grafts, $n = 10$) primary patency was 57% at 6 months. Eight of these patients were treated because of recurrent restenosis, and the authors noted that the interval between repeated angioplasty

went from 2 months prior to stent-graft placement to 4 months after. Further experience is needed, including randomization of covered versus uncovered stents, before we can determine if restenosis can be reduced with any type of covered stent.

■ Covered Stents for Acute Rupture During Angioplasty

The occurrence of angioplasty-induced rupture is estimated at 2% for synthetic grafts, 10% for Brescia-Cimino fistulas, and 18% for upper-arm fistulas.[39–41] Minor ruptures are most frequent and spontaneously seal without any clinical consequence. Moderate rupture can be defined as a leak with pain and swelling. These ruptures may lead to loss of the angioaccess because of compression by hematoma. When rupture is severe, acute extravasation is seen with a large hematoma adjacent to the shunt.

Endovascular treatment of acute rupture involves re-inflation of the balloon at low pressure upstream or at the level of the rupture for 15 to 20 minutes. This can solve the immediate problem of extravasation in many cases. However, the fact that a pseudoaneurysm is not

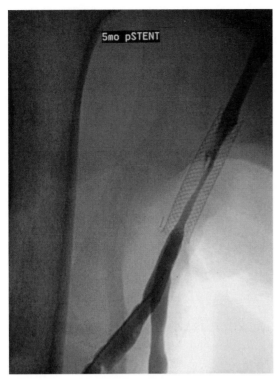

FIGURE 11–2. Recurrent stenosis owing to ingrowth of neointimal tissue through the interstices of a stent placed 5 months earlier to treat a venous anastomotic stenosis of a synthetic AV shunt.

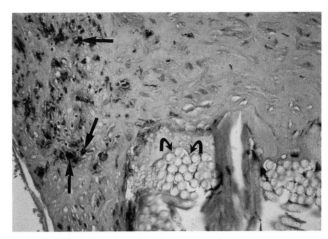

FIGURE 11–3. Histologic specimen shows neointimal hyperplasia and cellular infiltrates to the left of the polyethylene terephthalate (PET) fibers (curved arrows). Immunohistochemical labeling with antimacrophage antibody shows the presence of macrophages (straight arrows) among the smooth muscle cells, near the PET fibers.

pigs. The correlation of inflammation with neointimal hyperplasia has also been described in a number of different stent-graft applications, such as in coronary arteries, iliac arteries, and transjugular intrahepatic portosystemic shunts.[17,21,27–33] Because restenosis is linked to inflammation, stent-grafts that are based on inflammatory graft materials should be avoided.

Clinical inflammatory responses have been reported in humans, particularly in association with placement of PET covered stent-grafts. We observed one case of reversible inflammation with thickening of the arterial wall after placement of a Cragg Endopro stent-graft in an iliac artery.[34] In hemodialysis angioaccess intervention we have seen pain, swelling, and redness in all cases where Cragg Endopro stent-grafts were placed in forearm shunts.[35] This phenomenon was also observed after implantation of the same covered stent in the superficial femoral artery.[1] This so-called postimplantation syndrome has also been reported with exclusion of abdominal aortic aneurysms using the Stentor bifurcated stent-graft.[36] A common thread for all of these cases has been the use of PET as the stent-graft covering.[34] However, we have recently noted that implantation of the modified Passager PET stent-graft in dialysis shunts has not caused an inflammatory response, and we wonder if some preparations of PET are less inflammatory than others.

There are few data regarding restenosis of stent-grafts in human AV shunts. In one of our patients, restenosis in a Cragg Endopro stent-graft was analyzed following directional atherectomy of a stenosis within the stent-graft.[35] Histology included histochemical labeling that demonstrated the presence of smooth muscle cells and macrophages near the PET fibers (Fig. 11–3). In one other case published by Hausegger et al,[37] a Cragg Endopro was explanted after 9 months. Histology showed a 1- to 2-mm-thick layer of intimal hyperplasia.

In summary, this review of the literature suggests that the ePTFE covering may be a more effective graft barrier for use in dialysis shunt stent-grafts. ePTFE is certainly less inflammatory than PET and has been used successfully for decades as the predominant material for most synthetic arteriovenous shunts.

■ Clinical Results of Stent-Graft Placement in Dialysis Shunts

The only clinical reports of stent-graft use in dialysis shunts are with the Cragg Endopro. In 1996 we reported 14 patients treated over a 2-year period.[35] Patients underwent Cragg stent-graft placement for early restenosis ($n = 8$), rupture postangioplasty ($n = 3$), pseudoaneurysm ($n = 1$), and residual stenosis following angioplasty ($n = 2$). Fistulography and clinical examination during dialysis were used to follow patients. When the covered stents were implanted for restenosis, restenosis again occurred within 6 months in all cases (primary patency in the 14 patients was 28.5% ± 13.9% at 6 months). Figure 11–4 shows an example of restenosis 1

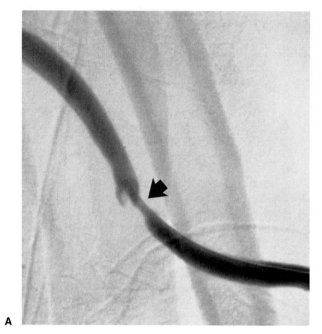

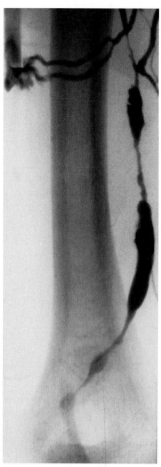

FIGURE 11–1. (A). Characteristic venous anastomotic stenosis involving a synthetic dialysis shunt (arrow). **(B)**. Multiple venous stenoses are noted within a native arteriovenous (AV) fistula.

Clearly, proliferative neointima within a stent-graft will be of little help in preventing restenosis at the venous anastomosis of a dialysis shunt. The degree of luminal neointimal proliferation and endothelialization of PET stent-grafts in humans, however, is not known. Although humans typically produce a limited neointima following placement of surgical PET grafts in larger arteries, there is no guarantee that PET stent-grafts used in dialysis shunts will not develop an exuberant neointima that may lead to restenosis.

Like PET materials, the healing response to ePTFE bypass grafts and stent-grafts has been predominantly characterized in animals using arterial models. Healing related to ePTFE includes the development of a luminal neointima that may be influenced by graft porosity. Golden et al[24] found that ePTFE grafts implanted in baboons developed a pattern of neointimal healing with endothelial cells and smooth muscle cells that was related to graft porosity. In high-porosity grafts with 60- and 90-μm internodal distances, there was a uniformly distributed neointima throughout the length of the graft with a complete luminal endothelial covering. Dolmatch et al[6] compared Memotherm stents with Memotherm stent-grafts prepared in a way that embedded the

stent within ePTFE. Using a porcine model of peripheral arterial neointima formation, they found less neointima in stent-grafts of medium and high porosity than in the corresponding bare stents. However, an ePTFE of low porosity had poor healing with an unstable neointima that consisted of organized thrombus. These data suggest that an ePTFE stent-graft may actually limit the process of neointimal stenosis and support the use of this type of device in AV dialysis shunts. Porosity, however, probably needs to fall within a certain range for a stable and nonproliferative neointima to form on the ePTFE.

Inflammation is characteristic of certain graft materials. In both surgical grafts and stent-grafts, PET produces a foreign body giant cell inflammatory reaction that is usually moderate in degree.[25] Furthermore, there are data that suggest a relationship between endovascular inflammation and secretion of powerful mitogenic factors that induce endothelial and smooth muscle cell proliferation.[26] The likelihood of a stent-graft developing stenosis or occlusion is generally high when an extensive inflammatory reaction occurs. This is supported by many reports with endovascular implants tested in different animal models including dogs, sheep, and

The Gore Hemobahn is a self-expanding ePTFE-covered nitinol stent with its graft material on the inner aspect of the stent. It is delivered through a 10-Fr sheath. To our knowledge, this device has been used only in peripheral arteries through European and U.S. multicenter clinical trials.

The final device is the Impra/Bard encapsulated ePTFE stent-graft. It consists of a Memotherm nitinol stent that is encapsulated within ePTFE. The ePTFE is carbon loaded, with the goal of reducing thrombogenicity by increasing the negative charge of ePTFE. This modification has been shown to reduce interaction of this graft material with platelets while increasing the adsorption of passivating proteins like albumin that may reduce the thrombogenic potential of ePTFE.[4,5] This device has been tested in pig iliac arteries[6] and will soon enter canine arteriovenous shunt testing followed by multicenter European and U.S. dialysis access studies.

■ Stent-Grafts for the Prevention of Anastomotic and Venous Outflow Stenoses

Neointimal growth at the venous anastomosis of a synthetic arteriovenous (AV) shunt (Fig. 11–1A) and in the venous outflow of both synthetic and native AV shunts (Fig. 11–1B) is a natural process. It occurs for a number of reasons including compliance mismatch, shear stress on the vein wall related to blood flow, vibratory effects, upstream and downstream cellular and molecular mechanisms, and vein wall injury at the time of surgical shunt formation.[7] The final result is a stenosis at the distal end of the shunt that reduces blood flow. Untreated, this leads to shunt thrombosis. Primary patency for a newly placed synthetic dialysis shunt ranges from 1 to 3 years, and the average hemodialysis patient can expect an episode of shunt thrombosis every 12 to 15 months.[8,9] The rationale for using stent-grafts to treat shunt-related stenoses is based on the assumption that cellular proliferation and intercellular matrix secretion will be decreased by the presence of a cellular barrier of polymeric graft, as proposed by Cragg and Dake.[10] They suggested that tissue ingrowth can be prevented by the tightness of the graft material.

One of the main interests for use of stent-grafts in hemodialysis access intervention is the potential for reducing the rate of postangioplasty restenosis. This is a clinically important problem because patency following angioplasty of a stenosed shunt is relatively poor. The recent National Kidney Foundation document regarding dialysis outcomes (Dialysis Outcomes Quality Initiative; DOQI) states that the anticipated primary patency rate following venous angioplasty of a synthetic dialysis shunt should be at least 40% at 6 months.[11] The DOQI document sets the standard even lower for thrombosed grafts following successful declotting, where venous angioplasty is expected to yield primary patency of only 40% at 3 months. These low expectations following angioplasty indicate that there is clearly room for improvement.

The mechanism for recurrent postangioplasty angioaccess stenosis is predominantly related to luminal narrowing caused by growth of neointimal hyperplasia with some contribution from postangioplasty elastic recoil.[12] Although elastic recoil may play a role as supported by an intravascular US study in AV shunts and other arteries, it does not explain all of the restenotic process, as patency rates following placement of a stent, however, are no better than results achieved with angioplasty alone.[13–15] When one looks at angiograms of stenosed stents in hemodialysis shunts, it is obvious that neointimal tissue, propagating through the interstices of the stent, is the dominant cause (Fig. 11–2).

As noted earlier, there are two types of graft materials that can be incorporated into a stent-graft for use in angioaccess: PET, a medical-grade textile that has been reviewed elsewhere in this text; and ePTFE. Soon after PET has been placed into the vascular system as a bypass conduit, a luminal fibrin layer forms. An external fibrous capsule begins to form as well. There is gradual ingrowth of fibroblasts through the interstices of the graft material.[16] The healing response for *endovascular* stent-graft implantation of PET graft material is different from that for surgically placed PET bypass grafts. This may be, in part, because endoluminal PET is placed in apposition to the biochemically active endothelial surface rather than within interstitial tissues where the PET conduit is often located.[17] Inflammatory and myointimal cells may pass directly into the interstices of the endoluminal PET from the vascular intima that is in contact with the outer graft surface.

From various animal models, it appears that PET stent-grafts are infiltrated and lined by a fibrocellular neointimal layer similar to that seen for surgical grafts. However, endothelialization occurs to a greater degree than for surgical grafts. In dogs[18] and minipigs,[19] neointimal tissue was found throughout PET stent-grafts with a complete endothelial surface by 6 weeks. Criado et al[20,21] studied stented PET grafts in dogs and demonstrated complete incorporation at 3 months. These implants developed a fibrocellular neointima that was approximately 250 μm thick, with endothelial coverage at 6 months. Eton et al,[22] in a dog model, noted incorporation with fibrocellular growth up to 0.9 mm thick after 6 months.[22] A greater degree of neointimal proliferation has been reported in a sheep model by Schurmann et al,[23] who noted more neointimal hyperplasia related to PET-covered stents when compared to bare stents.

11
···

Stent-Grafts in Hemodialysis Shunts

MARC R. SAPOVAL, LUC TURMEL-RODRIGUES, ALAIN C. RAYNAUD,
BERNARD M. BEYSSEN, AND JEAN-CLAUDE GAUX

Covered stents were originally conceived as an endovascular therapy for treatment of aneurysms and arterial stenoses. They have more recently been proposed in the treatment of conditions associated with angioaccess where they may prove useful for acute angioplasty-induced rupture, shunt pseudoaneurysms, and possibly in the treatment of restenosis after venous angioplasty. This chapter briefly presents the devices and materials that are likely to be used to treat hemodialysis shunts, and reviews the theoretical background and clinical results that have been obtained so far.

■ Different Stent-Grafts

Five devices are theoretically suitable for use in hemodialysis angioaccess:

The Passager (Boston Scientific Corp., Natick, MA)
The covered Jostent (Jomed Implantate, Rangendingen, Germany)
The Wallgraft (Boston Scientific Corp., Natick, MA)
The Hemobahn (W. L. Gore and Assoc., Scottsdale, AZ)
The Impra/Bard encapsulated stent-graft (Impra Inc., Tempe, AZ)

To our knowledge, only the first two have been clinically used for hemodialysis access intervention. Published data are available only for the Passager.

The Passager stent-graft was initially manufactured by Mintec (Cragg Endopro, La Ciotat, France) and has been slightly modified by the Boston Scientific Corp. It is made of a monofilament nitinol wire with thermal shape memory alloy, with wire that is 0.27 mm in diame-

ter. This wire is shaped into a tube configuration with a series of longitudinal zigzags. Every zigzag is attached to the next row with 7–0 polypropylene suture. The nitinol-polypropylene skeleton is covered with low-porosity woven polyethylene terephthalate (PET) graft material 0.1 mm thick. This stent-graft is self-expanding and can be delivered through a 9-French (Fr) sheath. Beside hemodialysis shunts, this stent-graft has been used for a variety of indications including the treatment of iliac artery stenoses and occlusions, popliteal aneurysms, and abdominal and thoracic aortic aneurysms.[1–3]

Another device that has recently been released in Europe is the covered Jostent. It is a stainless steel balloon-expandable expanded polytetrafluoroethylene (ePTFE)-covered stent delivered through a 7- or 8-Fr sheath. This stent-graft can be dilated from 4 to 12 mm in diameter. Owing to its lack of elasticity, however, it is not recommended for use in superficial vessels because there is a risk that extrinsic force may cause irreversible deformity of this device. Nevertheless, the ePTFE-covered Jostent may potentially be used in deeper venous outflow stenoses or possibly in central venous obstructions.

The Wallgraft is a PET-covered Wallstent that is currently in clinical trial for treatment of iliac artery occlusive and aneurysmal diseases. For sizes that are most suited to dialysis shunt use, it can be delivered through a 9-Fr sheath. Similarly to a Wallstent, it is difficult to determine its final implanted length because of the complex relationship between length and diameter. Potential advantages include its flexibility and self-expanding properties. There are no data regarding the use of this device in arteriovenous shunts or venous stenoses.

shunt stenosis. To do this, the new stent-grafts will need to combine several characteristics. They will need to have low thrombogenicity, high biocompatibility (with little or no inflammatory potential), high hemocompatibility, good radial strength, flexibility, and a mechanism that prevents migration and dislodgment. Although the challenges are great, we believe that in the future stent-grafts will be used to treat angioaccess stenoses and prolong the useful life of many of these shunts.

REFERENCES

1. Rousseau H, Gieskes L, Joffre F, et al. Percutaneous treatment of peripheral aneurysms with the Cragg EndoPro System. J Vasc Intervent Radiol 1996;7:35–39.
2. Pernes JM, Auguste MA, Hovasse D, Gignier P, Lasry B, Lasry JL. Long iliac stenosis: initial clinical experience with the Cragg endoluminal graft. Radiology 1995;196:67–71.
3. Mialhe C, Amicabile C, Becquemin J. Endovascular treatment of infrarenal abdominal aneurysms by the Stentor system: preliminary results of 79 cases. J Vasc Surg 1997;26:199–209.
4. Tsuchida H, Cameron BL, Marcus CS, Wilson SE. Modified polytetrafluoroethylene: indium 111-labeled platelet deposition on carbon-lined and high-porosity polytetrafluoroethylene grafts. J Vasc Surg 1992;16:643–649.
5. Babatasi G, Bara L, Galateau F, et al. An animal model for the evaluation of graft thrombosis in the acute phase on carbon-lined PTFE prosthesis. Int J Artif Organs 1994;17:643–650.
6. Dolmatch BL, Dong Y, Brennecke LH, Lieber ML. Evaluation of three polytetrafluoroethylene stent-grafts in a model of neointimal stenosis. J Vasc Intervent Radiol 1999;10(2)(suppl):253–254 (abstr.).
7. Fillinger MF, Reinitz ER, Schwartz RA, et al. Graft geometry and venous intimal-medial hyperplasia in arteriovenous loop grafts. J Vasc Surg 1990;11:556–566.
8. Coburn MC, Carney WJ. Comparison of basilic vein and polytetrafluoroethylene for brachial arteriovenous fistula. J Vasc Surg 1994;20:896–902.
9. Port FK. Morbidity and mortality in dialysis patients. Kidney Int 1994;46:1728–1737.
10. Cragg AH, Dake MD. Percutaneous femoropopliteal graft placement [see comments]. Radiology 1993;187:643–648.
11. Schwab S, Besarab A, Beathard G, et al. NKF-DOQI Clinical Practice Guidelines for Vascular Access. New York: National Kidney Foundation, 1997.
12. Isner JM. Vascular remodeling. Honey, I think I shrunk the artery [editorial; comment]. Circulation 1994;89:2937–2941.
13. Vorwerk D, Guenther RW, Mann H, et al. Venous stenosis and occlusion in hemodialysis shunts: follow-up results of stent placement in 65 patients. Radiology 1995;195:160–166.
14. Hoffer EK, Sultan S, Herskowitz MM, Daniels ID, Sclafani SJA. Prospective randomized trial of metallic intravascular stent in hemodialysis graft maintenance. J Vasc Intervent Radiol 1997;8:965–973.
15. Gray RJ. Percutaneous intervention for permanent hemodialysis access: a review. J Vasc Intervent Radiol 1997;8:313–327.
16. Lindenauer SM. The fabric vascular prosthesis. In: Rutherford RB, ed. Vascular Surgery. Philadelphia: WB Saunders, 1989:450–460.
17. Schurmann K, Vorwerk D, Kulisch A, Rosenbaum C, Biesterfeld S, Gunther RW. Puncture of stents implanted into veins and arteriovenous fistulas: an experimental study. Cardiovasc Intervent Radiol 1995;18:383–390.
18. Laborde JC, Parodi JC, Clem MF, et al. Intraluminal bypass of abdominal aortic aneurysm: feasibility study. Radiology 1992;184:185–190.
19. Piquet P, Rolland PH, Bartoli JM, Tranier P, Moulin G, Mercier C. Tantalum-Dacron co-knit stent for endovascular treatment of aortic aneurysms: a preliminary experimental study. J Vasc Surg 1994;19:698–706.
20. Criado E, Marston WA, Woosley JT, et al. An aortic aneurysm model for the evaluation of endovascular exclusion prosthesis. J Vasc Surg 1995;22:306–314.
21. Criado E, Marston WA, Reddick R, Woosley JT. Endothelial coverage of endovascular Dacron grafts in dogs [letter]. J Vasc Surg 1996;23:736–737.
22. Eton D, Warner D, Owens C, et al. Results of endoluminal grafting in an experimental aortic aneurysm model. J Vasc Surg 1996;23:819–829.
23. Schurmann K, Vorwerk D, Uppenkamp R, Klosterhalfen B, Bucker A, Gunther RW. Iliac arteries: plain and heparin-coated Dacron-covered stent-grafts compared with noncovered metal stents—an experimental study. Radiology 1997;203:55–63.
24. Golden MA, Hanson SR, Kirkman TR, Schneider PA, Clowes AW. Healing of polytetrafluoroethylene arterial grafts is influenced by graft porosity. J Vasc Surg 1990;11:838–844.
25. Harrison JH. Synthetic material as vascular prostheses II. A comparative study of Nylon, Dacron, Orlon, Ivalon sponge and Teflon in large blood vessels with tensile strength studies. Am J Surg 1958;95:16–24.
26. Greisler HP, Dennis JW, Endean ED, Ellinger J, Friesel R, Burgess W. Macrophage/biomaterial interactions: the stimulation of endothelialization. J Vasc Surg 1989;9:588–593.
27. Lincoff AM, Topol EJ, Chapekis AT, et al. Intracoronary stenting compared with conventional therapy for abrupt vessel closure complicating coronary angioplasty: a matched case-control study. J Am Coll Cardiol 1993;21:866–875.
28. Murphy JG, Schwartz RS, Edwards WD, Camrud AR, Vlietstra RE, Holmes DJ. Percutaneous polymeric stents in porcine coronary arteries. Initial experience with polyethylene terephthalate stents. Circulation 1992;86:1596–1604.
29. Holmes DR, Camrud AR, Jorgenson MA, Edwards WD, Schwartz RS. Polymeric stenting in the porcine coronary model: differential outcome of exogenous fibrin sleeves versus polyurethane-coated stents. J Am Coll Cardiol 1994;24:525–531.
30. Dake MD, Miller DC, Semba CP, Mitchell RS, Walker PJ, Liddell RP. Transluminal placement of endovascular stent-grafts for the treatment of descending thoracic aortic aneurysms. N Engl J Med 1994;331:1729–1734.
31. Vohra R, Drury JK, Shapiro D, Shenkin A, Pollock JG. Sealed versus unsealed knitted Dacron prostheses: a comparison of the acute phase protein response. Ann Vasc Surg 1987;1:548–551.
32. Lacroix H, Boel K, Nevelsteen A, Suy R. Early inflammatory response to gelatin- and collagen-sealed Dacron prostheses. Ann Vasc Surg 1995;9:152–154.
33. Ruiz CE, Zhang HP, Douglas JT, Zuppan CW, Kean CJ. A novel method for treatment of abdominal aortic aneurysms using percutaneous implantation of a newly designed endovascular device. Circulation 1995;91:2470–2477.
34. Sapoval MR, Gaux JC, Long AL, et al. Transient periprosthetic thickening after covered-stent implantation in the iliac artery. Am J Roentgenol 1995;164:1271–1273.
35. Sapoval MR, Turmel-Rodrigues LA, Raynaud AC, Bourquelot P, Rodrigue H, Gaux JC. Cragg covered stents in hemodialysis access: initial and mid term results. J Vasc Intervent Radiol 1996;7:335–342.
36. Blum U, Langer M, Spillner G, et al. Abdominal aortic aneurysms: preliminary technical and clinical results with transfemoral placement of endovascular self-expanding stent-grafts [see comments]. Radiology 1996;198:25–31.

treated for angioplasty-related rupture at the venous anastomosis of their graft. Stent-grafts were implanted for failure of balloon tamponade and/or Wallstent placement.[35] In all three cases, the stent-graft halted extravasation and maintained shunt patency. Follow-up in our three patients showed patency in two at a mean follow-up of 8.5 months. In the third case, the stent-graft was removed by the surgeon because of extensive local inflammation that was of concern for possible infection. No infection was found.

To summarize, rupture of a dialysis shunt during angioplasty should be managed conservatively, with initial balloon tamponade at low pressure. If there is persistent extravasation, Wallstent placement should be performed. Only when there is continued extravasation or when the degree of bleeding is pronounced should a stent-graft be placed. The best device that is available in Europe is the Passager, which has evoked inflammation in early work but now seems to be better tolerated, for unknown reasons. The Passager is also the device to use if treatment in the cannulation zone is required because it has a large mesh that allows it to be punctured.[45] However, the use of any device in the cannulation zone necessitates close monitoring because stent dislocation and recurrence of a pseudoaneurysm with associated skin ulceration have both been reported.[37]

■ Stent-Grafts for Dialysis Shunt Pseudoaneurysms

Most dialysis shunt pseudoaneurysms are not caused by angioplasty-related rupture but rather by bleeding from the cannulation site. These cannulation-related pseudoaneurysms are caused by disintegration of the synthetic graft material from repeated puncture, puncture with large needles, poor postdialysis compression, uremic platelet dysfunction, or typically a combination of these causes. Regardless of the etiology, all dialysis shunt pseudoaneurysms represent vascular ruptures, and are therefore unstable. But the ultimate decision to treat a pseudoaneurysm is based on its size, location, and the history of the angioaccess and of the patient. Treatment is mandated for any pseudoaneurysm that exhibits rapid growth, skin ulceration, rupture, or signs and symptoms of infection.

For the interventionalist who may be inclined to treat dialysis shunt pseudoaneurysms, two points are worth emphasizing. First, pseudoaneurysms are potentiated by outflow venous stenoses because these outflow lesions elevate the intrashunt pressure and increase the likelihood that bleeding will occur at the cannulation site or site of angioplasty rupture. A stenosis distal to the pseudoaneurysm should be identified and corrected, if possible. Second, the clinical examination is of utmost

importance prior to treating any pseudoaneurysm. The finding of infection or skin necrosis contraindicates any endovascular maneuvers and should prompt swift surgical treatment.

There has been a report of the successful treatment of dialysis shunt pseudoaneurysms with Wallstents in much the same way as these stents are used to treat acute ruptures.[43] This can be explained by the fact that the stent mesh of a Wallstent is tight and that fibrin and platelets can adhere to the stent struts and obstruct flow into the mouth of the pseudoaneurysm. This may lead to thrombosis of the pseudoaneurysm. It is logical, however, to propose covered stents in this setting. They have been used successfully,[35,37] but are not without secondary failure owing to repeated puncture of the stent-graft.[37] If possible, stent-graft placement in the cannulation zone should be avoided.

When possible, we prefer to wait several days following shunt declotting prior to placing a stent-graft across a pseudoaneurysm. In this way we are more comfortable that subclinical infection does not exist.

Finally, we believe that attempts should be made to avoid crossing collateral outflow pathways with stents or stent-grafts. Common pathways include the internal jugular vein (when placing a subclavian vein implant) and the cephalic vein (when placing an axillary vein implant). Although these suggestions may seem esoteric at this time, stent-grafts will undoubtedly become more available to the interventionalist for use in dialysis shunts in the near future. It will be important to appreciate the limitations of these devices as well as their successful applications.

■ Indications for Covered Stent Use and Future Developments

Based on our experience and a review of the published research and clinical series, covered stent implantation can be recommended in the following situations:

- Acute shunt rupture with failure of other methods to control bleeding
- Pseudoaneurysms, especially those distant from the cannulation zone
- Pseudoaneurysms not amenable to surgery, including those in the cannulation zone

Regarding treatment of stenoses, covered stent efficacy has not been adequately demonstrated with a large-enough series to recommend use for this application. Furthermore, experience is limited to the Passager stent-graft, a PET device that may have limited use because of graft-related inflammation and restenosis. However, it is possible that the modified Passager or other new devices will help solve the vexing issue of dialysis

shunt stenosis. To do this, the new stent-grafts will need to combine several characteristics. They will need to have low thrombogenicity, high biocompatibility (with little or no inflammatory potential), high hemocompatibility, good radial strength, flexibility, and a mechanism that prevents migration and dislodgment. Although the challenges are great, we believe that in the future stent-grafts will be used to treat angioaccess stenoses and prolong the useful life of many of these shunts.

REFERENCES

1. Rousseau H, Gieskes L, Joffre F, et al. Percutaneous treatment of peripheral aneurysms with the Cragg EndoPro System. J Vasc Intervent Radiol 1996;7:35–39.
2. Pernes JM, Auguste MA, Hovasse D, Gignier P, Lasry B, Lasry JL. Long iliac stenosis: initial clinical experience with the Cragg endoluminal graft. Radiology 1995;196:67–71.
3. Mialhe C, Amicabile C, Becquemin J. Endovascular treatment of infrarenal abdominal aneurysms by the Stentor system: preliminary results of 79 cases. J Vasc Surg 1997;26:199–209.
4. Tsuchida H, Cameron BL, Marcus CS, Wilson SE. Modified polytetrafluoroethylene: indium 111-labeled platelet deposition on carbon-lined and high-porosity polytetrafluoroethylene grafts. J Vasc Surg 1992;16:643–649.
5. Babatasi G, Bara L, Galateau F, et al. An animal model for the evaluation of graft thrombosis in the acute phase on carbon-lined PTFE prosthesis. Int J Artif Organs 1994;17:643–650.
6. Dolmatch BL, Dong Y, Brennecke LH, Lieber ML. Evaluation of three polytetrafluoroethylene stent-grafts in a model of neointimal stenosis. J Vasc Intervent Radiol 1999;10(2)(suppl):253–254 (abstr.).
7. Fillinger MF, Reinitz ER, Schwartz RA, et al. Graft geometry and venous intimal-medial hyperplasia in arteriovenous loop grafts. J Vasc Surg 1990;11:556–566.
8. Coburn MC, Carney WJ. Comparison of basilic vein and polytetrafluoroethylene for brachial arteriovenous fistula. J Vasc Surg 1994;20:896–902.
9. Port FK. Morbidity and mortality in dialysis patients. Kidney Int 1994;46:1728–1737.
10. Cragg AH, Dake MD. Percutaneous femoropopliteal graft placement [see comments]. Radiology 1993;187:643–648.
11. Schwab S, Besarab A, Beathard G, et al. NKF-DOQI Clinical Practice Guidelines for Vascular Access. New York: National Kidney Foundation, 1997.
12. Isner JM. Vascular remodeling. Honey, I think I shrunk the artery [editorial; comment]. Circulation 1994;89:2937–2941.
13. Vorwerk D, Guenther RW, Mann H, et al. Venous stenosis and occlusion in hemodialysis shunts: follow-up results of stent placement in 65 patients. Radiology 1995;195:160–166.
14. Hoffer EK, Sultan S, Herskowitz MM, Daniels ID, Sclafani SJA. Prospective randomized trial of metallic intravascular stent in hemodialysis graft maintenance. J Vasc Intervent Radiol 1997;8:965–973.
15. Gray RJ. Percutaneous intervention for permanent hemodialysis access: a review. J Vasc Intervent Radiol 1997;8:313–327.
16. Lindenauer SM. The fabric vascular prosthesis. In: Rutherford RB, ed. Vascular Surgery. Philadelphia: WB Saunders, 1989:450–460.
17. Schurmann K, Vorwerk D, Kulisch A, Rosenbaum C, Biesterfeld S, Gunther RW. Puncture of stents implanted into veins and arteriovenous fistulas: an experimental study. Cardiovasc Intervent Radiol 1995;18:383–390.
18. Laborde JC, Parodi JC, Clem MF, et al. Intraluminal bypass of abdominal aortic aneurysm: feasibility study. Radiology 1992;184:185–190.
19. Piquet P, Rolland PH, Bartoli JM, Tranier P, Moulin G, Mercier C. Tantalum-Dacron co-knit stent for endovascular treatment of aortic aneurysms: a preliminary experimental study. J Vasc Surg 1994;19:698–706.
20. Criado E, Marston WA, Woosley JT, et al. An aortic aneurysm model for the evaluation of endovascular exclusion prosthesis. J Vasc Surg 1995;22:306–314.
21. Criado E, Marston WA, Reddick R, Woosley JT. Endothelial coverage of endovascular Dacron grafts in dogs [letter]. J Vasc Surg 1996;23:736–737.
22. Eton D, Warner D, Owens C, et al. Results of endoluminal grafting in an experimental aortic aneurysm model. J Vasc Surg 1996;23:819–829.
23. Schurmann K, Vorwerk D, Uppenkamp R, Klosterhalfen B, Bucker A, Gunther RW. Iliac arteries: plain and heparin-coated Dacron-covered stent-grafts compared with noncovered metal stents—an experimental study. Radiology 1997;203:55–63.
24. Golden MA, Hanson SR, Kirkman TR, Schneider PA, Clowes AW. Healing of polytetrafluoroethylene arterial grafts is influenced by graft porosity. J Vasc Surg 1990;11:838–844.
25. Harrison JH. Synthetic material as vascular prostheses II. A comparative study of Nylon, Dacron, Orlon, Ivalon sponge and Teflon in large blood vessels with tensile strength studies. Am J Surg 1958;95:16–24.
26. Greisler HP, Dennis JW, Endean ED, Ellinger J, Friesel R, Burgess W. Macrophage/biomaterial interactions: the stimulation of endothelialization. J Vasc Surg 1989;9:588–593.
27. Lincoff AM, Topol EJ, Chapekis AT, et al. Intracoronary stenting compared with conventional therapy for abrupt vessel closure complicating coronary angioplasty: a matched case-control study. J Am Coll Cardiol 1993;21:866–875.
28. Murphy JG, Schwartz RS, Edwards WD, Camrud AR, Vlietstra RE, Holmes DJ. Percutaneous polymeric stents in porcine coronary arteries. Initial experience with polyethylene terephthalate stents. Circulation 1992;86:1596–1604.
29. Holmes DR, Camrud AR, Jorgenson MA, Edwards WD, Schwartz RS. Polymeric stenting in the porcine coronary model: differential outcome of exogenous fibrin sleeves versus polyurethane-coated stents. J Am Coll Cardiol 1994;24:525–531.
30. Dake MD, Miller DC, Semba CP, Mitchell RS, Walker PJ, Liddell RP. Transluminal placement of endovascular stent-grafts for the treatment of descending thoracic aortic aneurysms. N Engl J Med 1994;331:1729–1734.
31. Vohra R, Drury JK, Shapiro D, Shenkin A, Pollock JG. Sealed versus unsealed knitted Dacron prostheses: a comparison of the acute phase protein response. Ann Vasc Surg 1987;1:548–551.
32. Lacroix H, Boel K, Nevelsteen A, Suy R. Early inflammatory response to gelatin- and collagen-sealed Dacron prostheses. Ann Vasc Surg 1995;9:152–154.
33. Ruiz CE, Zhang HP, Douglas JT, Zuppan CW, Kean CJ. A novel method for treatment of abdominal aortic aneurysms using percutaneous implantation of a newly designed endovascular device. Circulation 1995;91:2470–2477.
34. Sapoval MR, Gaux JC, Long AL, et al. Transient periprosthetic thickening after covered-stent implantation in the iliac artery. Am J Roentgenol 1995;164:1271–1273.
35. Sapoval MR, Turmel-Rodrigues LA, Raynaud AC, Bourquelot P, Rodrigue H, Gaux JC. Cragg covered stents in hemodialysis access: initial and mid term results. J Vasc Intervent Radiol 1996;7:335–342.
36. Blum U, Langer M, Spillner G, et al. Abdominal aortic aneurysms: preliminary technical and clinical results with transfemoral placement of endovascular self-expanding stent-grafts [see comments]. Radiology 1996;198:25–31.

37. Hausegger KA, Tiessenhausen K, Klimpfinger M, Raith J, Hauser H, Tauss J. Aneurysms of hemodialysis access grafts: treatment with covered stents: a report of three cases. Cardiovasc Intervent Radiol 1998;21:334–337.

38. Farber A, Barbey MM, Grunert JH, Gmelin E. Access related venous stenosis and occlusions. Treatment with PTA and Dacron covered stents. Cardiovasc Intervent Radiol 1999; in press.

39. Quinn SF, Schuman ES, Demlow TA, et al. Percutaneous transluminal angioplasty versus endovascular stent placement in the treatment of venous stenoses in patients undergoing hemodialysis: intermediate results. J Vasc Interv Radiol 1995;6:851–855.

40. Turmel RL, Pengloan J, Blanchier D, et al. Insufficient dialysis shunts: improved long-term patency rates with close hemodynamic monitoring, repeated percutaneous balloon angioplasty, and stent placement. Radiology 1993;187:273–278.

41. Beathard GA. Percutaneous transvenous angioplasty in the treatment of vascular access stenosis. Kidney Int 1992;42:1390–1397.

42. Burger H, Kluchert BA, Kootstra G, Kitslaar PJ, Ubbink DT. Survival of arteriovenous fistulas and shunts for hemodialysis. Eur J Surg 1995;161:327–334.

43. Raynaud AC, Angel CY, Sapoval MR, Beyssen B, Pagny JY, Auguste M. Treatment of hemodialysis access rupture during PTA with Wallstent implantation. J Vasc Intervent Radiol 1998;9:437–442.

44. Funaki B, Szymski GX, Leef JA, Rosenblum JD, Burke R, Hackworth CA. Wallstent deployment to salvage dialysis graft thrombolysis complicated by venous rupture: early and intermediate results. Am J Roentgenol 1997;169:1435–1437.

45. Turmel RL, Blanchard D, Pengloan J, et al. Wallstents and Cragg-stents in hemodialysis grafts and fistulas: results for selective indications. J Vasc Intervent Radiol 1997;8:975–982.

12

Stent-Grafts in Transjugular Intrahepatic Portosystemic Shunt Procedures

ROBERT T. ANDREWS, RICHARD R. SAXON, JOSEF ROSCH, AND FREDERICK S. KELLER

In just over 10 years since its first clinical application, the transjugular intrahepatic portosystemic shunt (TIPS) or stented shunt (TIPSS) has become an established tool in the management of portal hypertension. Tens of thousands of TIPS procedures have been performed worldwide for the treatment of variceal hemorrhage, refractory ascites, or Budd-Chiari syndrome.[1–4] In experienced hands, the minimally invasive procedure can be accomplished in under an hour, using conscious sedation, with little or no blood loss. Technical success rates are excellent: a shunt is established in close to 100% of patients, with portal pressure reduced by an average of 24 mm Hg, and portosystemic pressure gradients reduced by 50%. Immediate cessation of acute variceal hemorrhage is seen in over 90% of patients, and progressive improvement in ascites is seen in over 60%. Symptoms, particularly variceal bleeding, recur in less than 20% of patients whose shunts remain viable. Procedural mortality is less than 2%, and morbidity is also low; elective patients are frequently discharged from the hospital within 2 days.

Surgical shunting, the historic "gold standard" for correcting portal hypertension, has greater procedural morbidity and mortality than TIPS, especially for patients in Child-Pugh class C.[5–7] In addition, surgical portosystemic shunts are more likely than TIPS to complicate subsequent liver transplantation.[8,9] Sclerotherapy and banding are endoscopic techniques for the control of variceal hemorrhage, but are ineffective in up to 20% of patients with acute bleeding. Several studies have also shown TIPS to be more effective than endoscopic alternatives in the prevention of rebleeding.[10–13] Furthermore, sclerotherapy is associated

with induced hemorrhage from mucosal ulceration, and both endoscopic procedures are difficult or impossible in patients with gastric varices. Serial paracentesis provides symptomatic relief from ascites refractory to medical therapy, but must be repeated frequently—sometimes on a weekly basis.[14,15] Neither the endoscopic techniques nor serial paracentesis addresses the underlying portal hypertension.

While the TIPS procedure can be safer and more efficacious than alternative treatments, it is limited by the need for periodic revision. Large studies, using different morphological and/or hemodynamic criteria, have reported shunt dysfunction in up to 85% of patients within 1 year.[1–4] Fortunately, these patients are rarely symptomatic; recurrent variceal bleeding is seen in just 25% of patients with anatomic TIPS stenosis.[1,16] Stenotic or occluded TIPS shunts are readily treated by balloon angioplasty or additional stent placement, and these interventions can achieve long-term assisted patency rates of over 90%. Although such efforts can be costly, are invasive, and require careful monitoring of the shunt by Doppler ultrasound or venography,[17–19] TIPS must currently be viewed as a multistage procedure.

The processes leading to TIPS dysfunction have been studied in detail, with no fewer than eight publications devoted to TIPS histology.[20–27] These examinations have identified an underlying set of pathophysiological processes that might be controlled by applying a semipermeable covering to the stent in the intrahepatic tract and draining hepatic vein. With this control achieved, long-term primary TIPS patency appears to be feasible. Following a review of the TIPS technique, this chapter addresses the anatomy, physiology, and histology of TIPS, and both the potential and realized impacts of TIPS stent-grafts.

■ TIPS Technique

The process of TIPS creation is discussed in detail elsewhere.[28] Briefly, using jugular access, the operator uses a long sheath-needle to establish intrahepatic communication between hepatic and portal vein branches, the parenchymal tract is dilated, and a vascular stent is deployed from the portal vein to the hepatic vein (Fig. 12–1). The procedure establishes a direct conduit from the high-pressure portal vein to the systemic circulation, thus providing a route for portosystemic decompression.

In most cases, the stent is initially dilated to 8 or 10 mm. Direct portal and right atrial pressures are then

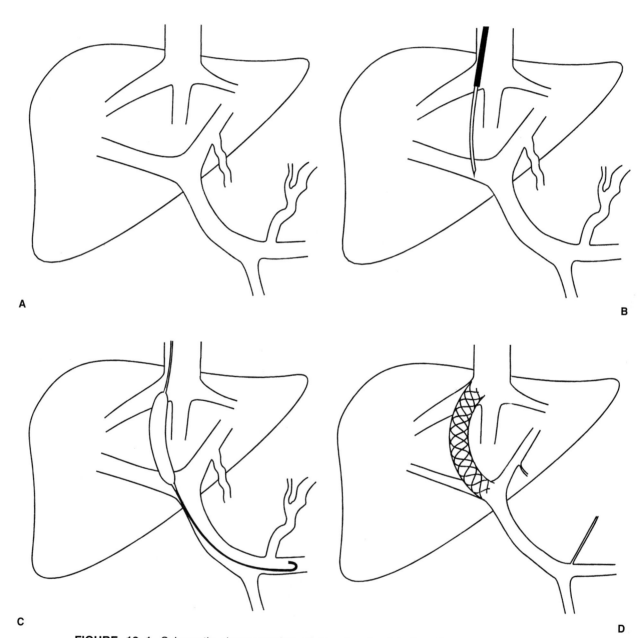

FIGURE 12–1. Schematic demonstration of transjugular intrahepatic portosystemic shunt (TIPS) creation. (**A**). Untreated portal hypertension results in a dilated (variceal) coronary vein and recanalized umbilical vein. (**B**). A transjugular sheath-needle is used to access the right portal vein from the right hepatic vein. (**C**). The parenchymal tract is dilated. (**D**). A stent is deployed to maintain shunt patency. Note decompression of the coronary and umbilical veins.

recorded, and a portosystemic gradient (PSG) calculated. Most authors consider a gradient of 10 to 15 mm Hg appropriate.[29,30] If the gradient is too high, symptoms may persist. If it is too low, the risk of hepatic encephalopathy is increased. The initial gradient can be reduced by dilating the shunt to a larger diameter or placing a second, parallel TIPS, and can be increased by the use of a constrained stent or other flow-limiting device introduced coaxially. Several constraining mechanisms have been described.[31,32,33]

A successful TIPS results in the arrest of variceal bleeding, prophylaxis against rebleeding, and the control of ascites. As indicated above, the recurrence of symptoms in patients with patent TIPSs is unusual. Thus, when rebleeding or an increase in ascites is seen, TIPS dysfunction should be suspected.

■ TIPS Dysfunction: Definition and Etiology

TIPS dysfunction must be distinguished from shunt-related complications. The latter, which are also seen after surgical shunting, include hepatic encephalopathy, right heart failure, and a deterioration of hepatic function.[1–3] These outcomes are ironically reflective of a TIPS that is working "too well," shunting blood from the portal system at rate in excess of that which can be tolerated by the patient. This chapter considers the opposite situation—loss of shunt patency, with inadequate shunt function.

In keeping with the classical surgical literature, primary patency is defined as the period from TIPS placement to shunt occlusion or the development of a significant stenosis. By the most stringent morphological and hemodynamic criteria, a significant stenosis is one that reduces the shunt diameter by 50%, increases the portosystemic gradient above 15 mm Hg, or causes decreased flow velocity by Doppler ultrasound, even if the presenting symptoms do not recur. Assisted patency is that period between initial shunt revision (by whatever means) and irreversible occlusion of the shunt. The period of assisted patency may encompass numerous revisions.

The etiology of TIPS dysfunction correlates strongly with the postprocedure time course.[16–18] Immediate occlusion is frequently the result of technical error. Most often, the stent is too short or is malpositioned, failing to bridge the entire parenchymal tract. Short-term failure (hours to days) is usually caused by acute thrombosis, and may be associated with biliary injury (see below). Mid-term and long-term dysfunctions, by comparison, are almost always the result of progressive stenosis within the parenchymal tract or the recipient hepatic vein. Such stenoses are an integral part of the biological response to

TIPS, and not under the direct control of the operator. It is by preventing or containing these responses that stent-grafts may serve to increase the primary patency of TIPS.

■ Anatomic and Physiological Considerations

TIPS has many features in common with other endovascular procedures. By disrupting the native vascular environment, angioplasty and/or stent placement incite a multifactorial process involving both physical and biological events. The normal response of arteries and veins to such perturbations has been extensively studied, and the prevailing theory can be summarized as follows: (1) injury to vascular endothelium occurs during dilatation; (2) the resulting surface irregularity and exposure of basement tissues induce platelet deposition; (3) platelet-derived growth factor (PDGF) and injury-mediated reparative processes induce the migration of synthetic smooth muscle cells (SMCs) into the thrombus; (4) the

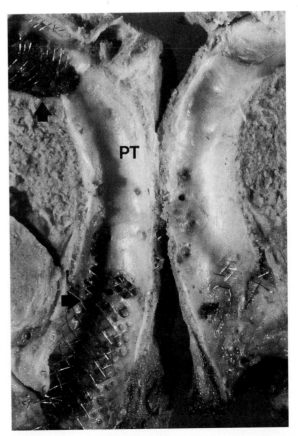

FIGURE 12–2. Longitudinal section of an explanted TIPS shunt (viewed in a posteroanterior projection). The stent is incompletely endothelialized in areas that spanned the hepatic and portal lumina (arrows). There is a smooth neointima covering the stent in the parenchymal tract (PT).

SMCs elaborate a protein matrix, creating an organized, stable neointima; and (5) the neointima is covered by a smooth layer of endothelium.[34–36] The eventual thickness of the neointimal layer varies directly with the degree of vascular injury and initial thrombus deposition.[37–41] When excessive, the process is known as neointimal hyperplasia (NH).

Stent placement further alters the endovascular environment, and may increase NH.[38,42] As foreign material, exposed stents are a site for platelet aggregation. Stent struts at the luminal aspect of the vascular wall also disturb laminar flow, creating eddy currents that further enhance platelet deposition.[43,44] The ongoing radial force generated by stents may exaggerate and prolong injury-mediated responses. In addition, the presence of a stent reduces vascular wall compliance. Some authors have suggested an inverse relationship between wall compliance and NH development, but the issue is debated in the literature.[45–49]

The TIPS shunt is an anatomically unique structure (Fig. 12–2), and physiological responses occurring within it vary significantly by location. In the portal and hepatic veins, the TIPS extends into an essentially normal vascular structure. The parenchymal tract, by contrast, is an internally scaffolded hepatic laceration with no native vascular endothelium. At both ends of the parenchymal tract, the stent passes through the disrupted vessel wall and crosses the vascular lumen. An understanding of the processes in each area of the shunt is imperative for the successful application of TIPS stent-grafts.

Portal Vein

At the portal end of a TIPS, interactions between the stent and vein are the dominant feature. The stent produces continuous radial force against the vein wall, reducing portal vein compliance and presenting an irregular foreign surface. However, there is little endothelial disruption, and vascular injury is insignificant. NH in the portal vein is consequently minimized, and the stent is rapidly covered by a thin, smooth neointima. Hemodynamically significant stenoses in the portal vein are exceedingly rare, occurring in fewer than 1% of patients.[16]

Hepatic Vein

Within the recipient hepatic vein, the usual responses described above are compounded by vascular trauma and by nonphysiological hemodynamic factors. The hepatic vein

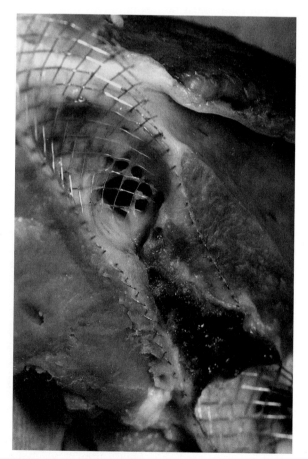

FIGURE 12–4. Longitudinal section of a TIPS stent at the level of the hepatic vein lumen. Note incomplete cellular coverage of the stent, with preservation of the native vascular channel. The triangular area of dark material represents bile staining in the stenotic parenchymal tract.

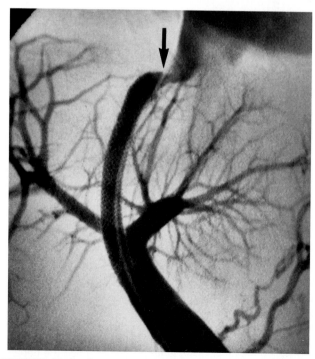

FIGURE 12–3. Stenosis at the hepatic venous outflow (arrow) in an otherwise patent TIPS.

may experience significant injury during TIPS creation, especially if the multiple needle passes are required to establish portal access. In addition, the vessel may be smaller in native diameter than is the final shunt, necessitating overdilatation of the vein. Once established, a TIPS significantly elevates blood flow velocity, volume, and pressure in the hepatic vein. Furthermore, inflow is directed toward the superior aspect of the vein above the shunt, resulting in a "jet effect" against the vessel wall. This small but continuous jet may result in mild but chronic injury. As a result of these factors, hemodynamically significant stenoses in the recipient hepatic vein are common, and their frequency increases with time (Fig. 12–3).

Transition Zones

As the TIPS stent exits the parenchymal tract and enters the portal and hepatic vein, it arches across the vascular lumen like a sieve. Examinations of TIPS stents and other stents placed across vascular branch points show a thin layer of neointima on the transluminal stent mesh, with flow maintained through the interstices (Fig. 12–4).[50,51] A classical TIPS, therefore, is a partial shunt; blood can flow through the TIPS or, by passing through the open mesh of the bare stent, through the normal course of the portal or hepatic veins. The degree of shunting varies inversely with the portosystemic gradient. Hemolysis can be seen in some cases, with cellular elements being damaged by the mesh, but it is uncommon for this process to reach clinical significance.[52]

Parenchymal Tract

In contrast to venous portions of the shunt, where endothelial disruption is minimal, blood flowing through the parenchymal tract is exposed on all sides to bare, severely injured liver parenchyma. The coagulation cascade is strongly activated. In addition, liver parenchyma protrudes irregularly through the interstices of the stent, reducing luminal diameter and creating an undulating surface that may further disrupt laminar flow.[20,23,25,53] These factors, possibly exaggerated by minimal wall compliance in the fibrotic liver, may increase the initial deposition of thrombus in the parenchymal portion of the

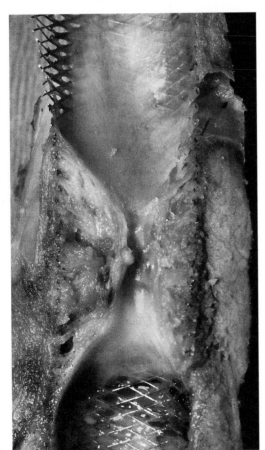
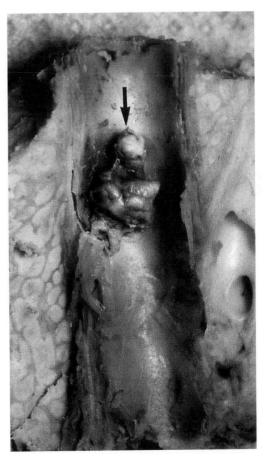

A   B

FIGURE 12–5. Longitudinal sections showing parenchymal tract stenosis. **(A)**. Diffuse narrowing involving the entire tract. **(B)**. Focal nodular stenosis (arrow) in a patient with a bile leak (not shown).

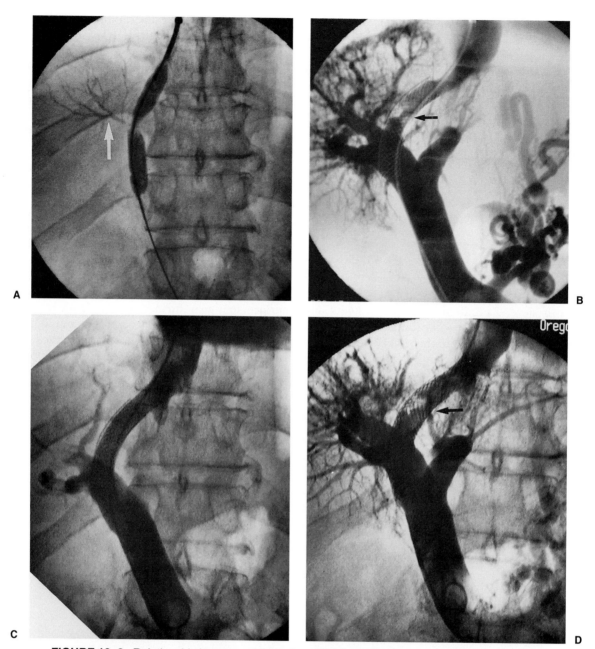

FIGURE 12–6. Relationship between a bile leak and TIPS dysfunction. (**A**). A bile leak was present at the time of initial TIPS creation, but was not recognized. (**B**). The patient returned with persistent ascites 3 months later, and was found to have a focal stenosis at the site of biliary injury (arrow). (**C**). Placement of a second stent gave an excellent angiographic result and reduced the portosystemic gradient from 23 to 12 mm Hg. (**D**). An identical restenosis (arrow) was present 1 month later, on venography performed after abnormal ultrasound.

shunt. As indicated above, greater thrombus deposition is associated with a more exuberant proliferative response. Because the parenchymal tract has no natural intimal covering, the reactive covering of the tract is referred to as pseudointima rather than neointima.

A high percentage of TIPS stenoses occur in the parenchymal tract, usually in the midterm (from a few days to 6 months) (Fig. 12–5). In the earlier period, the of-

fending material is thrombus, evolving in a continuum to hyperplastic pseudointima in the later period. The distribution of material may be diffuse or strikingly focal. Interestingly, if thrombus or pseudointimal hyperplasia recur after successful treatment of these stenoses by angioplasty or stent placement, the recurrence location in over 80% of patients is identical to that seen initially (Fig. 12–6).[16] In such cases, patients may require

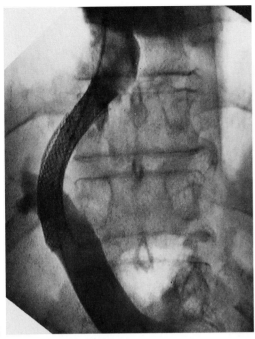

FIGURE 12–6. continued (E). A covered stent-graft was placed, and the patient has remained patent over the subsequent follow-up period of 9 months.

frequent revisions of the same site. While the specific nature of this process has not been definitively elucidated, biliary duct injury is strongly suspected by many authors as a contributing factor.

■ The Effect of Biliary Secretions

In addition to exposing bare liver parenchyma, the TIPS procedure creates macro- and microscopic biliary-vascular fistulae. Several authors have shown gross biliary-to-TIPS communication with venography, cholangiography, or the use of a specially designed dual-occlusion balloon (Fig. 12–7). Bile staining is commonly identified during the gross evaluation of explanted TIPS,[21–27] and histological examination often identifies encroachment of metaplastic biliary endothelium into the pseudointimal covering of the parenchymal tract.[22,23,54] In some cases the biliary endothelium forms neoducts or cysts. In others, it spreads through the pseudointima to form a biliary endothelial lining on the luminal surface of the TIPS shunt (Fig. 12–8). The endothelium is functional despite its ectopic location, and releases biliary secretions into the shunt.

LaBerge et al,[21] in 1993, were the first to suggest a correlation between biliary extravasation and pseudointimal proliferation. In a study of five stenotic or occluded TIPS, transected bile ducts and bile-stained pseudoin-

tima were identified in three (Fig. 12–9). LaBerge et al attributed the shunt failures to pseudointimal hyperplasia, and suggested that the hyperplasia was an inflammatory response stimulated by bile.

Subsequent reports have supported the relationship between biliary injury and pseudointimal hyperplasia. Jalan et al[23] studied 34 TIPS patients, and percutaneously biopsied the pseudointima of eight patients with stenoses greater than 70%. Four of these samples had bile staining, and two demonstrated incorporated biliary endothelium. Histological study of 10 explanted livers revealed four with mild or severe (>70%) stenosis. Biliary transections and bile staining were present in all four cases, and the authors reported a correlation between the degree of stenosis and the size of the transected duct. No stenoses were seen in the absence of bile staining. The authors agreed with LaBerge et al that an inflammatory response induced by bile was a significant contributing factor in shunt failure.

Saxon et al[22] reported similar findings but offered a slightly different explanation. They described comparative studies of TIPS histology in 13 swine and 21 human patients. Severe shunt compromise (occlusion or stenosis greater than 75%) was identified within the parenchymal tracts of nine porcine and eight human shunts. "Substantial" biliary fistulae were present in seven of the stenotic shunts from each group (77 and 88%, respectively). The associated pseudointimal hyperplasia was notable for invasion by metaplastic bile ducts containing active, mucin-secreting goblet cells (Fig. 12–10). In contrast, no evidence of significant biliary communication was found in two porcine and 13 human shunts that were widely patent at follow-up. The authors concluded that biliary duct injury was strongly associated with abnormalities in the parenchymal tract, and with TIPS failure. Unlike LaBerge et al and Jalan et al, however, Saxon et al suggested that the causative agent of shunt failure might be mucin, which is highly thrombogenic.[55,56] They postulated that exuberant mucin-induced thrombus might provide a physically larger matrix for subsequent ingrowth and hyperplasia of granulation tissue.

The mucin theory was supported by Teng et al.[26] In an in vitro study, they exposed cultured aortic smooth muscle cells to varying concentrations of bile, and found that SMC activity, as measured by the production of deoxyribonucleic acid (DNA) and protein, was significantly decreased at bile concentrations of 1% or greater. With concentrations of 2.5% or greater, 100% SMC mortality was observed within 3 days. In a concurrent in vivo study in 45 swine, the group found no significant correlation between bile leaks (seen in 13 animals) and neointimal thickness within the involved shunt. The authors concluded that bile does not cause NH, and may in fact be protective against the process. Like Saxon et al, Teng et al implicated mucin as the responsible agent.

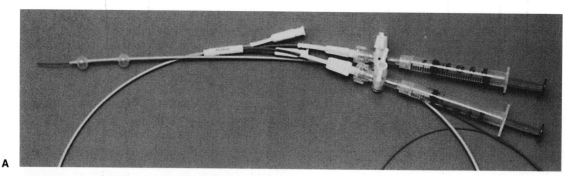

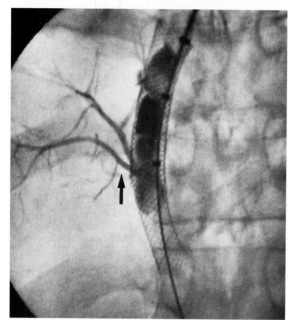

FIGURE 12–7. Dual-occlusion balloon. (**A**). This proprietary device consists of two balloons on opposite sides of an infusion port. (**B**). By excluding both inflow and outflow from a segment of the TIPS shunt, the device can be used to demonstrate an occult bile fistula (arrow).

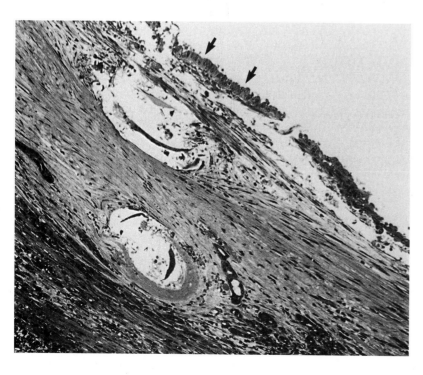

FIGURE 12–8. Photomicrograph of the lumen of a TIPS shunt, showing metaplastic biliary endothelium lining the shunt surface (arrows).

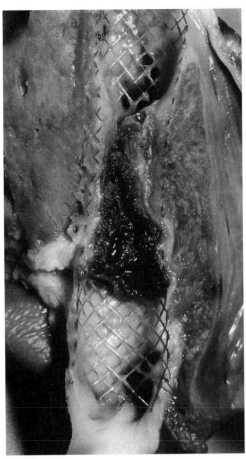

FIGURE 12–9. Dark staining of a stenotic TIPS shunt by bile pigments.

■ The Role of Stent-Grafts

Whether bile, mucin, or another as-yet-unknown agent or process is responsible for pseudointimal hyperplasia, it appears that the chances for long-term primary patency in TIPS would be improved by minimizing biliary contamination and reducing parenchymal injury. This would require great care and several modifications to the basic TIPS procedure. Careful imaging of the portal vein before and during parenchymal needle puncture might reduce the number of needle passes required to establish the shunt. It might also allow a more directed puncture, with a shorter tract and reduced chances for ductal transgression. After the tract is established, but before stent placement, major duct injury could be excluded using cholangiography, venography, or a dual-occlusion balloon. If a biliary injury is identified, the tract could be abandoned and a new site chosen. Such procedures, unfortunately, would be time-consuming, might require numerous tracts to be established and then abandoned, and would not exclude the presence of microscopic fistulae. Nor would such a process protect the hepatic vein from flow-related neointimal hyperplasia.

The application of a semipermeable covering to the TIPS stent is a promising alternative mechanism for controlling or eliminating stenoses in a TIPS shunt. A stent-graft physically separates flowing blood from exposed liver parenchyma and biliary secretions, while reducing the irregular protrusions of tissue through the stent struts. By so doing, the stent-graft may reduce

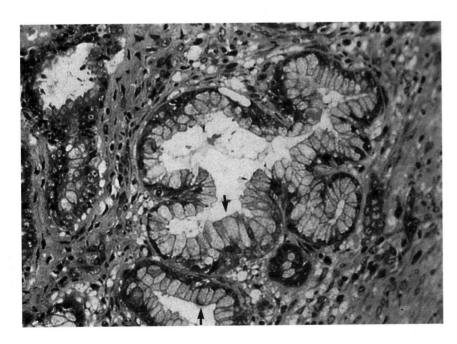

FIGURE 12–10. Photomicrograph of pseudointima showing goblet cells (arrows), which are actively producing thrombogenic mucin.

psudointimal hyperplasia by excluding biliary secretions, preventing direct migration of SMCs or pluripotential precursors from the liver, and providing a smoother, more regular surface area. In addition, the presence of a covering shields the hepatic vein from blood jetting through the top of the shunt. Such shielding might reduce neointimal hyperplasia in the hepatic vein by decreasing chronic injury-mediated processes.

■ Experimental and Clinical Stent-Graft Results

Animal Studies

Although TIPS stent-grafts had been considered for some time, it was not until 1995 that Nishimine et al[57] reported the first animal studies. Using a stent-graft comprised of expanded polytetrafluoroethylene (ePTFE) supported by Z-stents (Cook, Inc., Bloomington, IN)

and a Wallstent (Boston Scientific Vascular, Watertown, MA) (Fig. 12–11), the group placed covered TIPS in 13 swine, and compared their patency to bare-stent TIPS in the same number of control animals. Only one bare-stent TIPS (8%) remained patent at average follow-up of 3.6 weeks (±2.7). The control shunts were occluded in nine animals (69%), and had significant stenoses (50% or greater) in three others (23%). By comparison, six stent-grafts (46%) remained patent at an average follow-up interval of 7.8 weeks (±4.3). Of four others (31%) with significant stenoses, three were located in the uncovered hepatic vein and only one in the parenchymal tract. The latter occurred in a portion of the tract not fully covered by graft material. Biliary extravasation was found in two stent-grafts, only one of which was occluded. The biliary leak in the occluded stent-graft arose in a short, uncovered region of the parenchymal tract near the portal vein. In the patent stent-graft, bile was identified between the graft material and the parenchyma, but was excluded from contact with flowing blood.

Haskal et al[58] reported similar results in swine using a "boxcar" arrangement of Palmaz stents (Cordis Corp., Johnson and Johnson Interventional Systems, Warren, NJ) encapsulated by ePTFE (Fig. 12–12). Seven of eight stent-grafts remained patent over the 5-month study period, with one being occluded by the ingrowth of fibrous tissue from the hepatic vein. In contrast, only one of four bare stents in control animals remained patent at 6 weeks. One was occluded, and two others had significant stenoses (greater than 50%) in the parenchymal tract. Histologically, the authors found all of the stent-grafts to be surrounded by a thick layer of synthetic SMCs in a

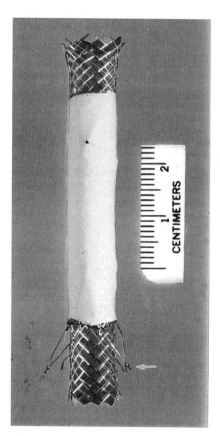

FIGURE 12–11. The stent-graft employed by Nishimine and Saxon. The device consists of a 4-cm length of polytetrafluoroethylene (PTFE) supported by two Z-stents. Radial force is supplied by a coaxially placed Wallstent. In this design, a third Z-stent with a distal flare is placed at the distal end of the graft (arrow), and is used to localize the portal vein wall.

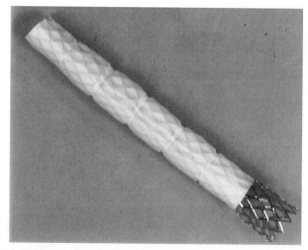

FIGURE 12–12. The "boxcar" stent-graft used by Haskal. This device consists of a series of Palmaz stents that are fully encapsulated by PTFE. The device can be cut to appropriate length by removing individual stent bodies.

collagen matrix. They indicated that this tissue was identical in appearance to that seen enveloping the bare stents of the control animals. Interestingly, no cases of bile staining or biliary duct proliferation were noted.

Haskal and Zaetta[59] reported good outcomes using ePTFE over a nitinol stent. Although this study was small (four stent-grafts and three controls), and has yet to be published, it found a reduced degree of stenosis among stent-graft animals (16%, n = 3) versus controls (59%, n = 3) at 60 days. One stent-graft animal had a late stenosis of 43%, which was attributed to incomplete tract coverage.

In contrast to the successes encountered with ePTFE-covered stent-grafts, those covered with other materials have fared poorly. Tanihata et al[60] used commercially available silicone-covered Wallstents to create TIPS shunts in 14 swine. Twelve shunts (86%) were occluded by thrombus at 3 weeks, and both patent shunts had stenoses greater than 50%. By 6 weeks, all shunts had occluded. Bloch et al[61] had almost identical results with polyurethane-coated, Dacron-covered Z-stents in six swine. Five (83%) were occluded by thrombus at 3 weeks, and all were occluded at 6 weeks. Haskal,[62] who covered Wallstents in polyethylene terephthalate (PET) in eight swine TIPS, found no advantage of the device over bare Wallstents stents in five controls. Histological evaluation revealed an exaggerated inflammatory response in all 28 stent-graft animals reported by these three authors.

Human Experience

Credit for the first published human application of a TIPS stent-graft belongs to Cohen et al,[63] who in 1996 reported using an ePTFE-covered Palmaz stent to treat a patient with early occlusion and a documented biliary fistula. At venography 2 months later, the shunt was widely patent, and the patient was asymptomatic throughout the reported clinical follow-up period of 4 months. Three additional case reports of stent-grafting have also been presented, describing improved TIPS patency in three patients and cessation of bleeding from portal lacerations in two others.[64–66]

The first prospective human trials of TIPS stent-grafts were reported by Saxon et al[67] in 1997. In their original series of six cases, Saxon et al treated patients with recurrent occlusion or parenchymal tract stenosis using a modified version of the ePTFE stent-graft that Saxon and Nishimine had developed in animals (Fig. 12–11). Patients had averaged 3.2 TIPS revisions prior to being enrolled, with 12 total episodes of recurrent variceal bleeding or ascites. Prior to stent-graft placement, the average primary patency in these patients had been 50 days (range 9–100). The average assisted patency had been 53 days (range 1–180). After stent-grafting, the primary patency in five patients averaged 229 days (range 27–324) (one patient who was critically ill at the time of stent-graft placement died of multiorgan system failure 6 days later, before repeat venography). More importantly, with a mean clinical follow-up period of 290 days (range 6–384), none of the five patients had a recurrence of ascites or variceal bleeding.

Long-term outcomes of this patient group have not yet been published, but were available to us for review. Three of the stent-grafts were still primarily patent at the time of liver transplantation, at an average of 577 days (±84). Another was primarily patent on last follow-up at 846 days. The fifth patient had been found on follow-up venography at 176 days to have an asymptomatic parenchymal tract stenosis of 70%. Double-occlusion venography detected an occult bile fistula, and a second stent-graft was placed. The revised shunt was secondarily patent on last follow-up at 579 days (755 days total). This patient had a recurrence of ascites, but no other cases of recurrent symptoms have been noted.

In another as-yet-unpublished study, the same group of researchers placed de novo stent-grafts into eight patients undergoing initial TIPS creation.[68] The device was identical to that used by Nishimine and Saxon in swine. Seven of the eight shunts (88%) remained primarily patent when evaluated a mean of 324 days after TIPS (range 137–460); five were patent at transplantation, the sixth at autopsy (this patient died 326 days after TIPS from complications of a cholecystectomy); and the seventh at the most recent venography, 460 days after TIPS creation. Only one of eight patients (13%) developed a stenosis, and this was in the hepatic vein outflow 127 days after TIPS. The patient underwent percutaneous transluminal angioplasty (PTA) without additional stent placement. A follow-up ultrasound performed at 227 days showed asymptomatic slow flow through the shunt, but the patient refused venography. She died of progressive hepatic failure 2 days later, and the family refused autopsy.

The only other published prospective trial of TIPS stent-grafts is that of Ferral et al.[69] The group used the PET covered Cragg Endopro stent (Mintec, Bahamas) to create de novo stent-graft TIPS in 13 patients. Two patients, both of whom were critically ill at the time of TIPS placement, died within 1 week, and another died at 4 months of hepatic failure. The shunt was patent on autopsy in one case (24 hours), but was not reported in the other two. Among the remaining patients, there were two occlusions (at 2 and 3 months), one of which could not be recanalized. The second was attributed to a kink in the portal end of the stent, and was successfully revised with balloon dilatation. The primary patency of surviving patients at 6 months was 77%, with secondary patency of 92%.

In summarizing the experimental and clinical data, several significant points can be made. First, it seems clear that stent-grafts have the potential for reducing interventions for those TIPS patients who have had recurrent stenosis in the parenchymal tract. Second, it is likely that this improvement is due to the exclusion of biliary secretions, SMCs, or some other as-yet-undetermined agent from the shunt. Third, even when the parenchymal tract is completely covered, and thus protected from pseudointimal hyperplasia, stenosis of the hepatic vein outflow remains problematic. Fourth, materials used in the construction of the stent-graft have a significant impact upon TIPS patency.

■ Stent-Graft Positioning

The length of a stent-graft in TIPS is critical to its success. As indicated by the above experiences, failure to fully cover the entire parenchymal tract and hepatic venous outflow will increase the likelihood of new or recurrent stenosis. Of course, carrying the graft all the way to the inferior vena cava (IVC) will necessarily result in occlusion of the normal outflow from the recipient hepatic vein, but the surgical literature indicates that segmental hepatic venous occlusion is inconsequential.[70,71] In any case, hepatic vein stenosis or occlusion complicating a bare-stent TIPS creates a physiologically identical situation. Thus, most authors agree that the theoretical (and unsupported) risk of segmental hepatic vein occlusion by a stent-graft is more than balanced by the benefit of improved shunt patency.

Excessive stent-graft length should also be avoided. Most patients, even those with severe portal hypertension, derive significant hepatic oxygenation from the portal vein. In addition, antegrade flow through the portal provides "first-pass" clearance of toxins absorbed by the mesenteric venous system. A covered graft extending to the main portal would exclude parenchymal portal branches, thus increasing the likelihood of both hepatic ischemia and encephalopathy after TIPS. (These risk are lower in patients with baseline reversal of portal flow, as they have already been forced to compensate for the loss of parenchymal inflow.)

Any TIPS stent—bare or covered—that extends into the main portal vein or the IVC can complicate liver transplantation by making venous clamp placement and transection difficult or impossible.[72–75] The ideally configured and positioned stent-graft, then, would have a bare anchoring segment in the portal system (not extending into the main portal), and a covered segment spanning the entire distance from portal wall to the IVC.

Nishimine and Saxon positioned their de novo stent-grafts by placing a flared Z-stent at the portal end of the covered segment.[57,67] They deployed this stent in the main portal, and then withdrew the entire device while observing the flare fluoroscopically. When the flared stent reached the portal puncture site, the flare began to compress. At this point, withdrawal was discontinued and the stent fully deployed. Saxon used a modification of this device for his study of stent-grafts placed during TIPS revision; because he could use in-situ stents to provide a real-time reference to the portal vein wall, the flared stent was unnecessary for accurate positioning of the distal graft. Saxon directly measured tract and hepatic vein lengths by kinking a guidewire and then selected a graft of appropriate length (1-cm increments were available from 4 to 7 cm).

Like Nishimine and Saxon, Ferral et al[69] used a device of predetermined length. They chose among 3-, 6-, and 10-cm-long stent-grafts by observing the distance between waists on their balloon during predilatation of the parenchymal tract. Positioning was based on contrast injections through the delivery sheath.

Haskal et al[58] used a direct portal venogram to identify the portal and hepatic vein puncture sites, and made direct measurements of the tract length using the kinked-guidewire technique. Their device could be modified to approximate the desired length by cutting away individual stents from the "boxcar" device. Each stent body was 12 mm in length. The entire device was then positioned and deployed by referencing the portogram.

■ Stent-Graft Design

The ideal stent-graft for TIPS applications should have a low profile, be easily delivered over a guidewire, be flexible enough to accommodate the natural curve of a TIPS tract, and have adequate radial force to resist parenchymal recoil. In addition, the device should either be capable of length adjustment (to accommodate tracts of varying lengths) or be inexpensive enough to allow a full range of predetermined lengths to be maintained on hand. Finally, there must be a mechanism for indicating point of transition from bare to covered stent at the caudal (portal) end of the stent-graft.

Stent Features

The stents most commonly employed in TIPS have been the Wallstent and the Palmaz stent.[1] Both are bare metal designs, with an open-mesh configuration in the deployed state.[76,77] The Wallstent has superior flexibility[78] and conforms easily to the curved tract generated during TIPS creation. The original Palmaz, by comparison, is inflexible, requiring a straighter, more central tract (newer designs of this device, now commercially available, may overcome the flexibility problems of the original). The Palmaz has higher radial force than the Wallstent[78] and may provide better long-term patency.[79] In addition, the Palmaz stent can easily be dilated beyond its original size, while the Wallstent has a predetermined maximal diameter. Thus, the Palmaz device facilitates fine-tuning of the shunt diameter to achieve the desired portosystemic gradient. Other open-mesh stent designs have been used in TIPS with mixed success, but the number of cases is small.[1,53,80,81] None has offered a clear advantage over the stents discussed above.

Graft Material

As in other locations, the graft material used for TIPS stent-grafts must be biologically stable and biocompatible. The lack of significant inflammatory response is particularly important, given the moderate diameter of the shunt and the relatively rigid tissue surrounding it. If the graft material generates a vigorous inflammatory or thrombogenic response, there is simply no space in which to accommodate it while maintaining luminal flow. Graft permeability is also critical in TIPS. The material must be capable of excluding both cellular elements (metaplastic biliary endothelium, SMCs) and fluids (bile, mucin) from the shunt lumen.

Several graft materials are available in a configuration that allows bonding or suturing to a stent.[82,83] ePTFE has had the greatest use in both animal and human TIPS trials and has provided the best shunt patency.[57,58,67] Presumably, this success is due to the relatively low level of inflammation induced by ePTFE and its low permeability. Silicone, though less permeable than PTFE, incites a significant biological response, resulting in primary thrombosis.[60] PET, commonly known as Dacron, can be woven or knitted. In both forms, however, its permeability is greater than that of PTFE. In addition, PET incites an aggressive inflammatory response similar to that of silicone. Another material, polyurethane (PU), has excellent biocompatibility, but is not stable over long periods. A modified form, polycarbonate polyurethane (PCPU), is both biocompatible and stable. It has been postulated that a composite of PCPU-PET would combine the biocompatibility of PCPU with the structural support of PET. The results of Bloch et al,[61] however, suggest that such may not be the case in TIPS applications. A new material, yet to be tested on a large scale, is collagen derived from small bowel submucosa (Med Institute; West Lafayette, LA). Experimental collagen-covered Z-stents have been used with great success in the venous system,[84] and we are currently initiating trials in TIPS.

■ When Should a Stent-Graft Be Used?

Early data clearly indicate that TIPS patency can be improved by a well-designed, well-positioned stent-graft. In addition, stent-grafts have been used to control peritoneal bleeding after extrahepatic portal vein laceration during TIPS.[64] The remaining question is whether the additional efforts and potential complications of stent-grafting are justified in all TIPS patients. That is, should stent-grafts be used in all TIPS cases, or only in those cases complicated by unsatisfactory results?

Since most patients with bare TIPSs will eventually develop parenchymal tract or hepatic vein stenoses, it can be logically argued that most patients will eventually have an unsatisfactory result that requires intervention. Each subsequent procedure will result in costs of several thousand dollars. Thus, any additional time and cost associated with de novo stent-grafting are likely to be balanced by the reduced need for subsequent interventions and long-term surveillance. With this in mind, we believe that primary stent-grafting will become standard practice once an easily managed device is available.

Special Considerations

Absolute and relative contraindications for TIPS stent-graft placement are generally the same as those for bare TIPS, including known or suspected bacteremia, bacterial cholangitis, cavernous transformation of the portal vein, and symptomatic central venous or pulmonary hypertension. Polycystic disease of the liver and intrahepatic ductal dilatation are contraindications for bare TIPS, but a stent-graft might allow the procedure to be performed safely in both situations.

The risk of infection during placement of a stent-graft may be greater than that during a standard TIPS. Procedure times and catheter manipulations may be increased, the volume of implanted material is greater, and the semipermeable nature of the graft may inhibit the action of antibiotics and cellular and/or humoral immune processes. We routinely use a formal surgical scrub prior to stent-grafting, and all patients receive either ampicillin with sulbactam (1.5 g IV) or cefotetan (1 g IV). In our experience with 18 stent-graft patients, only one—who had a history of Caroli syndrome—manifested postprocedural infection. He required chronic suppression with oral ciprofloxacin until his death of unrelated liver failure 5 months later. Ferral et al[69] use cefazolin (1 g IV) an hour before TIPS and then an additional 1 g IV q8h for three doses afterward. They reported no infections.

Operator experience is a critical factor in considering the appropriateness of TIPS stent-grafting. TIPS is among the most technically challenging procedures undertaken by interventional radiologists. The risk of procedural complications (including failure to establish a shunt) is inversely related to operator experience. Stent-graft placement adds another measure of difficulty to the procedure, and increases the likelihood of complications. It can thus be argued that those with limited experience or low patient volume, if they perform TIPS at all, should continue to limit themselves to bare stents. When and if patients develop a stenosis, they could be referred to another facility for placement of a stent-graft.

■ Conclusion

In early clinical reports, it was speculated that the TIPS procedure would entirely replace surgical and endoscopic alternatives for the management of portal hypertension. By converting TIPS from a multistaged procedure requiring diligent monitoring to a one-step intervention, stent-graft technology may finally allow that dream to become a practical reality. The technical challenges of creating a durable, easily delivered stent-graft should not be diminished, but we believe that such a device will be commercially available in the near future.

REFERENCES

1. Barton RE, Rosch J, Saxon RR, et al. TIPS: short- and long-term results: a survey of 1750 patients. Semin Intervent Radiol 1995;12(4):364–367.
2. LaBerge JM, Ring EJ, Gordon RL, et al. Creation of transjugular intrahepatic portosystemic shunts with the Wallstent endoprosthesis: results in 100 patients. Radiology 1993;187:413–420.
3. Rossle M, Haag K, Ochs A, et al. The transjugular intrahepatic portosystemic stent-shunt procedure for variceal bleeding. N Engl J Med 1994;330:165–171.
4. Rossle M, Siegerstetter V, Huber M, et al. The first decade of the transjugular intrahepatic portosystemic shunt (TIPS): state of the art. Liver 1998;18:73–89.
5. Coy DL, Blei AT. Portal hypertension. In: Haubrich WS, Schaffner, F, Berk JE, eds. Gastroenterology. 5th ed. Philadelphia: WB Saunders, 1995:1955–1987.
6. Rikkers LF. Surgical complications of cirrhosis and portal hypertension. In: Sabiston DC, Lyerly HK, eds. Textbook of Surgery: The Biological Basis of Modern Surgical Practice. 15th ed. Philadelphia: WB Saunders, 1997:1088–1103.
7. Rikkers LF. The changing spectrum of treatment for variceal bleeding. Ann Surg 1998;228(4):536–546.
8. Menegaux F, Keeffe EB, Baker E, et al. Comparison of transjugular and surgical portosystemic shunts on the outcome of liver transplantation. Arch Surg 1994;129(10):1018–1023.
9. Aboujoud MS, Levy MF, Rees CR, et al. A comparison of treatment with transjugular intrahepatic portosystemic shunt or distal splenorenal shunt in the management of variceal bleeding prior to liver transplantation. Transplantation 1995;21(2):226–229.
10. Cabrera J, Maynar M, Granados R, et al. Transjugular intrahepatic portosystemic shunt versus sclerotherapy in the elective treatment of variceal hemorrhage. Gastroenterology 1996;110(3):832–839.
11. Jalan R, Forrest EH, Stanley AJ, et al. A randomized trial comparing transjugular intrahepatic portosystemic stent-shunt with variceal band ligation in the prevention of rebleeding from esophageal varices. Hepatology 1997;26(5):1115–1122.
12. Cello JP, Ring EJ, Olcott EW, et al. Endoscopic sclerotherapy compared with percutaneous transjugular intrahepatic portosystemic shunt after initial sclerotherapy in patients with acute variceal hemorrhage. A randomized, controlled trial. Ann Intern Med 1997;126(11):858–865.
13. Chau TN, Patch D, Chan YW, et al. "Salvage" transjugular intrahepatic portosystemic shunts: gastric fundal compared with esophageal variceal bleeding. Gastroenterology 1998;114(5):981–987.
14. Porayko MK, Wiesner RH. Management of ascites in patients with cirrhosis. What to do when diuretics fail. Postgrad Med 1992;92(8):155–158, 161–166.
15. Bataller R, Arroyo V, Gines P. Management of ascites in cirrhosis. J Gastroenterol Hepatol 1997;12(11):723–733.
16. Saxon RR, Ross PL, Mendel-Hartvig J, et al. Tips patency and the importance of stenosis location in the development of recurrent symptoms. Radiology 1998;207:683–693.
17. Haskal ZJ, Pentecost MJ, Soulen MC, et al. Transjugular intrahepatic portosystemic shunt stenosis and revision: early and midterm results. AJR 1994;163:439–444.
18. Hausegger KA, Sternthal HM, Klein GE, et al. Transjugular intrahepatic portosystemic shunt: follow-up and secondary interventions. Radiology 1994;191:177–181.
19. Haskal ZJ, Carroll JW, Jacobs JE, et al. Sonography of transjugular intrahepatic portosystemic shunts: detection of elevated portosystemic gradients and loss of shunt function. J Vasc Intervent Radiol 1997;8:549–556.
20. LaBerge JM, Ferrell LD, Ring EJ, et al. Histopathologic study of transjugular intrahepatic portosystemic shunts. J Vasc Intervent Radiol 1991;2(4):549–556.
21. LaBerge JM, Ferrell LD, Ring EJ, et al. Histopathologic study of stenotic and occluded transjugular intrahepatic portosystemic shunts. J Vasc Intervent Radiol 1993;4(6):779–786.
22. Saxon RR, Mendel-Hartvig J, Corless CL, et al. Bile duct injury as a major cause of stenosis and occlusion in transjugular intrahepatic portosystemic shunts: comparative histopathologic analysis in humans and swine. J Vasc Intervent Radiol 1996;7(4):487–497.
23. Jalan R, Harrison DJ, Redhead DN, et al. Transjugular intrahepatic portosystemic stent-shunt (TIPSS) occlusion and the role of biliary venous fistulae. J Hepatol 1996;24:169–176.
24. Ducoin H, El-Khoury J, Rousseau H, et al. Histopathologic analysis of transjugular intrahepatic portosystemic shunts. Hepatology 1997;25(5):1064–1069.
25. Terayama N, Matsui O, Kadoya M, et al. Transjugular intrahepatic portosystemic shunt: histologic and immunohistochemical study of autopsy cases. Cardiovasc Intervent Radiol 1997;20(6):457–461.
26. Teng GJ, Bettman MA, Hoopes PJ, et al. Transjugular intrahepatic portosystemic shunt: effect of bile leak on smooth muscle cell proliferation. Radiology 1998;208:799–805.
27. Sanyal AJ, Contos MJ, Yager D, et al. Development of pseudointima and stenosis after transjugular intrahepatic portasystemic shunts: characterization of cell phenotype and function. Hepatology 1998;28(1):22–32.
28. Rösch J, Uchida BT, Barton RE, et al. Coaxial catheter-needle system for transjugular portal vein entrance. J Vasc Intervent Radiol 1993;4:145–147.
29. Viallet A, Marleau D, Huet M, et al. Hemodynamic evaluation of patients with intrahepatic portal hypertension. Relationship between bleeding varices and the portohepatic gradient. Gastroenterology 1975;69(6):1297–1300.
30. Casado M, Bosch J, Garcia-Pagan JC, et al. Clinical events after transjugular intrahepatic portosystemic shunt: correlation with hemodynamic findings. Gastroenterology 1998;114(6):1296–1303.
31. Haskal ZJ, Middlebrook MR. Creation of a stenotic stent to reduce flow through a transjugular intrahepatic portosystemic shunt. J Vasc Intervent Radiol 1994;5(6):827–829, discussion 829–830.
32. Hauenstein KH, Haag K, Ochs A, et al. The reducing stent: treatment for transjugular intrahepatic portosystemic shunt-induced refractory hepatic encephalopathy and liver failure. Radiology 1995;194(1):175–179.
33. Gerbes AL, Waggershauser T, Holl J, et al. Experiences with novel techniques for reduction of stent flow in transjugular intrahepatic portosystemic shunts. Z Gastroenterol 1998;36(5):373.

34. Robinson KA, Roubin G, King S, et al. Correlated microscopic observations of arterial responses to intravascular stenting. Scanning Microsc 1989;3(2):665–679.

35. Palmaz JC. Intravascular stenting: from basic research to clinical application. Cardiovasc Intervent Radiol 1992;15:279–284.

36. Bai H, Masuda J, Sawa Y, et al. Neointima formation after vascular stent implantation: spatial and chronological distribution of smooth muscle cell proliferation and phenotypic modulation. Atherosclerosis Thrombosis 1994;14(11):1846–1853.

37. Schwartz RS, Huber KC, Murphy MB, et al. Restenosis and the proportional neointimal response to artery injury: results in a porcine model. J Am Coll Cardiol 1992;19(2):267–274.

38. Karas SP, Gravanis MB, Santoian EC, et al. Coronary intimal proliferation after balloon injury and stenting in swine: an animal model of restenosis. J Am Coll Cardiol 1992;20:467–474.

39. Carter AJ, Laird JR, Farb A, et al. Morphologic characteristics of lesion formation and time course of smooth muscle cell proliferation in a porcine proliferative restenosis model. J Am Coll Cardiol 1994;25(5):1398–1405.

40. Unterberg C, Sandrock D, Nebendahl K, et al. Reduced acute thrombus formation results in decreased neointimal proliferation after coronary angioplasty. J Am Coll Cardiol 1995;26:1747–1754.

41. Kubota Y, Kimihiko K, Uchida H, et al. Pharmacological treatment of intimal hyperplasia after metallic stent placement in the peripheral arteries: an experimental study. Invest Radiol 1995;30(9):532–537.

42. Hanke H, Hassenstein S, Kamenz J, et al. Prolonged proliferative response of smooth muscle cells after experimental intravascular stenting: a stent wire phenomenon (abstr). Circulation 1992; 86(suppl I):I-186.

43. Berry JL, Moore JE, Newman VS, Routh WD. In vitro flow visualization in stented arterial segments. 1995 advances in bioengineering. Abstracts of the 1995 International Mechanical Engineering Congress and Exposition, San Francisco, California, 1995:231–232.

44. Newman VS, Berry JL, Routh WD, et al. Effects of vascular stent surface area and hemodynamics on intimal thickening. J Vasc Intervent Radiol 1996;7:387–393.

45. Fontaine AB, Spigos DG, Eaton G, et al. Stent-induced intimal hyperplasia: are there fundamental differences between flexible and rigid stent designs? J Vasc Intervent Radiol 1994;5(5):739–744.

46. Rogers C, Edelman ER. Endovascular stent design dictates experimental restenosis and thrombosis. Circulation 1995;91(12):2995–3001.

47. Okuhn SP, Connelly DP, Calakos N, et al. Does compliance mismatch alone cause neointimal hyperplasia? J Vasc Surg 1989;9(1): 35–45.

48. Abbott WM, Megerman J, Hasson JE, et al. Effect of compliance mismatch on vascular graft patency. J Vasc Surg 1987;5(2):376–382.

49. Back M, Kopchok G, Mueller M, et al. Changes in arterial wall compliance after endovascular stenting. J Vasc Surg 1994;19(5):905–911.

50. Desgranges P, Hutin E, Kedzia C, et al. Aortic stents covering the renal arteries ostia: an animal study. J Vasc Intervent Radiol 1997;8 (1 pt 1):77–82.

51. Malina M, Lindh M, Ivancev K, et al. The effect of endovascular aortic stents placed across the renal arteries. Eur J Vasc Endovasc Surg 1997;13(2):207–213.

52. Jalan R, Redhead DN, Allan PL, Hayes PC. Prospective evaluation of haematological alterations following the transjugular intrahepatic portosystemic stent-shunt (TIPSS). Eur J Gastroenterol Hepatol 1996;8(4):381–385.

53. Rosch J, Uchida BT, Putnam JS, et al. Experimental intrahepatic portacaval anastomosis: use of expandable Gianturco stents. Radiology 1987;162(2):481–485.

54. Stout LC, Lyon RE, Murray NG, et al. Pseudointimal biliary epithelial proliferation and Zahn's infarct associated with a 6 1/2-month-old transjugular intrahepatic portosystemic shunt. Am J Gastroenterol 1995;90(1):126–130.

55. Pineo GF, Regoeczi E, Hatton MW, et al. The activation of coagulation by extracts of mucus: a possible pathway of intravascular coagulation accompanying adenocarcinomas. J Lab Clin Med 1973; 82(2): 255–266.

56. Pineo GF, Brain MC, Gallus AS, et al. Tumors, mucus production, and hypercoagulability. Ann NY Acad Sci 1974;230:262–270.

57. Nishimine K, Saxon RR, Kichikawa K, et al. Improved transjugular intrahepatic portosystemic shunt patency with PTFE-covered stent-grafts: experimental results in swine. Radiology 1995;196: 341–347.

58. Haskal ZJ, Davis A, McAllister A, Furth EE. PTFE-encapsulated endovascular stent-graft for transjugular intrahepatic portosystemic shunts: experimental evaluation. Radiology 1997;205:682–688.

59. Haskal Z, Zaetta J. Comparison of a novel ePTFE-based endovascular stent-graft versus the Wallstent for transjugular intrahepatic portosystemic shunts in a porcine model. JVIR 9 (1, Part 2) supplement 201.

60. Tanihata H, Saxon RR, Kubota Y. Transjugular intrahepatic portosystemic shunt with silicone-covered Wallstents: results in a swine model. Radiology 1997;205:181–184.

61. Bloch RD, Pavcnik D, Uchida BT. Polyurethane-coated dacron-covered stent-grafts for TIPS: results in swine. Cardiovasc Intervent Radiol 1998;21(6):497–500.

62. Haskal Z. Comparison of polyethylene terephthalate (PET) covered Wallstents versus uncovered Wallstents for TIPS in an animal model. JVIR 9 (1, Part 2) supplement 201.

63. Cohen GS, Young HY, Ball DS. Stent-graft as treatment for TIPS-biliary fistula. J Vasc Intervent Radiol 1996;7(5):665–668.

64. Krajina A, Hulek P, Ferko A, et al. Extrahepatic portal vein laceration in TIPS treated with stent-graft placement. Hepatogastroenterology 1997;44:667–670.

65. DiSalle RS, Dolmatch BL. Treatment of TIPS stenosis with ePTFE graft-covered stents. Cardiovasc Intervent Radiol 1998;21:172–175.

66. Beheshti MV, Dolmatch BL, Jones MP. Technical considerations in covering and deploying a Wallstent endoprosthesis for the salvage of a failing transjugular intrahepatic portosystemic shunt. J Vasc Intervent Radiol 1998;9:289–293.

67. Saxon RR, Timmermans HA, Uchida BT, et al. Stent-grafts for revision of TIPS stenoses and occlusions: a clinical pilot study. J Vasc Intervent Radiol 1997;8:539–548.

68. Saxon RR. Unpublished data.

69. Ferral H, Alcantara-Peraza A, Kimura Y. Creation of transjugular intrahepatic portosystemic shunts with use of the Cragg Endopro system I. J Vasc Intervent Radiol 1998;9:283–287.

70. Beppu M, Fukazaki T, Mitani K, et al. Hepatic segmentectomy with segmental hepatic vein sacrifice. Arch Surg 1990;125:1170–1175.

71. Cho KJ, Geisinger KR, Shields JJ, et al. Collateral channels and histopathology in hepatic vein occlusion. AJR 1982;139:703–709.

72. Wilson MW, Gordon RL, LaBerge JM, et al. Liver transplantation complicated by malpositioned transjugular intrahepatic portosystemic shunts. J Vasc Intervent Radiol 1995;6(5):695–699.

73. Mazziotti A, Morelli MC, Grazi GL, et al. Beware of TIPS in liver transplant candidates. Transjugular Intrahepatic Portosystemic Shunt. Hepatogastroenterology 1996;43(12):1606–1610.

74. Lerut JP, Laterre PF, Goffette P, et al. Transjugular intrahepatic portosystemic shunt and liver transplantation. Transplant Int 1996;9(4):370–375.

75. Clavien PA, Selzner M, Tuttle-Newhall JE, et al. Liver transplantation complicated by misplaced TIPS in the portal vein. Ann Surg 1998;227(3):440–445.

76. Rousseau H, Puel J, Joffre F, et al. Self-expanding endovascular prosthesis: an experimental study. Radiology 1987;164(3): 709–714.

77. Palmaz JC. Balloon-expandable intravascular stent. AJR 1988;150: 1263–1269.

78. Lossef SV, Lutz RJ, Mundorf J, Barth KH. Comparison of mechanical deformation properties of metallic stents with use of stress-strain analysis. J Vasc Intervent Radiol 1994;5(2):341–349.

79. Siegerstetter V, Krause T, Rossle M, et al. Transjugular intrahepatic portosystemic shunt (TIPS). Thrombogenicity in stents and its effect on shunt patency. Acta Radiol 1997;38(4 pt 1): 558–564.

80. Rossi P, Bezzi M, Salvatori FM, et al. Self-expanding stents in transjugular intrahepatic portosystemic shunt: experience with nitinol Strecker stents. Eur Radiol 1996;6(5):741–747.

81. Ugolotti U, Larini P, Marcata C, et al. Is the tantalum Strecker stent suitable for TIPS creation? Short- and mid-term results in 20 consecutive patients. Cardiovasc Intervent Radiol 1997;20(1):38–42.

82. Palmaz JC. Review of polymeric graft materials for endovascular graft applications. J Vasc Intervent Radiol 1998;9:7–13.

83. Dolmatch BL. Tissue reaction to endoluminal graft materials and graft-covered stents. Ninth annual International Symposium on Vascular Diagnosis and Intervention, 1997:279–282.

84. Pavcnik D. Unpublished data.

13

Stent-Grafts for Peripheral Arterial Injury

CLAUDIE S. MCARTHUR AND MICHAEL L. MARIN

Both penetrating and blunt trauma may lead to arterial occlusion, dissection, pseudoaneurysm, and arteriovenous fistula (AVF) formation. The technical aspects of current operative therapy for traumatic arterial injuries may be complicated by several factors. The inaccessibility of the vascular lesion (i.e., central vessel involvement), anatomic distortion that results in venous hypertension with excessive bleeding, and inherent problems with operating in a traumatized and often contaminated field are among these limiting factors. Furthermore, the presence of multiple trauma or severe medical comorbidities may increase the incidence of surgical complications and mortality.[1]

Dotter[2] first presented the concept of using endovascular stent-grafts for the management of such traumatic injuries as early as 1969. Over the past 8 years endovascular grafting has been evaluated as an alternative to conventional surgical repair in the management of aneurysms and other vascular lesions. The application of this form of therapy to the treatment of vascular trauma is reasonable for several reasons. The use of endovascular stent-grafting has been shown to be associated with a decrease in anesthetic requirement, blood loss, and extent of dissection.[3] The less invasive nature of the surgery without the need for a surgical incision makes this intrinsically attractive to both patient and physician. High-velocity missiles can produce a significant amount of tissue damage even if not suspected on initial examination based on the classically small size of the entrance and exit wounds.[4] The inherent problems of graft placement in the setting of severe tissue damage, gross contamination, and scar tissue formation make the use of a remote insertion site particularly advantageous in the trauma patient.[5]

At present, the largest experience with endovascular graft therapy for the management of vascular trauma has been with the treatment of arterial pseudoaneurysms and AVFs.[3,5,6–11] Still in the early phase of its development, this method of repair is limited to the stable patient, usually the victim of penetrating injury, either a knife or gunshot wound, or iatrogenic injury. Any patient demonstrating pulse deficits and severe ischemia or active hemorrhage requires urgent conventional operative repair.[7] Similarly, the patient with an expanding hematoma or multiple traumatic injuries cannot be considered a candidate for endovascular graft therapy. Stented grafts have been extensively studied and have demonstrated excellent technical success rates.[12] In its use for arterial trauma, endovascular stent-grafting has been safe and efficacious in preliminary investigations.[3] This chapter focuses on the specific application of this technology to the trauma patient. It presents the potential benefits and disadvantages of the methods, reviews the current status of the field and available data, and addresses the future role of this technology within the field of trauma surgery.

■ Techniques

Clinical experience has demonstrated the wide variety of options for device use in the treatment of traumatic lesions.[3,8,12,13] In their current design, stented grafts

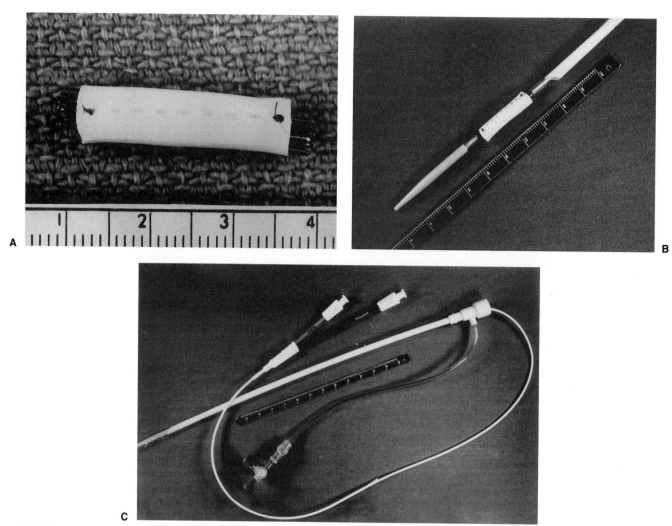

FIGURE 13–1. (**A**). Palmaz covered stent. A segment of polytetrafluoroethylene (PTFE) is attached to a stainless steel balloon-expandable Palmaz stent using two 5–0 prolene "U" stitches. (**B**). Covered stent crimped to an 8-mm ×3-cm balloon-dilatation catheter. The catheter has been backloaded into a 12-Fr sheath, the cut end of the sheath dilator has been fitted to the tip of the catheter. (**C**). The stent-graft is mounted on an angioplasty balloon and placed into sheath prior to insertion.

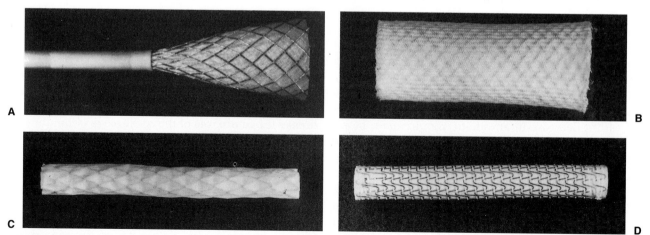

FIGURE 13–2. (**A**). Corvita self-expanding stent of braided wire covered with polycarbonate elastomer fibers. (**B**). The PET covered Wallgraft®. (**C**). Passager nitinol thermal-expanding stent covered with an ultrathin woven polyester fabric. (**D**). Hemobahn graft constructed from an ultrathin expanded PTFE (ePTFE) tube externally supported by nitinol wire arranged in a helical coil fashion.

for treating traumatic arterial injuries are composed of a stent rendered nonporous by an outer covering. The covering, either expanded polytetrafluoroethylene (ePTFE) or polyethylene terephthalate (PET), does not appear to influence outcome for stent-grafts placed in large vessels.[7] Some have used radially expandable thin-walled PET grafts;[12] others have used autogenous vein (jugular or saphenous) sutured to a Palmaz stent (Fig. 13–1).[12,14] At our institution, we have used Palmaz balloon-expandable metallic stents in conjunction with thin-walled ePTFE graft material to perform arterial repair of pseudoaneurysm and AVFs. Precise delivery to the site of injury is performed under fluoroscopic guidance. Heparin is used during insertion, but long-term anticoagulation has not been necessary.

An alternative device is the Corvita stent-graft, which is fabricated from a self-expanding stent of braided wire. The Corvita stent-graft was the first commercially available endograft to enter into clinical trials. The stent is covered with polycarbonate polyurethane fibers (Fig. 13–2A). This stent-graft has the distinct advantage of allowing it to be cut to the desired length in the operating room prior to loading into a special delivery sheath. The sheath has a special pusher catheter that is used for maintaining the graft in position while the outer sheath is being retracted. The Wallgraft has a similar design with a PET outer covering (Fig. 13–2B). A third system that has been used to treat traumatic lesions is the Passager endograft system. This system uses a nitinol thermal-expanding stent covered with an ultrathin woven polyester fabric (Fig. 13–2C).

Additional endograft devices that have been successfully used for traumatic lesions include the Hemobahn graft produced by W. L. Gore and Associates (Flagstaff, AZ) (Fig. 13–2D). This device is also fabricated from an ultrathin ePTFE tube externally supported by nitinol wire arranged in a helical coil fashion.

■ Carotid Injuries

Internal carotid artery (ICA) pseudoaneurysms are often the result of a previous dissection either occurring spontaneously or in association with an identifiable traumatic episode.[15] The significant risk of life-threatening stroke or hemorrhage warrants strong consideration for treatment of these lesions even if asymptomatic.[15] Treatment options include ICA ligation in the absence of contralateral disease and open surgical repair, and recently endovascular techniques have been developed to address this problem.[6,15] Conventional open repair is often technically difficult or impossible when exposure at the skull base is required.[4,6,15] In such a situation endovascular repair provides a potential alternative. Several centers have reported the use of noncovered stents to treat

such aneurysms.[15–18] However, in the case of larger wide-mouthed aneurysms,[18] the aneurysms were not totally excluded by the Palmaz stents alone and continue to be at risk for rupture. Endovascular stent-grafts seem a more reasonable option in the case of large ICA aneurysms.

Our institution recently described the successful use of an endovascular stented graft using a Palmaz balloon-expandable stent covered with an ePTFE thin-wall vascular graft (Impra, Tempe, AZ) for the treatment of a 2-cm ICA pseudoaneurysm located at the skull base (Fig. 13–3).[6] Access may be obtained by either a femoral approach or direct operative exposure of the common carotid artery at the base of the neck. Open exposure of the proximal carotid permits flow arrest, reducing the risk of embolization secondary to luminal manipulations. Because the aneurysm is excluded from the systemic circulation, there should be no intracranial thromboembolic events. The patient remains asymptomatic on oral anticoagulation with full exclusion of the aneurysm after 1 year. Parodi[19] reported two cases of traumatic carotid artery pseudoaneurysms treated with autogenous vein covered stents in conjunction with oral anticoagulation, with the rationale of providing a less thrombogenic surface. Success in these patients was limited to one failure related to external compression of the Palmaz stent at the level of the base of the skull. Determination of the potential benefit of using autogenous vein versus a synthetic covered stented graft in such patients will need to be addressed in a controlled study. Whether exclusion of the aneurysm will prevent future expansion and potential rupture of the pseudoaneurysm will require long-term evaluation.

■ Femoral Artery Trauma

With the rapid expansion of interventional procedures and rising incidence of civilian-based trauma, AVFs and pseudoaneurysms of the femoral arteries have become common vascular complications. Small AVFs may resolve spontaneously, but larger fistulas do not generally have the same benign prognosis.[20,21] Current recommendations are surgical treatment for the prevention of complications including hemorrhage, thrombosis, compression of local neurovascular structures, venous hypertension, and congestive heart failure.[5] Surgical repair is often technically difficult due to bleeding secondary to venous hypertension associated with the arterialized vascular bed.[5] We reported the first successful endovascular stent-graft repair of a traumatic AVF of the superficial femoral artery and vein with a balloon-expandable stented ePTFE graft in an 18-year-old man injured by a bullet (Fig. 13–4).[5] An ePTFE covered Palmaz stent was used to repair the AVF. At 5 months follow-up, the endograft was still patent.

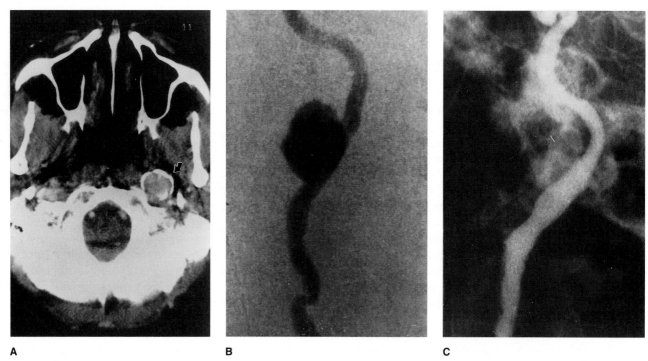

A   **B**   **C**

FIGURE 13–3. (**A**). Transaxial CT scan revealing a 2-cm calcified round lesion in the left parapharyngeal space (arrow). (**B**). Digital subtracted arteriogram. Note the internal carotid artery pseudoaneurysm. (**C**). Follow-up left carotid arteriogram. The covered stent is patent. The pseudoaneurysm is not opacified. The internal carotid artery is widely patent.

Subsequently, two groups have reported on the successful treatment of traumatic femoral pseudoaneurysms and AVFs.[3,12] One reported patient had an infected pseudoaneurysm of the common femoral artery that was treated with a vein covered Palmaz stent.[12] The five patients reported all had successful treatment of the lesion without complications with primary patencies of 100% at 17.4 months mean follow-up.

■ Axillary-Subclavian Artery Trauma

Penetrating axillary and subclavian artery trauma may result in the formation of a dissection, pseudoaneurysm, or AVF. Posttraumatic pseudoaneurysms of the subclavian and axillary arteries are rare, and like aneurysms of other arteries can rupture, thrombose, or embolize (Fig. 13–5).[22,23] Other mechanisms of injury include compression with contusion, avulsion, and traction from stretch or rotational stress.[24] The surgical approaches developed to repair such lesions include clavicular resection, median sternotomy, and thoracotomy, but these are each associated with significant potential for morbidity.[25] The approaches require extensive dissection often with large volumes of blood loss and prolonged hospital stay. Although the optimal management of such injuries is unclear, the role of endovascular stent-grafting

for such lesions has expanded over the past few years.[3,9,12,26–29] In a collective review of 18 recent cases of axillary or subclavian artery trauma managed with endovascular stent-graft therapy, a technical success rate of 94% was reported.[8] Primary patency in these patients was 85% at a mean follow-up period of 18 months. The associated complication rate was 6%. Mean length of hospital stay was 3.3 days. Another group recently reported their experience with one patient with an embolizing traumatic subclavian artery aneurysm. The aneurysm was repaired with a polyester covered nitinol stent with concomitant vein bypass of embolic brachial artery occlusion. At 24 months follow-up, both bypasses were patent.[28] These are encouraging results when one considers the morbidity associated with conventional surgery, and the observed cost-effectiveness of the procedure in this series.

■ Aorta or Iliac Artery Trauma

Patients sustaining blunt trauma to the abdominal aorta usually do not survive owing to the impact of the direct compressive force and associated injuries. In one review, the mortality rate associated with blunt abdominal aortic injury was 24%.[30] Injuries may include intimal dis-

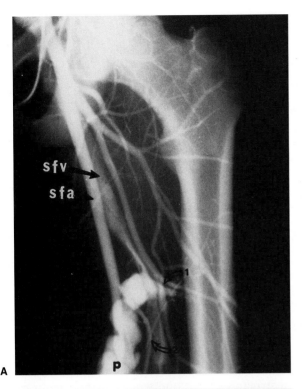

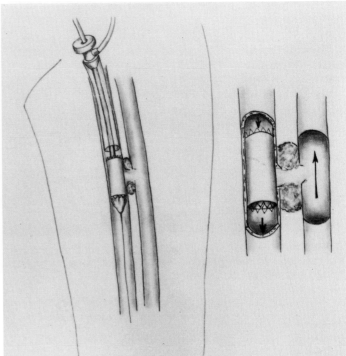

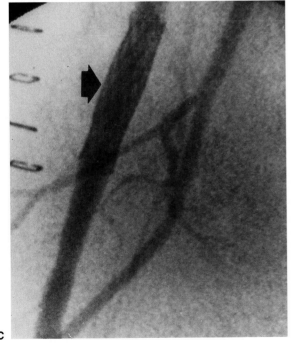

FIGURE 13–4. (**A**). Femoral arteriogram after gunshot wound to the left thigh. An arteriovenous fistula associated with a large pseudoaneurysm (p) is seen between the left superficial femoral artery (sfa) and the superficial femoral vein (sfv). Selective catheterization of the deep femoral artery (1) and the sfa branch (2) showed that these vessels were not injured. (**B**). Following deployment, the stented graft occludes the arteriovenous fistula. (**C**). Completion arteriogram demonstrates patency of the sfa, proper positioning of the stented graft (arrow), and no evidence of the arteriovenous fistula or extravasation. Note the metal clips placed in the skin before the procedure to facilitate fluoroscopic localization of the arteriovenous fistula and proper placement of the stented graft.

ruption with dissection, intramural hematoma, and pseudoaneurysms, ranging from simple contusion to frank rupture.[31,32] Endovascular stent-graft repair of such injuries has emerged as a therapeutic option in the case of stable aortoiliac injuries. Most of the experience has been with penetrating injuries of these vessels, either iatrogenic, related to surgery or catheterization procedures, or bullet injuries (Fig. 13–6).[8,10,33] In the presence of associated injuries or hemodynamic instability, conventional open repair should be undertaken. Fifteen patients in recent reports underwent endovascular stent-graft repair of traumatic injuries to the abdominal aorta or iliac arteries that were either AVFs or pseudoaneurysms.[3,11,12,26] Technical success of the procedures was 100% with primary patencies of 100% at a mean follow-up period of 10.5 months.[8]

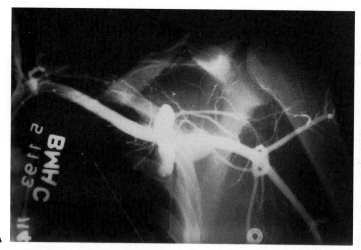
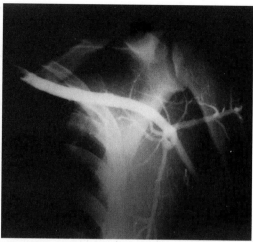

FIGURE 13–5 . **(A).** Axillary-subclavian artery arteriogram of a patient with a large pseudoaneurysm after a stab wound to the chest resulted in a hemopneumothorax. **(B).** Following transluminal insertion of the stent-graft device, the pseudoaneurysm was repaired and flow was restored.

Isolated injuries to the iliac vessels have also been successfully treated with endovascular grafting.[34,35] Rupture of the iliac artery occurs in one in every 200 angioplasty procedures.[36,37] In these cases, emergent repair is likely to be necessary as in Formichi et al's[34] report on endovascular stent-graft repair of the acute rupture of the external iliac artery during angioplasty. There, temporary hemostasis was obtained using balloon tamponade, followed by exchange for a Cragg Endopro System covered endoprosthesis to seal the injury. At >18 months follow-up, the endograft was still patent without endoleak.

■ Thoracic Aortic Trauma

Most blunt thoracic aortic injuries are caused by deceleration injuries, most often related to motor vehicle accidents.[38,39] Patients who sustain trauma to the thoracic aorta, whether blunt or penetrating, do not usually survive.[40] The few patients who survive the immediate injury often develop a chronic aortic aneurysm.[41,42] Open thoracic surgery for repair of a chronic traumatic aneurysm is associated with a reported mortality rate of 5 to 18% owing mainly to bleeding, heart failure, or renal failure, with associated morbidity rates as high as 50%.[42,43] In the case of acute aortic injury, the frequency of multiple traumatic injuries further increases the mortality rate.[44–46] The presence of medical comorbidities also contributes to a poorer prognosis.[47]

Owing to the lack of prospective data regarding the optimal management of these injuries, controversy exists as to the indications for operative therapy. Minor injuries, including mural hematoma and intimal flap, usu-

ally resolve on their own.[48] Pseudoaneurysms, even small ones, rarely remain stable over time, with a high risk of rupture, embolization, fistulization, or compression of adjacent structures.[48,49] Nonoperative management can be considered only for simple lesions, for some patients with severe neurologic deficits, or arterial injuries not actively bleeding.[48,50,51] In these patients, antihypertensive therapy with nitroprusside or labetalol is recommended until a decision on aortic repair is reached.[52] Nevertheless, Finkelmeier et al[42] reported that 33% of his patients with untreated chronic aortic aneurysm died of complications attributed to the aortic lesion, with 75% of deaths secondary to aneurysm rupture.

Endovascular stent-grafting of traumatic thoracic injuries has begun to assume a role in the management of these injuries (Fig. 13–7).[53–56] Using this technique, the need for aortic clamping is obviated. This could potentially decrease the incidence of paraplegia, the incidence of which has been reported as between 4 and 32% in surgery for thoracoabdominal aortic aneurysm.[57] Although several factors have been implicated in the pathophysiology of paraplegia in thoracic aortic surgery,[57] duration of spinal cord ischemia is undoubtedly a major factor.[58] The endovascular approach does not allow for the reimplantation of intercostal arteries. However, in the case of nonpenetrating thoracic aortic injury, the location of the lesion is at the isthmus approximately 90% of the time[39,59]; therefore, the area of repair usually does not involve segments with branches to the spinal cord.[53]

In addition, respiratory failure is the most common complication following surgery for thoracic aortic aneurysms.[60] The elimination of thoracotomy, especially in patients with existing pulmonary disease, will likely

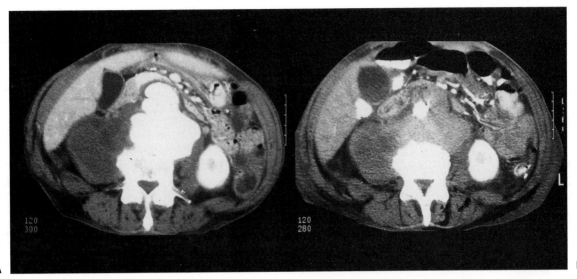

FIGURE 13–6. (A). Computed tomography (CT) scan demonstrating pseudoaneurysm of the infrarenal abdominal aorta with extravasation of contrast noted in the retroperitoneum. **(B).** CT demonstrating full exclusion of pseudoaneurysm with contrast evident within lumen of endograft. Also demonstrated is thrombosis of pseudoaneurysm.

decrease the incidence of this complication, with a major impact on hospital cost reduction. The potential decrease in other complications related to the decrease in operative blood loss, minimal invasiveness of this form of therapy, and reduced need for general anesthesia, particularly in patients with relatively prohibitive risk factors for open repair, is likely to be demonstrated in large studies with long-term follow-up.

Several limitations must be addressed. With most of these injuries occurring at the isthmus just beyond the origin of the subclavian artery, the length of the proximal neck may be insufficient for adequate fixation of the stented graft if precise deployment is not achieved, which may result in either endoleak (incomplete aneurysm exclusion) or occlusion of the upper extremity inflow. Preprocedural left subclavian to carotid transposition has been useful to increase the proximal endograft landing zone. Also, the relative rigidity of the stent-grafts currently used limits their ability to conform to the curved aortic contour of the distal arch or proximal descending aorta.[53]

Another problem that could potentially limit benefits of a minimally invasive procedure may arise in the case of a large traumatic aneurysm, whereby compression of adjacent structures (e.g., mainstem bronchus) is unrelieved by simple surgical graft interposition. Removal of large amounts of intramural thrombus around a mainstem bronchus are necessary to relieve lung atelectasis.[61] Furthermore, heparin is required to prevent thrombosis related to the obstruction of blood flow related to the large delivery sheath, which in the acute trauma patient with coexisting injuries, is potentially hazardous.

To date, four groups have reported on experience with endovascular stent-graft repair of thoracic aortic trauma. One group reported a single case of a previously paralyzed patient who sustained a bullet wound injury to the descending thoracic aorta at the level of T11. The pseudoaneurysm was discovered 3 months after the injury, and was repaired using a PET (Dumont, Wilmington, DE) covered nitinol stent inserted via a retroperitoneal approach to the iliac artery. Follow-up studies failed to demonstrate the presence of an endoleak or pseudoaneurysm.[55] A second group reported on 10 patients who underwent repair of a traumatic thoracic aortic aneurysm.[53] In their study, using modified Z-stents covered with either woven PET or ePTFE graft material, 9 of 10 aneurysms were located at the level of the isthmus. In this report, three major complications were noted. One patient developed an endoleak that was successfully treated with coil embolization. The second patient developed thrombosis of the subclavian artery, which was treated by subclavian-carotid bypass. The last patient required stenting of the left mainstem bronchus to relieve left lung atelectasis. There were no other major or minor complications, such as paraplegia, embolization, respiratory failure, renal failure, or myocardial infarction. The third report was of two patients with distal descending thoracic aortic pseudoaneurysms who underwent successful stent-graft repair whereby only the T11 intercostal artery was sacrificed by endoluminal exclusion.[56]

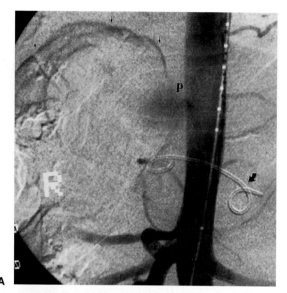

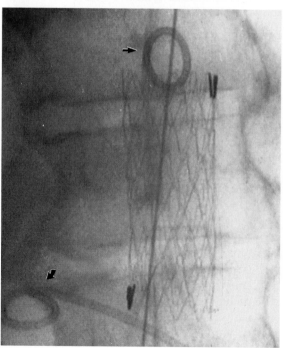

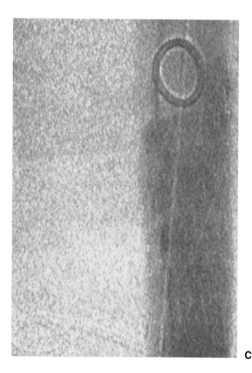

FIGURE 13–7. (A). Digital subtracted arteriogram of thoracic aorta 1 month after placement of double-J stent (curved arrow) for internal drainage of a pancreatic pseudocyst demonstrates large aortic pseudoaneurysm (p) (outlined by arrows). **(B).** Thoracic aorta after deployment of stent-graft. Note double-J stent (curved arrow) and diagnostic pigtail catheter (straight arrow). **(C).** Completion arteriogram demonstrates full exclusion of pseudoaneurysm without extravasation of contrast.

Our recent series of thoracic aortic stent-grafting using balloon-expandable and self-expandable endovascular grafts in 14 patients included five traumatic injuries.[62] In this series, graft insertion was technically successful in 11 of 14 patients (79%), with procedural failures related to graft migration and endoleaks. Self-expanding devices were found to be associated with greater success, most likely related to the avoidance of asystole in obtaining precise device position. There were two deaths as a result of microembolization and multiorgan system failure. Average length of hospital stay was 2.9 days. The use of endovascular stent-graft repair for traumatic thoracic aortic injuries, despite significant limitations to its application, will likely be shown to be of great benefit for select patients in future studies.

■ Anastomotic Pseudoaneurysms

Anastomotic pseudoaneurysms present a major challenge to the vascular surgeon. First, based on a lack of routine surveillance following graft insertion, detection is difficult, and the true incidence is unknown. Reported incidences vary from 0.2 to 15%.[63–65] Second, conventional operative repair is technically challenging, requiring dissection in a previously dissected field, sometimes requiring total graft excision.[63,66] Reported conventional operative mortality for aortoiliac anastomotic aneurysms is as high as 21% in elective situations,[67] with major complication rates reported between 8 and 73%.[67,68] These pseudoaneurysms are at risk for the development of the same complications as true aneurysms, and early diagnosis and treatment are necessary. It seems that an ideal method of repair in these cases would employ the use of endovascular stent-grafting (Figs. 13–8 and 13–9). Recently, 10 patients with 12 noninfected aortic or iliac anastomotic aneurysms underwent endovascular stent-graft repair, all of whom had serious comorbid medical illnesses.[69] Endovascular grafts were successfully inserted in all patients, with one wound complication and one postoperative myocardial infarction. Graft patency was observed at a follow-up of 16.1 months.

Potential limitations of the use of endovascular grafts for this indication will need to be addressed. A suitable neck length of between 1 and 2 cm is often difficult to achieve in a para-anastomotic aneurysm without placing a graft across the renal arteries when dealing with a proximal aortic anastomosis. Also, this approach would not be applicable to the previously repaired vessel with a proximal end-to-side anastomosis. Retrograde perfusion of the aneurysm would maintain an endoleak, preventing effective therapy.[69] Long-term effectiveness of this mode of repair is not known.

■ Discussion

Since Parodi et al's[70] first report of the use of endovascular stent-grafting for the treatment of aneurysms, the use of endovascular surgery has broadened to include the treatment of arterial trauma, although experience is limited. Endoluminal grafts have been studied for the treatment of occlusive and aneurysmal arterial disease with variable success.[71] In comparison with standard operative repair of traumatic injuries, this new, less invasive method appears to be associated with less blood loss and a reduced requirement for anesthesia. Less dissection in a traumatized field is of particular advantage in the case of arteriovenous fistulas with venous hypertension, where standard surgical repair is notoriously difficult and associated with large operative blood losses in the setting of either acute or chronic traumatic injury. When successfully applied, the procedure has the advantage of its simplicity and decreased operative time. As vascular surgeons are increasingly faced with older patients who have severe comorbid illnesses that can increase operative morbidity and mortality, the use of a minimally invasive approach is necessary.

Despite the potential benefits, eventual long-term utility will rely on the ability to overcome the limitations associated with this mode of therapy.[72] It is presumed that the full exclusion of aneurysms will lead to the elimination of rupture potential. It is possible that arterial pressure that is transmitted to the thrombosed excluded circulation will lead to eventual aneurysm expansion and rupture. The fact that a decrease in the excluded aneurysm size has been observed is encouraging[10,12]; however, rupture has been observed following stent-graft repair of an aneurysm following a demonstrated decrease in size.[73] The effects of a stent embedded in the wall of a vessel in preventing future expansion is not known.[19] Long-term follow-up is necessary to determine this risk.

Another problem in the use of this technology in the potential for the development of intimal hyperplasia at the junction of the artery and stent-graft. The Palmaz stent has been shown to be associated with only minimal intimal hyperplasia in experimental studies evaluating stenting of occlusive or stenotic iliac lesions.[74]

Difficulty in obtaining access accounts for occasional problems,[19] and extended incisions resulting in prolonged procedures from more invasive approaches complicate the technical ease of the operation.

Microembolization is a serious problem encountered with endovascular surgery. In Parodi's[19] study, three of four patients who developed embolic complications died as a result. These procedures all involved technical difficulties in patients with large aneurysms. Possible reasons for the increased potential for embolization in larger aneurysms were suggested by Parodi, including both the negotiation of the guidewire inside a large chamber with embolic material within it and multiple manipulations resulting from miscalculation of aneurysm length.

In addition, device limitations exist and are the focus of current investigative work. Stent compression has been reported in the case stent-graft repair of axillary-subclavian injury[8] owing to compression between the clavicle and first rib. In these situations, the use of less rigid self-expanding devices has been advocated.

REFERENCES

1. Messina LM, Brothers TE, Wakefield TW, et al. Clinical characteristics and surgical management of vascular complications in patients undergoing cardiac catheterization: interventional versus diagnostic procedures. J Vasc Surg 1991;13:593–600.
2. Dotter CT. Transluminally-placed coilspring endarterial tube grafts. Long-term patency in canine popliteal artery. Invest Radiol 1969;4:329–332.
3. Marin ML, Veith FJ, Panetta TF. Transluminally placed endovascular stented graft repair for arterial trauma. J Vasc Surg 1994;20:466–473.
4. Perry MO. Vascular injuries in the neck and thoracic outlet. In: Veith FJ, Hobson RW, Williams RA, et al., eds. Vascular Surgery: Principles and Practice. 2nd ed. New York: McGraw-Hill, 1994:967–975.
5. Marin ML, Veith FJ, Panetta TF. Percutaneous transfemoral insertion of a stented graft to repair a traumatic femoral arteriovenous fistula. J Vasc Surg 1993;18:299–302.

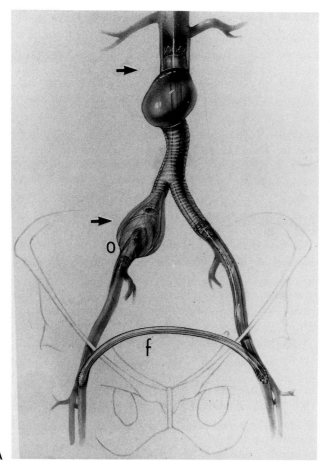
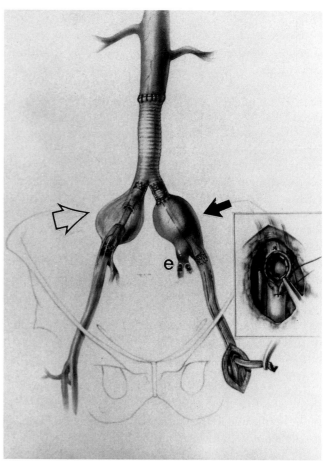

A

B

FIGURE 13–8. (**A**). Anastomotic aneurysms of the proximal aortic anastomosis and right common iliac artery (arrows) subsequent to the placement of a bifurcated aortic graft. These lesions may be treated with the endoluminal placement of an aorto-iliac graft with femorofemoral bypass (f) and occlusion of the right common iliac artery (o, occluder). (**B**). Iliac anastomotic aneurysms with both false anastomotic aneursym (white arrow) and true anastomotic aneurysm (black arrow). These lesions may be treated with both right and left stent-grafts as shown. Note that embolization of the left hypogastric (e) is necessary as the aneurysm extends distal to the bifurcation of the common iliac artery.

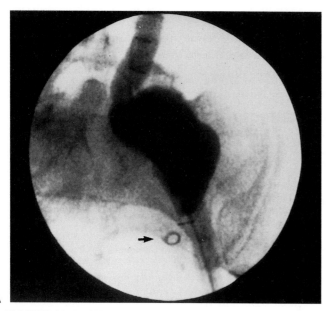
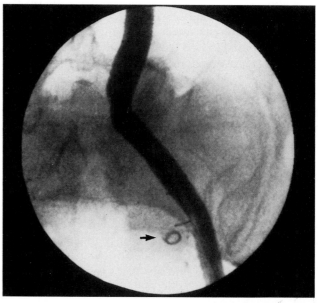

A

D

FIGURE 13–9. (**A**). Intraoperative arteriogram of a distal anastomotic aneurysm of the left iliac anastomosis of a bifurcated aortic graft placed 9 years prior to procedure. (**B**). Arteriogram after placement of endovascular stent across pseudoaneurysm demonstrates exclusion of the aneurysm. Note the coils placed preoperatively in the left hypogastric artery (**A** and **B**, arrow).

6. Reiter BP, Marin ML, Teodorescu VJ, et al. Endoluminal repair of an internal carotid artery pseudoaneurysm. J Vasc Intervent Radiol 1998;9:245–248.

7. Marin ML, Veith FJ Endovascular stents and stented grafts for the treatment of aneurysms and other arterial lesions. Adv Surg 1996; 29:93–109.

8. Ohki TO, Veith FJ, Marin ML, et al. Endovascular approaches for traumatic arterial lesions. Semin Vasc Surg 1997;10(4):272–285.

9. Patel AV, Marin ML, Veith FJ. Endovascular graft repair of penetrating subclavian artery injuries. J Endovasc Surg 1996;3(4):382–388.

10. Marin ML, Veith FJ, Cynammon J, et al. Initial experience with transluminally placed endovascular grafts for the treatment of complex vascular lesions. Ann Surg 1995;222(4):449–465.

11. Ohki T, Marin ML, Veith FJ. Use of endovascular grafts to treat nonaneurysmal arterial disease. Ann Vasc Surg 1997;11:200–205.

12. Parodi JC. Endovascular repair of abdominal aortic aneurysms and other arterial lesions. J Vasc Surg 1995;21:549–557.

13. Becker GJ, Benenati JF, Zemel G, et al. Percutaneous placement of a balloon-expandable intraluminal graft for life-threatening subclavian arterial hemorrhage. J Vasc Intervent Radiol 1991;2:225–229.

14. Dorros G, Joseph G. Closure of a popliteal arteriovenous fistula using an autologous vein covered Palmaz stent. J Endovasc Surg 1995;2:177–181.

15. Hurst RW, Haskal ZJ, Zager E, et al. Endovascular stent treatment of cervical internal carotid artery aneurysms with parent vessel preservation. Surg Neurol 1998;50:313–317.

16. Ditmars ML, Klein SR, Bongard FS. Diagnosis and management of zone III carotid injuries. Injury 1997;8:515–520.

17. Horowitz MB, Miller G, Meyer Y, et al. Use of intravascular stent in the treatment of internal carotid and extracranial vertebral artery pseudoaneurysms. AJNR 1996;17:693–696.

18. Marks MP, Dake MD, Steinberg GK, et al. Stent placement for arterial and venous cerebrovascular disease: preliminary experience. Radiology 1994;191:441–446.

19. Parodi JC. Endovascular repair of aortic aneurysms, arteriovenous fistulas, and false aneurysms. World J Surg 1996;20:655–663.

20. Allen BT, Munn JS, Stevens SL, et al. Selective non-operative management of pseudoaneurysms and arteriovenous fistulae complicating femoral artery catheterization. J Cardiovasc Surg 1992;33:440–447.

21. Mills JL, Wiedeman JE, Robison JG, et al. Minimizing mortality and morbidity from iatrogenic arterial injuries: the need for early recognition and prompt repair. J Vasc Surg 1986;4:22–27.

22. Rich NM, Hobson RW, Jarstfer BS, et al. Subclavian artery trauma. J Trauma 1973;13:485–496.

23. Cosell JS, Crawford ES. Surgical treatment of aneurysms of the intrathoracic segment of the subclavian artery. Chest 1987;91:704–708.

24. Babatasi G, Massetti M, Le Page O, et al. Endovascular treatment of a traumatic subclavian artery aneurysm. J Trauma 1998;44(3):545–547.

25. McCann RL. Basic data related to peripheral artery aneurysms. Ann Vasc Surg 1990;4:411–414.

26. Schmitter SP, Marx M, Bernstein R, et al. Angioplasty-induced subclavian artery dissection in a patient with internal mammary artery graft: treatment with endovascular stent and stent-graft. AJR 1995;165:449–451.

27. Gomez-Jorge JT, Guerra JJ, Scagnelli T, et al. Endovascular management of a traumatic subclavian arteriovenous fistula. J Vasc Intervent Radiol 1996;7:599–602.

28. Meyer T, Merkel S, Lang W. Combined operative and endovascular treatment of a post-traumatic embolizing aneurysm of the subclavian artery. J Endovasc Surg 1998;5:52–55.

29. May J, White G, Waugh R, et al. Transluminal placement of a prosthetic graft-stent device for treatment of subclavian artery aneurysm. J Vasc Surg 1993;18:1056–1059.

30. Roth SM, Wheeler JR, Gregory RT, et al. Blunt injury of the abdominal aorta: a review. J Trauma 1997;42(4):742–755.

31. Michaels AJ, Gerndt SJ, Taheri PA, et al. Blunt force injury of the abdominal aorta. J Trauma 1996;41(1):105–109.

32. Marty-Ane C, Alric P, Prudhomme M, et al. Intravascular stenting of traumatic abdominal aortic dissection. J Vasc Surg 1996;23:156–161.

33. White R, Donayre C, Walot I, et al. Endograft repair of an aortic pseudoaneurysm following gunshot wound injury: impact of imaging on diagnosis and planning of intervention. J Endovasc Surg 1997;4:344–351.

34. Formichi M, Raybaud G, Benichou H, et al. Rupture of the external iliac artery during balloon angioplasty: endovascular treatment using a covered stent. J Endovasc Surg 1998;5:37–41.

35. Allgayer B, Theiss W, Naundorf M. Percutaneous closure of an arteriovenous iliac fistula with a Cragg endoluminal graft. AJR 1996;166:673–674.

36. Weibull H, Bergqvist D, Jonsson K, et al. Complications after percutaneous transluminal angioplasty in the iliac, femoral and popliteal arteries. J Vasc Surg 1987;5:681–686.

37. Schubart PJ, Porter JM. Arterial complications associated with the use of balloon catheters. In: Bernhar VM, Towne JB, eds. Complications in Vascular Surgery. 2nd ed. New York: Grune & Straton, 1984:87–109.

38. Feliciano SV, Mattox KL. Thoracic and abdominal vascular trauma. In: Veith FJ, Hobson RW, Williams RA, Wilson SE, eds. Vascular Surgery: Principles and Practice. New York: McGraw-Hill, 1984:947–966.

39. Pretre R, Chilcott M. Blunt trauma to the heart and great vessels. N Engl J Med 1997;336:626–632.

40. Cornwell EE, Kennedy F, Berne TV, et al. Gunshot wounds to the thoracic aorta in the 90s: only prevention will make a difference. Am Surg 1995;61:721–723.

41. Spencer FC, Guerin PF, Blake HA, et al. Report of fifteen patients with traumatic aneurysm of thoracic aorta. J Thorac Cardiovasc Surg 1961;41:1–22.

42. Finkelmeier BA, Mentzer RM, Kaiser DL, et al. Chronic traumatic thoracic aneurysm. J Thorac Cardiovasc Surg 1982;84:257–266.

43. Bacharach JM, Garratt KN, Rooke TW. Chronic traumatic thoracic aneurysm: report of two cases with the question of timing for surgical intervention. J Vasc Surg 1993;17:780–783.

44. Mattox KL, Feliciano DV, Burch J, et al. Five thousand seven hundred sixty cardiovascular injuries in 4459 patients: epidemiologic evaluation 1958 to 1987. Ann Surg 1989;209:698–707.

45. Li RC Jr, Trunkey DD, Blaisdell FW. Acute abdominal aortic injury: an analysis of operative and postoperative management. Arch Surg 1974;109:706–711.

46. Synder WH III, Thal ER, Perry MO. Peripheral and abdominal vascular injuries. In: Rutherford RB, ed. Vascular Surgery. 2nd ed. Philadelphia: WB Saunders, 1984:460–500.

47. McCombs PR, Roberts B. Acute renal failure following resection of abdominal aortic aneurysm. Surg Gynecol Obstet 1979;148:175–178.

48. Frykberg ER, Crump JM, Dennis JW, et al. Non-operative observation of clinically occult arterial injuries: a prospective evaluation. Surgery 1991;109:85–96.

49. Pretre R, LaHarpe R, Cheretakis K, et al. Blunt injury to the ascending aorta: three patterns of presentation. Surgery 1996;119:603–610.

50. George SM Jr, Croce MA, Fabian TC, et al. Cervicothoracic arterial injuries: recommendations for diagnosis and management. World J Surg 1991;15:134–140.

51. Cogbill TH, Moore EE, Meissner M, et al. The spectrum of blunt injury to the carotid artery: a multicenter perspective. J Trauma 1994;37:473–479.

52. Walker WA, Pate JW. Medical management of acute traumatic rupture or the aorta. Ann Thorac Surg 1990;50:965.

53. Kato N, Dake MD, Miller DC, et al. Traumatic thoracic aortic aneurysm: treatment with endovascular stent-grafts. Radiology 1997;205:657–662.

54. Semba CP, Kato N, Kee ST. Acute rupture of the descending thoracic aorta: repair with use of endovascular stent-grafts. J Vasc Intervent Radiol 1997;8:337–342.

55. Desgranges P, Mialhe C, Cavillon A. Endovascular repair of post-traumatic thoracic pseudoaneurysm with a stent graft. AJR 1997;169:1743–1745.

56. Deshpande A, Mossop P, Gurry J, et al. Treatment of traumatic false aneurysm of the thoracic aorta with endoluminal grafts. J Endovasc Surg 1998;5:120–125.

57. Hamilton IN Jr, Hollier LH. Adjunctive therapy for spinal cord protection during thoracoabdominal aortic aneurysm repair. Semin Thorac Cardiovasc Surg 1998;10:35–39.

58. Duhaylongsod FG, Glower DD, Wolfe WG. Acute traumatic aortic aneurysm: the Duke experience from 1970–1990. J Vasc Surg 1992;15:331–343.

59. Galan G, Penalver JC, Paris F, et al. Blunt chest injuries in 1696 patients. Eur J Cardiothorac Surg 1992;6:284–287.

60. Money SR, Rice K, Crockett D, et al. Risk of respiratory failure after repair of thoracoabdominal aortic aneurysms. Am J Surg 1994;168:152–155.

61. Yuzuru S. Endovascular stent-grafts for traumatic thoracic aortic aneurysm. Radiology 1998;209:283–284.

62. Temundom T, D'Ayala M, Marin M. Endovascular grafts in the treatment of thoracic aortic aneurysms and pseudoaneurysms. 1998 submitted for publication.

63. Szilagyi D, Smith R, Elliot J, et al. Anastomotic aneurysms after vascular reconstruction: problems of incidence, aetiology, and treatment. Surgery 1975;78:800–816.

64. Mikati A, Marache P, Watel A, et al. End-to-side aortoprosthetic anastomoses: long-term computed tomography assessment. Ann Vasc Surg 1990;4:584–591.

65. Van der Akker P, Brand R, van Schlifgaarde R, et al. False aneurysms after prosthetic reconstructions for aortoiliac obstructive disease. Ann Surg 1989;210:658–666.

66. Crawford E, Manning L, Kelly T. "Redo" surgery after operations for aneurysm and occlusion of the abdominal aorta. Surgery 1977;81:41–52.

67. Allen R, Schneider J, Longenecker L, et al. Paraanastomotic aneurysms of the abdominal aorta. J Vasc Surg 1993;18:424–432.

68. Treiman G, Weaver F, Cossman D, et al. Anastomotic false aneurysms of the abdominal aorta and the iliac arteries. J Vasc Surg 1988;8:268–273.

69. Yuan JG, Marin ML, Veith FJ, et al. Endovascular grafts for noninfected aortoiliac anastomotic aneurysms. J Vasc Surg 1997;26:210–221.

70. Parodi JC, Palmaz JC, Barone HD. Transfemoral intraluminal graft implantation for abdominal aortic aneurysms. Ann Vasc Surg 1991;5:491–499.

71. Marin M, Veith F, Cynamon J, et al. Transfemoral endovascular stented graft treatment of aorto-iliac and femoropopliteal occlusive disease for limb salvage. Am J Surg 1994;168:156–162.

72. White R, Donayre C, Walot I, et al. Preliminary clinical outcome and imaging criterion for endovascular prosthesis development in high-risk patients who have aortoiliac and traumatic arterial lesions. J Vasc Surg 1996;24:556–571.

73. Lumsden A, Allen R, Chaikof E, et al. Delayed rupture of aortic aneurysm following endovascular stent graftings. Am J Surg 1995;170:174–178.

74. Palmaz J, Laborde J, Rivera F, et al. Stenting of the iliac arteries with the Palmaz stent: experience from a multicenter trial. Cardiovasc Intervent Radiol 1992;15:291–297.

14

Gastrointestinal Stents and Stent-Grafts

GREGORY ZUCCARO, JR.

■ Esophageal Stents

Rationale for Stenting

Stents are employed in the esophagus and across the gastroesophageal junction as a means of palliation for malignant obstruction. There are several clinical circumstances in which stenting is employed. One is to increase the luminal diameter of the esophagus in cases of intrinsic malignancy, so that patients are able to maintain adequate nutrition and swallow their oral secretions. Both the first-generation plastic stents and current self-expanding metal stents allow for patients to take soft foods and liquids without much difficulty. More solid foods may also be ingested if dentition and mastication are adequate. Another indication for stenting is to seal off a malignant fistula between the airway and the esophagus, as may be seen as a complication of proximal esophageal or tracheobronchial cancers. Stents may less commonly be employed in palliation of dysphagia from extrinsic compression of the esophagus.

Alternatives to Stenting

Stents are only employed in palliation of malignant dysphagia in patients who are not candidates for more curative interventions such as surgery or chemoradiotherapy. In most cases, palliation is chosen due to the presence of metastatic disease, multiple comorbid illnesses, and/or advanced age.

There are several treatment modalities available for the palliation of esophageal or gastroesophageal junctional malignancies. Periodic endoscopic dilation alone

can be performed. Typically, dilation is performed after a guidewire is placed through the stricture into the stomach with combined endoscopic and fluoroscopic guidance. Then progressively larger dilators are passed over the wire. There are several factors that influence the maximum diameter of dilation achieved, including the initial diameter of the stricture, the degree of resistance felt as progressively larger dilators are used, and the presence or absence of previous radiation therapy. Palliation of dysphagia is often satisfactory after dilation alone, but not unexpectedly the response is short lived.[1] Dilation of a malignant stricture is associated with increased risk of perforation compared to routine dilation of benign, peptic strictures or rings.[2] This dilation may also be performed immediately prior to esophageal stent placement.

Sclerosants may be injected into the obstructing tumor under endoscopic guidance. There have been three clinical series reporting on the success of injection therapy with 95% alcohol.[3–5] The technique involved multiple injections of 0.5 to 1.0 cc in multiple areas of the neoplasm. In general, there is improvement in the ability to swallow, and the benefit may last for a month or longer. Potential complications include fever, chest pain requiring narcotic analgesia, mediastinitis, and esophageal perforation.

Thermal methods are commonly utilized to ablate exophytic portions of an obstructing malignancy. Laser therapy can be accomplished with the Nd:YAG (neodynium:yttrium-aluminum-garnet) laser. A quartz fiber is passed down the operating channel of the endoscope and is used to apply the laser energy to the exophytic portions of the tumor. Laser energy may be applied in an anterograde or retrograde fashion. Retrograde therapy affords the operator the optimal visualization and the ability to keep the esophageal lumen in view. However, for tight malignant strictures, treating in retrograde fashion requires dilation of the malignant stricture prior to laser therapy, thereby exposing the patient to the risk of perforation from dilation. In a comparative trial of laser versus injection therapy (polidocanol) for palliation of malignant esophageal obstruction, there was excellent initial response for both modalities, with 82% response for injection and 89% for laser. There was one perforation, in the injection group. Several treatment sessions were required for each modality.[6]

Photosensitizing agents that preferentially accumulate in malignant tissue may be administered prior to laser therapy for malignant dysphagia. Porfimer sodium is a commonly utilized agent. In photodynamic therapy with this agent, light at 630 nm is generated by a tunable dye laser and application performed via a probe inserted through the operating channel of the endoscope 2 to 4 days after injection of the photosensitizing agent. This technique is effective in restoring luminal patency in the esophagus. A disadvantage of this technique is that the photosensitivity is not limited to the tumor alone, and therefore patients must avoid direct sunlight for 30 to 45 days or risk dermal burns. This is a significant issue in patients whose life expectancy is relatively short. In one comparative trial, Nd:YAG and photodynamic therapy had equal success in relieving malignant dysphagia at 1 week and 1 month after treatment.[7] Some adverse effects were somewhat more frequent in the photodynamic therapy group, including fever, pleural effusion, and photosensitivity. However, perforation was more common in the Nd:YAG group. Another smaller trial showed photodynamic therapy to be superior to Nd:YAG laser in both initial and mean duration of relief of malignant dysphagia.[8]

Esophageal Stenting

From the above discussion, the potential advantages of esophageal prosthesis, or stents, are evident. A stent, properly positioned, affords the opportunity for relatively longer-term palliation compared with some of the methods described above. Placement of the prosthesis generally can be achieved with one endoscopic procedure. The relief of malignant dysphagia is immediate. The procedure may now be done on an outpatient basis in most cases. Avoidance of direct sunlight, stricture, and other disadvantages of photodynamic therapy do not occur. While there are potential adverse effects of prosthesis placement, and failures can occur, it is the preferred method of palliation of esophageal malignancy in our institution.

Early Prostheses

The first esophageal prostheses were made of rigid materials such as Tygon or Celestin (Fig. 14–1). The prostheses did vary, but frequently they were approximately 15 mm in diameter. They were fashioned by the endoscopist and technician to the appropriate length based on the individual tumor to be stented. Early models were straight, but as experience increased the ends were fashioned with funnels or flanges to decrease stent migration. Placement methods varied and were often fashioned by the individual endoscopist rather than utilizing a standard, commercially available system. Most frequently, this would be done with a pusher tube mounted over a fluoroscopically placed guidewire or onto the insertion tube of the endoscope. Tumors in the middle and distal esophagus were the optimal candidates; extremely proximal tumors could not be stented satisfactorily as the proximal end of the stent would be too close to the cricopharyngeus, an intolerable situation for the patient. This stent has been modified considerably over time. Currently, rigid stents are made of materials such as silicone or polyvinyl chloride. Many have an inner coil or metal spring for increased strength. Some have more tapered proximal margins for better patient tolerance for palliation of the proximal malignancy.

A summary of some of the larger clinical trials utilizing the rigid prosthesis in the palliation of esophageal

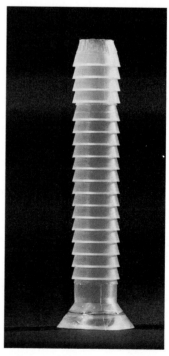

FIGURE 14–1. A rigid esophageal prosthesis. These devices have largely been replaced by the self-expanding metal stent.

TABLE 14–1. Clinical Series Utilizing Rigid Esophageal Prostheses for Palliation of Esophageal Cancer

Series	No. of Patients	Success Rate (%)	Perforation Rate (%)	Necrosis/Delayed Perforation (%)	Tumor Ingrowth or Obstruction (%)	Stent Migration	Death Rate (%)
Tytgat[18]	297	97	8	4	9	19	1
Atkinson et al[19]	25	96	8	NR	0	12	4
Palmer[20]	75	100	0	0	1	0	0
Ogilvie et al[21]	118	100	13	8	6	4	8

NR, not reported.

cancer is presented in Table 14–1. Overall, in experienced hands these devices provided reasonable palliation of malignant dysphagia. There were several potential complications. These could be divided into early (related to insertion of prosthesis and first few days afterward) and later complications. The early complications included perforation of the malignant stricture, and airway compromise due to the rigid, large diameter tube. Perforation might occur with dilation of the malignant stricture; these devices called for dilation of the malignant stenosis to 16 mm or greater to create enough space for deployment. Perforation could also occur with the placement of the tube due to its rigidity. Airway compromise could occur in palliation of proximal esophageal tumors, or where a pulmonary malignancy led to a fistula to the esophagus, as the mass effect of the malignancy could cause the prosthesis to compress the trachea. Later complications included migration of the prosthesis out of the malignant stricture,

pressure necrosis, bleeding, and obstruction due to tumor growth at the proximal or distal aspects of the stent, or from a food bolus lodged in the prosthesis.

In a clinical trial comparing these early rigid stents with Nd:YAG laser in the palliation of malignant dysphagia, it was found that midesophageal tumors were equally palliated by either technique, but for tumors of the esophagogastric junction the placement of a prosthesis was superior.[9] More treatment sessions were required for the laser therapy, but laser was associated with a lower perforation rate; the perforation rate for the rigid prosthesis was 13%. Survival was no different in the two groups (Fig. 14–2).

Self-Expanding Metal Stents

These prostheses are wire or metal stents in a mesh or coil configuration, which are implanted at a relatively

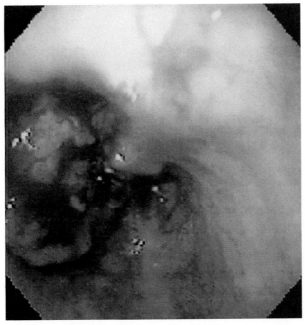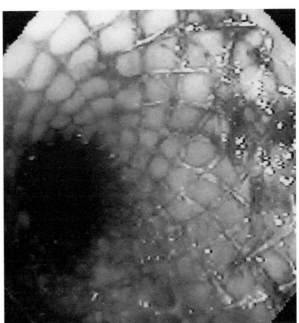

FIGURE 14–2. (A). An obstructing esophageal cancer; the patient also has distant metastases. **(B).** A self-expanding metal stent has been placed to palliate the dysphagia.

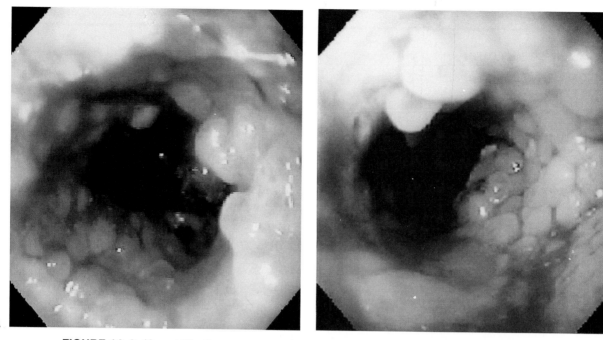

FIGURE 14–3. (A and **B).** Squamous pseudoepithelial hyperplasia has formed at the proximal aspect of a previously placed self-expanding metal stent. This is felt to be an inflammatory response to the stent.

smaller diameter and then expand to full diameter after implantation within the malignant stricture (Fig. 14–3). There are several commercially available self-expanding metal stents, each made of different materials, each with different tensile strengths. Among the materials utilized in the construction of these stents are stainless steel, titanium, and cobalt/chromium alloys. These stents may be uncovered, or covered with a silicone coating. The main theoretical advantage of coating a self-expanding stent is to retard obstruction due to tumor ingrowth (Fig. 14–4). However, it has been felt that uncovered stents may be preferable because they are less likely to migrate distally after placement. Attributes of some of these stents are listed in Table 14–2.

There are several potential advantages to the self-expanding metal stents (Table 14–3). One of the greatest is the lower diameter of the stent prior to deployment. This lower diameter allows for much less aggressive dilation compared with rigid stents prior to placement. Also, the delivery systems are far less difficult to use in the deployment of these stents.

There are several clinical trials comparing self-expanding metal stents with rigid prostheses. In a comparison of 41 patients randomized to palliation with a 16-mm plastic prosthesis (Wilson-Cook, Winston-Salem, NC) or an uncovered self-expanding to 16 mm Wallstent (Schneider AG, Bulach, Switzerland), there was equal excellent palliation of malignant dysphagia.[10] However, complications occurred in 43% of the patients receiving the plastic prosthesis, compared with

0% in the self-expanding stent group. The plastic stent group, therefore, had a greater number of days in the hospital and larger number of reinterventions. Despite the greater commercial cost of the self-expanding

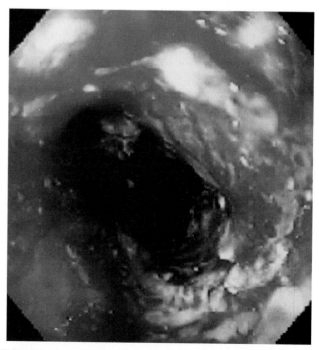

FIGURE 14–4. Tumor ingrowth (seen at the 12 o'clock to 3 o'clock aspect of the lumen) has caused a recurrence of dysphagia in a patient with a previously placed self-expanding metal stent. Note visible stent at the 4 to 6 o'clock aspect of the lumen.

TABLE 14–2. Characteristics of Self-Expanding Metal Stents

Stent Type	Flanges	Length (cm)	Coating (cm)	Delivery Catheter Size (Fr)	Minimum Lumen Diameter (mm)	Maximum Flange Diameter (mm)	Cost*
Ultraflex (Microvasive)	Proximal	10,15	None	15	18	23	$1,195
Ultraflex (Microvasive	Proximal	10,15	Yes 7,12	15	18	23	$1,295
Wallstent esophageal (Schneider)	Proximal, distal	8,10,13	Premalume 4,6,9	38	18	20–28	$1,495–$1,895
Wallstent esophageal II (Schneider)	Proximal, distal	10,15	Permalume 8,13	18	19	20–28	$1,695–$1,895
Wallstent enteral (Schneider)	None	6,9	None	10	18,20,22	18,20,22	$1,195–$1,825
Z-Stent (Wilson-Cook)	Proximal, distal	6,8,10, 12,14	Polyurethane 6, 8,10,12,14	31	18	21–25	$1,045–$1,125
Esophacoil (Instent) (Bard)	Proximal, distal	10,15	Coil	32	16–18	21–24	$1,500
Plastic stents (multiple manufacturers)	Proximal distal	4.4–16.4	N/A	N/A	12	25	$32–$134

*Does not include cost of reusable delivery components.
From ASGE Technology Assessment document, May 1997.

stents, a cost analysis favored use of the self-expanding metal stents for the palliation of malignant dysphagia. Another comparison of 39 patients randomized to a plastic prosthesis (Wilson-Cook) or self-expanding un-coated Ultraflex metal stent (Boston Scientific, Water-town, MA) showed similar success in deployment and initial dysphagia relief.[11] Again, there was a significant difference in the complication rate (21% plastic stent, 0% metal stent) and mortality (16% plastic stent, 0% metal stent). Still another series of 75 patients random-ized to latex plastic stents or coated self-expanding metal stents again demonstrated a significantly greater major complication rate with placement of the plastic stents.[12] All of these trials were prospective and random-ized. There is one retrospective analysis that indicated no significant difference in procedure-related mortal-ity, relief of dysphagia, or survival from installation of plastic versus a variety of self-expanding metal stents.[13]

Self-expanding metal stents have been compared with other modalities in the palliation of esophageal cancer. In one prospective trial randomizing patients to plastic stents, self-expanding metal stents, or laser therapy, pa-tients undergoing stent placement had superior relief of dysphagia compared to the laser group.[14] A small prospective trial compared laser therapy alone with laser therapy followed by self-expanding metal stent place-ment.[15] It appeared that stent placement did lengthen the dysphagia-free interval.

Many patients undergoing placement of self-expand-ing metal stents may have had previous chemoradio-therapy, or will undergo radiation therapy after stent placement. There has been some suggestion in the liter-ature that stent placement under these circumstances may be associated with an increased complication rate compared with patients undergoing stent placement without radiation therapy. One series reported a 36% rate of serious complications in patients with previous chemoradiotherapy associated with placement of a self-expanding metal stent compared with a 3% rate in pa-tients without prior chemoradiotherapy.[16] Two retro-spective trials, however, report that patients undergoing stent placement had a similar rate of complications

TABLE 14–3. Clinical Experience with Most Commonly Utilized Self-Expanding Metal Stents

Stent	Dysphagia Relief	Stent Obstruction (%)	Stent Migration (%)
Ultraflex[22–27]	Good	18	5
Z Stent[13,28–33]	Good	11	9
Wallstent[10,34–37]	Good	5–15	3

whether or not they had undergone prior chemoradiotherapy.[13,17]

■ Pancreatobiliary Stents

Rationale for Stenting

The most common reason for placing a stent in the bile duct or pancreatic duct is in the palliation of malignant obstruction. However, there are other reasons for the placement of stents, including therapy for inflammatory or postoperative benign strictures, palliation of large, obstructing common bile duct stones, and therapy for chronic pancreatitis. Endoscopic placement of biliary duct stents was first described in 1980.[38] At endoscopic retrograde cholangiopancreatography (ERCP), ductal anatomy can be defined, brushing or biopsy obtained from a suspicious stricture, and a stent placed over a guidewire through the use of stiffening and pushing catheters. Percutaneous transhepatic cholangiography (PTHC) also provides biliary (but not pancreatic) ductal anatomy, the ability to brush strictures, and the ability to stent strictures. In some centers, patients with distal malignant strictures (e.g., due to pancreatic cancer) are managed with ERCP, and those with more proximal strictures with proximal dilation (e.g., bifurcation cancers) are managed with PTHC. However, this is not universally true, and it depends on multiple factors, including available local expertise, the primary manager of the patient, the degree of proximal ductal dilation, and the status of the liver (e.g., presence or absence of metastatic disease).

Stent Composition

The most commonly utilized stents placed in the pancreatobiliary tree at ERCP are composed of plastic. The advantage of the plastic stents is that they are easily placed, can be removed when necessary, and can be constructed with flanges or pigtails to anchor them in the appropriate position. The very great disadvantage of the plastic stents is that they have a tendency to clog, leading to a recurrence of biliary obstruction and jaundice, often associated with symptoms and signs of acute cholangitis. Careful electron microscopy studies have indicated that these stents clog via the formation of a bacterial biofilm along the interior of the stent, followed by deposition of crystals of calcium palmitate, calcium bilirubinate, and cholesterol, leading to clogging of the stent.[39] Interestingly, side holes have sometimes been added to the design of the plastic stent in an attempt to increase patency. However, careful in vitro studies have indicated that stents with side holes have a greater tendency to form occlusive sludge than those without the side holes.[40] Use of antibiotics, bile salts, and other materials does not typically decrease the likelihood of stent occlusion. Although it is impossible to predict the life span of a plastic stent within the biliary tree, most endoscopists routinely change these stents every 3 to 4 months to prevent complete occlusion and cholangitis.

Another in vitro model of stent occlusion studied the impact of stent design and material on the likelihood of sludge formation within a stent. In this model, as expected, perfusion of the stent with a bacteria-laden bile was more likely to result in sludge formation than perfusion with sterile bile. Stent made of Teflon materials were less likely to form sludge compared with plastics such as polyurethane and polyethylene.[41] However, in a prospective trial comparing polyethylene plastic stents with Teflon stents in the palliation of malignant obstruction of the biliary tree, there was no significant difference demonstrated in stent patency or survival.[42]

Metal stents are also available for use, and can be deployed at ERCP or PTHC (Fig. 14–5). The most common design is that of an expandable metal mesh, but one design is that of a more tightly wound coil. In some of these designs, the stent shortens and expands off the introducing catheter simultaneously, making deployment somewhat more challenging compared with plastic stents. As these stents typically are difficult or impossible to remove or reposition after deployment, extreme care is necessary. Also, the inability to remove most of these stents once they are placed makes their use less attractive in the treatment of benign strictures. In contrast to the metal stents for the esophagus discussed above, metal stents for the biliary tree are typically not covered, as there is concern of migration, or occlusion of the cystic duct or other ducts if a covered stent is employed. However, at the time of this writing there are ongoing endoscopic trials of covered metal stents for stenting of biliary strictures, but these stents are not commercially available for endoscopic placement.

Therapy for Malignant Strictures

Stenting for palliation of malignant obstruction of the distal biliary tree, most commonly due to pancreatic cancer, has been clearly established to be highly effective. One trial randomized patients to surgical biliary bypass versus endoscopic stenting for palliation of malignant distal biliary obstruction. Jaundice was relieved in over 90% of the patients, and while survival in the two groups did not differ, the overall number of hospital days was greater in the surgery group.[43] Endoscopic stenting for more proximal cancers can also be accomplished. However, achieving cannulation and stent placement for both the right and left systems in the case

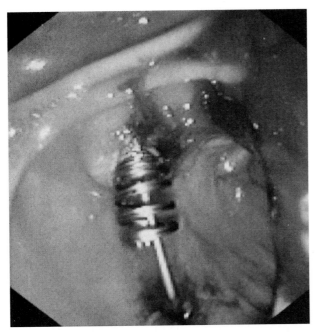 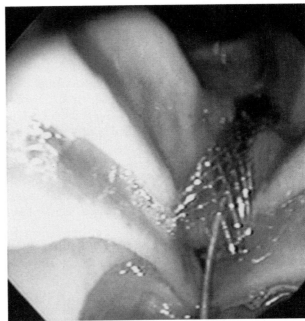

A   B

FIGURE 14–5. Coil-type (**A**) and mesh-type (**B**) self-expanding metal stents being placed in the biliary tree; note the guidewire over which the stent is placed.

of a bifurcation cancer requires considerable endoscopic skill and experience, and in general the success rates are not as high as for distal cancers without a combined endoscopic and radiologic approach.[44]

Metal stents are considerably more expensive than their plastic counterparts. Several recent prospective trials have focused on the appropriate use of plastic versus metal stents for the palliation of malignant biliary obstruction (Fig. 14–6). In one such trial of 105 patients with irresectable malignant obstruction of the distal bile duct, metal stents had significantly longer patency compared with plastic stents. Stent occlusion in the metal group was due to tumor ingrowth, and in the plastic group due to occlusion with sludge. A 28% decrease in endoscopic procedures was found when metal stents were utilized.[45] Another trial of 62 patients with malignant biliary obstruction had metal or plastic stents placed endoscopically or by combined endoscopic-percutaneous route. At 1 month after stent placement, both groups were similar. However, as expected, as the observation period extended, more stent failures occurred in the plastic group, as did the rate of cholangitis. Hospital days for stent-related failure was greater in the plastic stent group. Despite the higher initial cost of the metal stents, overall costs were greater in the plastic stent group.[46] Another trial examined palliation of malignant obstruction using a plastic stent left in place until signs/symptoms of dysfunction occurred, versus a plastic stent routinely changed every 3 months, versus placement of a metal stent. The initial overall success rate for stent placement and palliation was 97%. Complication-

free survival time was least for the group with the plastic stent not routinely changed. Metal stents were most cost-effective when the life expectancy of the patient was greater than 6 months.[47]

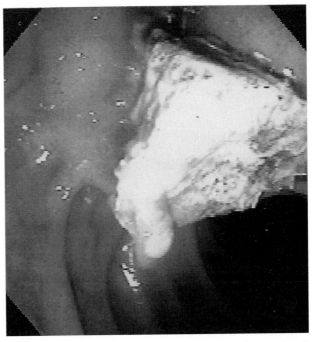

FIGURE 14–6. Debris has clogged the lumen of a previously placed self-expanding metal biliary stent.

Therapy for Benign Biliary Tract Disease

There are several circumstances where stents are placed in the biliary tract for benign disease. Complications of laparoscopic or open cholecystectomy include cystic duct leaks and strictures of the extrahepatic biliary tree. Plastic stents placed in the extrahepatic biliary tree may promote spontaneous closure of cystic duct leaks.[48] Postoperative strictures may be managed with endoscopic and/or percutaneous dilation followed by stenting for 6 to 12 months in an attempt to restore biliary flow.[49] The patient with an extrahepatic dominant stricture in primary sclerosing cholangitis is often best managed with balloon dilatation, but short-term plastic stent placement may augment the effect.[50,51] Anastomotic strictures after liver transplantation may be managed with dilation with or without stent placement.[52] On rare occasions a patient with contraindications to surgery and large, symptomatic common bile duct stones unsuccessfully removed at ERCP may be successfully managed by placement of plastic stents in the bile duct to prevent obstruction and cholangitis.[53] There have been reports of the use of metal stents for patients with benign biliary strictures.[54] However, the inability to remove the majority of these stents makes them a less attractive alternative to plastic stents for treatment of most benign conditions.

Stents in the Pancreatic Duct

Stenting the pancreatic duct is less common than biliary stenting. Plastic stents may cause changes suggestive of chronic pancreatitis when left in the main pancreatic duct for more than several weeks.[55] Stents may be temporarily placed in the main pancreatic duct at ERCP, to facilitate cannulation of the biliary tree via precut sphincterotomy.[56] These stents may also be placed to prevent post-ERCP pancreatitis in patients at increased risk for this complication.[57] Pancreatic stents may facilitate the performance of pancreatic duct papillotomy in therapy for pancreatic divisum or pancreatic sphincter dysfunction.[58] In these cases, the stents used are typically of small caliber (e.g., 5 French), and are designed with a paucity of flanges so that they will fall out of the duct within 1 to 2 weeks (Fig. 14–7). Larger-caliber plastic stents are utilized to endoscopically drain mature pancreatic pseudocysts, in a transpapillary, transgastric, or transduodenal approach.[59] Stents may be placed in the pancreatic duct for longer periods, as in the palliation of pain from chronic pancreatitis with resultant ductal strictures.[60] However, the exact role of stent therapy for chronic pancreatitis is far from completely understood (Fig. 14–8).

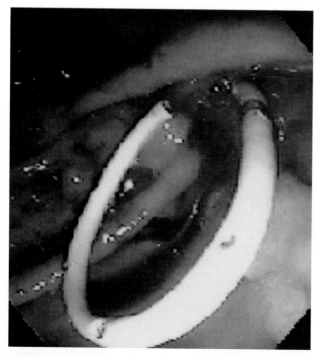

FIGURE 14–7. A single pigtail 5-French plastic stent placed in the pancreatic duct prior to biliary sphincterotomy. Such stenting is helpful in preventing post–endoscopic retrograde cholangiopancreatography (ERCP) pancreatitis in some cases. The stent must not be left for long, as long-term pancreatic duct stenting may lead to ductal changes of chronic pancreatitis.

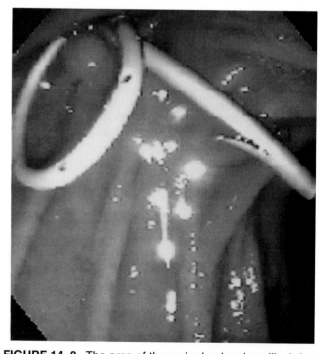

FIGURE 14–8. The area of the main duodenal papilla 4 days after ampullectomy for tubular adenoma of the main duodenal papilla. Stents were placed in the distal bile duct and pancreatic duct immediately after the ampullectomy to prevent cholangitis or pancreatitis. The endoscopy 4 days later was to remove the stents. Note that the straight biliary stent has migrated out of the papilla somewhat; these stents are typically placed such that the visible flange abuts the main papilla.

■ Stents for Obstruction of the Gastric Outlet, Proximal Small Bowel, and Rectosigmoid

Malignant obstruction in these regions of the gastrointestinal tract are most frequently palliated with surgery. However, in patients with significant comorbid illnesses and/or extremely limited life expectancy, metal stents may be used to palliate the obstruction. The technique is most frequently an endoscopic one, usually with fluoroscopic guidance. The stricture is approached with a therapeutic flexible endoscope. Most frequently, the degree of obstruction is such that the endoscope will not pass. The stricture may be dilated with balloons, followed by endoscopic passage through the stricture to assess its exact length and facilitate placement of the stent. If this approach is felt to expose the patient to unacceptably high risk of bleeding or perforation, an alternative method involves placement of a hollow catheter into the malignant stricture, administration of contrast to visualize the length and contour of the stricture, followed by stent placement. In either case, the stent is typically deployed over the guidewire with endoscopic and fluoroscopic guidance. There have been reports of successful palliation of malignant obstruction of the gastric outlet, proximal small bowel, and rectosigmoid.[61,62]

REFERENCES

1. Heit HA, Johnson LF, Siegel SR, Boyce HW. Palliative dilation for dysphagia in esophageal carcinoma. Ann Intern Med 1978;89:629–631.
2. Van Dam J, Rice TW, Sivak MV, et al. Malignant esophageal stricture is predictive of tumor stage and is a contraindication for endosonography using dedicated endoscopes. Cancer 1993;71:2190–2197.
3. Nwokolo CU, Payne-James JJ, Silk DBA, Loft DE. Palliation of malignant dysphagia by ethanol induced tumour necrosis. Gut 1994;35:299–303.
4. Payne-James JJ, Spiller RC, Misiewicz JJ, Silk DBA. Uses of ethanol-induced tumor necrosis to palliate dysphagia in patients with esophagogastric cancer. Gastrointest Endosc 1990;36:43–46.
5. Chung SCS, Leong HT, Choi CYC, Leung JWC, Li AKC. Palliation of malignant oesophageal obstruction by endoscopic alcohol injection. Endoscopy 1994;25:275–277.
6. Angelini G, Fratta Pasini A, Ederle A, Castagnini A, Talamini G, Bulghin G. Nd:YAG laser versus polidocanol injection for palliation of esophageal malignancy: a prospective, randomized study. Gastrointest Endosc 1991;37:607–610.
7. Lightdale CJ, Heier SK, Marcon NE, et al. Photodynamic therapy with profimer sodium versus thermal ablation with Nd:YAD laser for palliation of esophageal cancer; a multicenter randomized trial. Gastrointest Endosc 1995;42:507–512.
8. Heir SK, Rothman KA, Heier LM, Rosenthal LM. Photodynamic therapy for obstructing esophageal cancer: light dosimetry and randomized comparison with Nd:YAG laser therapy. Gastroenterology 1995;109:63–72.
9. Loizou LA, Grigg D, Atkinson M, Robertson C, Brown SA. A prospective comparison of laser therapy and intubation in endoscopic palliation for malignant dysphagia. Gastroenterology 1991;100:1303–1310.
10. Knyrim K, Wagner HJ, Bethge N, Keymling M, Vakil N. A controlled trial of an expansible metal stent for palliation of esophageal obstruction due to inoperable cancer. N Engl J Med 1993;329:1302–1307.
11. DePalma G, deMateo E, Romano G, Fimmano A, Rondinone G, Catanzano C. Plastic prosthesis versus expandable metal stents for palliation of inoperable esophageal thoracic carcinoma: a controlled prospective study. Gastrointest Endosc 1996;96:478–482.
12. Siersema PD, Hop WCJ, Dees J, Tilanus HW, van Blankenstein M. Coated self-expanding metal stents versus latex prostheses for esophagogastric cancer with special reference to prior radiation and chemotherapy: a controlled, prospective study. Gastrointest Endosc 1998;47:113–120.
13. Kozarek RA, Ball TJ, Brandabur JJ, Patterson DJ, Low D, Hill L, Raltz S. Expandable versus conventional prosthesis: easier insertion may not preclude subsequent stent-related problems. Gastrointest Endosc 1996;43:204–208.
14. Adam A, Ellul J, Watkinson AF, Tan BS, Morgan RA, Saunders MP, Mason RC. Palliation of inoperable esophageal carcinoma: a prospective randomized trial of laser therapy and stent placement. Radiology 1997;202:344–348.
15. Tranberg KG, Stael van Holstein C, Ivancev K, Cwikiel W, Lunderquist A. The YAG laser and Wallstent endoprosthesis for palliation of cancer in the esophagus or gastric cardia. Hepatogastroenterology 1995;42:139–144.
16. Kinsman KJ, DeGregorio BT, Katon RM, et al. Prior radiation and chemotherapy increase the risk of life-threatening complications after insertion of metallic stents for esophago gastric malignancy. Gastronintest Endosc 1996;43(3):196–203.
17. Raijman I, Siddique I, Lynch P. Does chemoradiation therapy increase the incidence of complications with self-expanding metal coated stents in the management of malignant esophageal strictures? Am J Gastroenterol 1997;92:2192–2196.
18. Tytgat GN. Endoscopic methods of treatment of gastrointestinal and biliary stenoses. Endoscopy 1980#ppl:57–58.
19. Atkinson M, Ferguson R, Parker GC. Tube introducer and modified Celestin tube for use in palliative intubation of oesophagogastric neoplasms at fibreoptic endoscopy. Gut 1978;19:669–671.
20. Palmer ED. Peroral prosthesis for the management of incurable esophageal cancer. Am J Gastroenterol 1973;59:487–498.
21. Ogilvie AL, Dronfield MW, Ferguson R, Atkinson M. Palliative intubation of oesophagogastric neoplasms at fibreoptic endoscopy. Gut 1982;23:1060–1067.
22. Cwikeil W, Stridbeck H. Esophageal stent placement in malignant disease. J Vasc Intervent Radiol 1993;4:125–126.
23. Sass N, Hagenmuller F. First endoscopic implantation of memory metal stents in the esophagus. Endoscopy 1992;24:622.
24. Raijman I, Walden D, Kortan P, et al. Expandable esophageal stents: initial experience with a new nitinol stent. Gastrointest Endosc 1994;40:614–621.
25. Maynar M, Ribero L, Pulido-Duque J, et al. Palliative treatment of malignant dysphagia with elastalloy esophageal endoprosthesis (Strecker): preliminary results (abstract). Society of Cardiovascular and Interventional Radiology Meeting 1993;4:174.
26. Alhalel IR, Bourke MJ, Elfant AB, et al. Palliation of malignant dysphagia with expandable esophageal stents (EES) in intrinsic vs. Extrinsic disease (abstract). Gastrointest Endosc 1995;41:345.
27. Grund K, Sotrek D, Naruhn M. Flexible metal stents in the esophagus. Gastrointest Endosc 1993;39:278.
28. Kozarek R, Ball T, Patterson D. Metallic self-expanding stent application in the upper gastrointestinal tract: caveats and concerns. Gastrointest Endosc 1992;38:1–6.
29. Wu W, Katon R, Saxon R, et al. Silicon-covered self-expanding metallic stents for the palliation of malignant esophageal obstruc-

tion and esophagorespiratory fistulas: experience in 32 patients and a review of the literature. Gastrointest Endosc 1994;40:22–33.

30. Solt J, Papp Z. Coated metallic self-expanding (Gianturco Z) stent implantation in malignant esophagogastric stenosis. Endoscopy 1994;26:368–372.

31. Song H, Choi K, Cho B, et al. Esophagogastric neoplasms: palliation with a modified Gianturco stent. Radiology 1991;180:349–354.

32. Song H, Choi K, Kwon H, et al. Esophageal strictures: treatment with a new design of modified Gianturco stent. Radiology 1992;184:729–744.

33. Weigert N, Neuhaus H, Rosch T, et al. Treatment of esophagorespiratory fistulas with silicone self-expanding metal stents. Gastrointest Endosc 1995;41:490–496.

34. Ell C, Hochberger J, May A, Fleig W, Hahn E. Coated and uncoated self-expanding metal stents for malignant stenosis in the upper GI tract: preliminary clinical experiences with Wallstents. Am J Gastroenterol 1994;89:1496–1500.

35. Neuhaus H, Hoffman W, Dittier H, et al. Implantation of self-expanding metal stents for palliation of malignant dysphagia. Endoscopy 1992;24:405–410.

36. Fleischer D, Bull-Henry K. A new coated self-expanding metal stent for malignant esophageal strictures. Gastrointest Endosc 1992;38:494–496.

37. Vermeijden J, Bartelsman J, Fockens P, Meijer R, Tytgat G. Self-expanding metal stents for palliation of esophagocardial malignancies. Gastrointest Endosc 1995;41:58–63.

38. Soehendra N, Reijnders-Frederix V. Palliative bile duct drainage: a new endoscopic method of introducing a transpapillary drain. Endoscopy 1980;12:8–11.

39. Speer AG, Cotton PD, Rode J, et al. Biliary stent blockage with bacterial biofilm. A light and electron microscopy study. Ann Intern Med 1988;108:546–553.

40. Coene PP, Groen AK, Cheng J, Out MM, Tytgat GN, Huibregtse K. Clogging of biliary endoprostheses: a new perspective. Gut 1990;31:913–917.

41. Dowidar N, Kolmos HJ, Matzen P. Experimental clogging of biliary endoprostheses. Role of bacteria, endoprosthesis material and design. Scand J Gastroenterol 1992;27:77–80.

42. van Berkel AM, Boland C, Redekop WK, et al. A prospective randomized trial of Teflon versus polyethylene stents for distal malignant biliary obstruction. Endoscopy 1998;30:681–686.

43. Shepherd HA, Royle G, Ross AP, Diba A, Arthur M, Colin-Jones D. Endoscopic biliary endoprosthesis in the palliation of malignant obstruction of the distal common bile duct: a randomized trial. Br J Surg 1988;75:1166–1168.

44. Faulkner J, Kozarek RA, Traverso LW. The role of ERCP in diagnosis and treatment of cholangiocarcinoma. Gastroenterology 1993; 104:A382.

45. Davids PH, Groen AK, Rauws EA, Tytgat GN, Huibregtse K. Randomised trial of self-expanding metal stents versus polyethylene stents for distal malignant biliary obstruction. Lancet 1992;340: 1488–1492.

46. Knyrim K, Wagner HJ, Pausch J, Vakil N. A prospective, randomized, controlled trial of metal stents for malignant obstruction of the common bile duct. Endoscopy 1993;25:207–212.

47. Prat F, Chapat O, Ducot B, et al. A randomized trial of endoscopic drainage methods for inoperable malignant strictures of the common bile duct. Gastrointest Endosc 1998;47:1–7.

48. Davids PH, Rauws EA, Tytgat GN, Huibregtse K. Postoperative bile leakage: endoscopic management. Gut 1992;33:1118–1122.

49. Berkelhammer C, Kortan P, Haber GB. Endoscopic biliary prostheses as treatment for benign postoperative bile duct strictures. Gastrointest Endosc 1989;35:95–101.

50. van Milligen de Wit AW, Rauws EA, van Bracht J, et al. Lack of complications following short-term stent therapy for extrahepatic bile duct strictures in primary sclerosing cholangitis. Gastrointest Endosc 1997;46:344–347.

51. van Milligen de Wit AW, van Bracht J, Rauws EA, Jones EA, Tytgat GN, Huibregtse K. Endoscopic stent therapy for dominant extrahepatic bile duct strictures in primary sclerosing cholangitis. Gastrointest Endosc 1996;44:293–299.

52. Rossi AF, Grosso C, Zanasi G, et al. Long-term efficacy of endoscopic stenting in patients with stricture of the biliary anastomosis after orthotopic liver transplantation. Endoscopy 1998;30:360–366.

53. Maxton DG, Tweedle DE, Martin DF. Retained common bile duct stones after endoscopic sphincterotomy: temporary and long-term treatment with biliary stenting. Gut 1995;36:446–449.

54. Deviere J, Cremer M, Baize M, Love J, Sugai B, Vandermeeren A. Management of common bile duct stricture caused by chronic pancreatitis with metal mesh self-expandable stents. Gut 1994;35: 122–126.

55. Smith MT, Sherman S, Ikenberry SO, Hawes RH, Lehman GA. Alterations in pancreatic ductal morphology following polyethylene pancreatic stent therapy. Gastrointest Endosc 1996;44: 268–275.

56. Fogel EL, Sherman S, Lehman GA. Increased selective biliary cannulation rates in the setting of periampullary diverticula: main pancreatic duct stent placement followed by pre-cut biliary sphincterotomy. Gastrointest Endosc 1998;47:396–400.

57. Sherman S, Ruffolo TA, Hawes RH, Lehman GA. Complications of endoscopic sphincterotomy. A prospective series with emphasis on the increased risk associated with sphincter of Oddi dysfunction and nondilated bile cuts. Gastroenterology 1991;101: 1068–1075.

58. Lehman GA, Sherman S. Diagnosis and therapy of pancreas divisum. Gastrointest Endosc Clin North Am 1998;8:55–77.

59. Beckingham IJ, Krige JE, Bornman PC, Terblanche J. Endoscopic management of pancreatic pseudocysts. Br J Surg 1997;84:1638–1645.

60. Laugier R, Renou C. Endoscopic ductal drainage may avoid resective surgery in painful chronic pancreatitis without large ductal dilatation. Int J Pancreatol 1998;23:145–152.

61. Tack J, Gevers AM, Rutgeerts P. Self-expandable metallic stents in the palliation of rectosigmoidal carcinoma: a follow-up study. Gastrointest Endosc 1998;48:267–271.

62. Nevitt AW, Vida F, Kozarek RA, Traverso LW, Raltz SL. Expandable metallic prostheses for malignant obstructions of gastric outlet and proximal small bowel. Gastrointest Endosc 1998;47:271–276.

15

Tracheobronchial Stents and Stent-Grafts

ASOK DASGUPTA AND ATUL C. MEHTA

Diverse etiologies, both malignant and benign, may lead to central airway obstruction. Every situation should be considered for surgical correction with a curative intent, yet in a majority of cases recourse to some sort of palliation remains the only therapeutic option. Today, management of tracheobronchial obstruction has evolved into a multidisciplinary approach that involves thoracic surgeons, otolaryngologists, oncologists, interventional radiologists, pulmonologists, and radiation oncologists. The development of newer accessories and therapeutic modalities and their adaptation to the rigid as well as flexible endoscopes has significantly enhanced the role of the interventional bronchoscopists in the management of such lesions.[1-3] As outlined in Table 15–1, selection of any particular modality is influenced not only by the acuity of presentation and the nature and location of the lesion, but also by the skill of the interventionist and the availability of the particular modality. With growing experience, tracheobronchial stents have become an integral part of this therapeutic armamentarium.

A stent is a cylindrical structure placed endoluminally to provide artificial support and maintain patency of hollow tubular organs. Although its roots can be traced as far back as the late 19th century,[4] it is only recently that its use has been popularized. Stents are broadly classified as either tube stents or metallic stents[5-10] (Table 15–2). Synthetic coverings are often incorporated into the metallic stents to minimize their inherent drawbacks. The tube stents, in contrast, are by and large made of silicone. This chapter focuses on the design and use of both the silicone and the covered metallic stents.

■ Indications

Airway stents are advocated for the treatment of either focal narrowing, extrinsic compression, or diffuse involvement as seen with tracheobronchomalacia. The indications for stent placement are listed in Table 15–3. However, the use of a particular stent may differ somewhat based on its design and the nature of the obstruction. Specifically, because of the relative difficulty encountered in removing metallic stents, their use should be avoided in situations where the need for stent placement is short-lived. Furthermore, the expansile characteristics of some of the metallic stents precludes their use when the airway obstruction is due to extrinsic compression from a vascular aneurysm, because of the potential risk of perforation[55] (Fig. 15–1).

Insertion techniques for silicone and metallic stents are discussed elsewhere.[9,10,27]

Tube Stents

Silicone is a synthetic rubber made from silicone elastomeres that contains polymers with alternate silicon and oxygen. It was introduced in the 1940s. The modern-day silicone stents are derived from the Montgomery T-tube (Boston Medical Products, Inc., Waltham, MA), first described in 1965 and still enjoying substantial clinical use (Fig. 15–2). Designed for treatment of subglottic stenosis, it is introduced through a tracheostomy. The proximal limb of the T-tube lies above the tracheostomy within the subglottic stenosis and below the vocal cord. The distal limb lies below the tracheostomy and extends into the distal trachea, while

Stent-Grafts: Current Clinical Practice. Edited by Dolmatch and Blum. Thieme Medical Publishers, Inc., New York © 2000.

TABLE 15–1. Palliative Therapeutic Options in Major Airway Obstruction

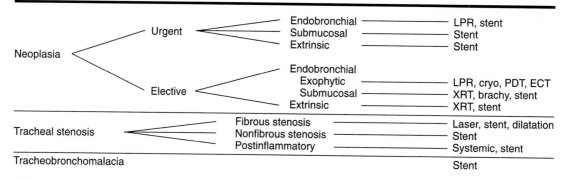

LPR, laser photoresection; PDT, photodynamic therapy; XRT, external beam radiation; brachy, brachytherapy; cryo; cryotherapy; ECT, electrocautery.

TABLE 15–2. Types of Stents

Synthetic tube stents[a]

Montgomery T-tube	Silicone; requires tracheostomy; simultaneous relief of obstruction at subglottic and distal trachea
Neville prosthesis	Silicone; frequent complications; hardly used
Westaby modification	Silicone, tube with distal bifurcation straddles carina; introduced by RB/laryngoscopy; Westaby-Shepard Y tube
Dumon	Silicone, external studs, Y tube newly added; most widely used stent
Hood	Silicone tube with flanges, smooth walled, can be cautomized to L or Y shape
Orlowski	Polyvinyl chloride (PVC) with metal armor inside, long stent with side branch for right main bronchi; requires a long stent despite a short area of stenosis
Nova	Thin silicone sheet rolled like a cigarette, metal armor (nitinol); expands to its original size after deployment
Freitag	Silicone with anterolateral wall metallic hoop reinforcement, Y shaped to prevent migration; difficult to introduce
Polyflex	Polyester filament mesh stent with silicone layer; prototype only

Metallic stents[b]

Palmaz	Stainless steel, balloon expandable; limited clinical experience mainly in children; lack of self-expansion may potentiate migration or obstruction
Strecker	Tantalum or nitinol, balloon expandable; limited clinical data; used in Europe; lack of self-expansion may potentiate migration or obstruction
Gianturco	Stainless steel, zigzag wire, self-expandable, single stent or double; most commonly used metallic stent world wide for variety of pathology; available in covered form
Wallstent	Cobalt based alloy, self-expandable; growing experience; available in covered form with silicone
Ultraflex	Nitinol (nickel-titanium alloy), self expandable, "shape memory" properties; only available in bare form commercially; limited published literature and follow-up data

[a]From refs. 5, 7–14, 17.

[b]From refs. 19–24, 38–40, 49, 55–61, 68–71.

RB, rigid bronchoscope.

TABLE 15–3. Indication for the Use of Tracheobronchial Stents

I. *Malignant neoplasm*
   a. Extrinsic compression or submucosal disease
      i. Prior to external beam or brachytherapy in acutely symptomatic patient
      ii. Residual obstruction immediately following LPR, PDT, cryotherapy, or electrocautery for endobronchial disease to maintain airway patency
      iii. Where all other palliative modalities have been exhausted
   b. Tracheobronchial esophageal fistula (TEF): in conjunction with esophageal stent[29–31]
II. *Benign disease*
   a. Posttraumatic (prolonged or traumatic intubation,[32] post-LPR or balloon bronchoplasty)
      i. Fibrotic scar
      ii. Bottleneck stricture
   b. Postinfectious
      i. Endobronchial tuberculosis[33–35]
      ii. Histoplasmosis-fibrosing mediastinitis
      iii. Herpes virus, diphtheria, pseudodiphthericum, *Klebsiella rhinoscleromatis*[36]
      iv. Opportunistic infection in immunocompromised host[5]
   c. Postinflammatory
      i. Wegener's granuloma[37]
      ii. Lye ingestion[19]
   d. Post–lung transplantation[24,38–42]
      i. Anastomotic stenosis
      ii. Tracheobronchomalacia
   e. Tracheobronchomalacia
      i. Focal—following tracheostomy, radiation therapy
      ii. Diffuse—idiopathic, relapsing polychondritis,[43,44] Mounier-Kuhn syndrome[45]
   f. Benign tumors
      i. Amyloidosis[46]
      ii. Papillomatosis[47]
   g. Congenital TEF
   h. Miscellaneous
      i. Kyphoscoliosis[48]
      ii. Extrinsic compression from aneurysm[19,49–51]
      iii. Extrinsic compression from achalasia and mega-esophagus[52]
III. *Following esophageal stent placement[31,53]*

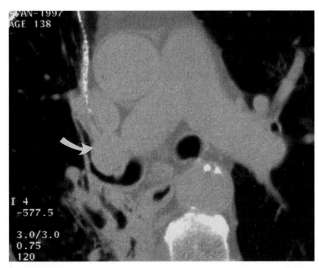

FIGURE 15–1. Poststenotic dilatation of the right pulmonary artery (RPA) producing extrinsic compression of the right main bronchus (RMB)—a contraindication for a self-expandable metallic stent.

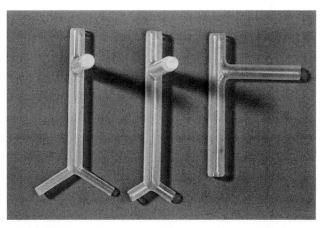

FIGURE 15–2. Montgomery T-tube and its modifications.

the side tube protrudes through the tracheostomy. Closure of the side tube prevents drying of the inspired air and helps to vocalize, whereas opening it permits cleaning and prevents the formation of inspissated mucus plugs.[11] A number of modifications ensued over the next few years. Neville et al[12] introduced a silicone stent that was sutured into place during open thoracotomy and tracheal reconstruction. Westaby et al[13] designed a T-tube in which the distal limb was elongated and bifurcated to saddle the carina. Cooper and colleagues[15] eliminated the side tube thus, converting it into a cylinder, which could be introduced through a laryngoscope or rigid bronchoscope.

Numerous experimentation with the original Montgomery T-tube ultimately led Dumon to introduce a new silicone cylindrical stent made of molded silicone (Fig. 15–3), with external studs being placed at regular intervals over its exterior (Dumon stent, Novatech, Aubagne, France, distributed by Bryan Corp., Woburn, MA).[14] The function of these studs is to improve stent-airway interface and thus prevent migration. Insertion of this stent usually requires the use of the rigid bronchoscope and special introducer system. Its advantage lies in the fact that it is easily inserted and removed. Moreover, unlike metallic stents, it can be easily grasped with a forceps and its position adjusted. However, there are certain limitations. The wall thickness of these stents creates a low internal to external diameter ratio such that the area of the available inner channel is reduced. Silicone stents are not quite pliable and are thus unable to adapt to any tortuous airways. They are also unsuitable for use in short and conical stenosis where there is a higher incidence of migration. The latter is also potentiated by inappropriate sizing and following radiation therapy, sometimes even requiring external fixation.[61,62] Other

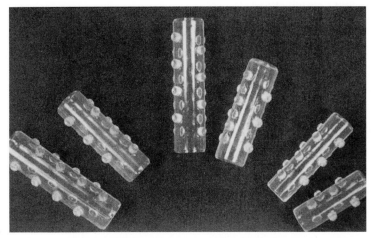

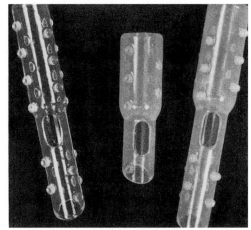

A   **B**

FIGURE 15–3. Dumon endobronchial stent (**A**) and its modified version for the right main stem bronchus (**B**). Note the side port, which is aligned with the right upper lobe bronchus. (Reprinted with permission from Dumon JF. A dedicated tracheobronchial stent. Chest 1990;97:328–332.)

potential serious complications include thick secretions and granuloma formation. Both endotracheal intubation (friction with endotracheal tube) and laser therapy (fire hazard)[63] requires the elective removal of the stent. Similar to our own experience with metallic Wallstents, the incidence of complications are much more pronounced in the subglottic region and when used for benign stenosis.[52,63] Despite this, the Dumon stent remains the most widely used stent worldwide and against which the performance of all other stents are measured (Table 15–4).[52,58,63–67] Dumon et al[52] published their experience with this prosthesis over a 7-year period involving 1,058 patients and 1,574 stents. Stents were placed for both malignant and benign lesions. The main complications reported were migration (9.5%), granuloma formation (7.9%), and obstruction by secretions (3.6%). Rare complications included ulceration of the tracheal or bronchial wall leading to hemorrhage, mediastinal perforation, esophagobronchial fistula, secondary tumor obstruction from growth both above and below the stent, infection, septic shock, and aphonia. Dumon et al also noted a higher complication rate with tracheal stenosis compared to malignant disease: 18.6% versus 6.0% for migration, 17.2% versus 1.4% for granuloma formation, and 5.7% versus 1.4% for obstruction.

Experimentation with incorporation of metals has led to the development of some hybrid stents. One such stent, designed by Freitag (Dynamic Stent, Rusch AG, Kernan, Germany), is a silicone Y stent with its anterior and lateral wall reinforced by steel struts.[16,68–71] The nonreinforced posterior thinner silicone membrane is collapsible and thus mimics the dynamics of a normal trachea. One of the Y limbs is cut short to accommodate the shorter right main stem bronchi and prevent obstruction of the upper lobe bronchus (Fig. 15–4). The stent is well tolerated and suitable for disease at the ca-

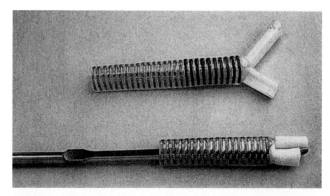

FIGURE 15–4. Dynamic Y stent designed by Freitag with its delivery device in place. (Reprinted with permission from Freitag L, Tekalf E, Stamatis G, Greschuchna D. Clinical evaluation of a new bifurcated dynamic airway stent: a 5 year experience with 135 patients. Thorac Cardiovasc Surg 1997;45: 6–12.)

rina, but it is available in only three sizes. Although the stent's design avoids secretion accumulation and facilitates expectoration, several cases of stent migration have occurred. Another such stent is the Nova stent (Novadis, Saint-Victoret, France), which is made up of a thin silicone sheet containing small nitinol hoops (Fig. 15–5). The stent is inserted, rolled up like a cigarette, and the metal hoops help expansion to the preset diameter. Silicone bands at either end prevent migration. There are no published data at this time, but this stent is currently being tested in patients with malignancy in Europe.[10]

Two other stents warrant special mention. The first one was described by Noppen and colleagues in 1996 (Reynder's Stent, Reynder's Medical Supply, Lennik, Belgium). This stent is a Tygon synthetic cylindrical tube (Fig. 15–6) that is thermatically molded to a screw-thread prosthesis, imparting a rigidity that is far more evident

TABLE 15–4. Wallstent Experience: Demographics and Complications

	Brichon[26] 1992	Rousseau[28] 1993	Carre[25] 1994	Tan[32] 1996	Bolliger[30] 1996*	Monnier[31] 1996*	Wang[33] 1997	Dasgupta[†] 1998
No. of patients	11	36	8	7	27	40	11	45
No. of stents	15	39	9	9	36	50	15	64
Etiology	Ltx	MP	Ltx	Ca	Ca	Ca	Ca	MP
Deployment	F 11	F 39	F 8	R 9	F 23/R4	R 40	F 11	F 45
Complications								
Retained secretions	0	0	0	0	5	15	2	0
Granuloma form[n]	2	0	1	0	4	4	1	6
Migration	0	0	0	0	6	5	1	0
Inappropriate length (laser, no.)	1 (la,1)	1 (la,1)	2 (la,2)	6	NR	3	6 (la,3)	8 (la,3)
Mean follow-up (mos.)	8	10	15	5	2	3	2–10	11

*Series with covered Wallstents.

[†]Includes 51 stents reported earlier, ref. 27.

Ltx, lung transplantation; MP, mixed pathology; Ca, carcinoma; F, flexible bronchoscope; R, rigid bronchoscope; la, laser ablation of stent filaments; NR, not reported.

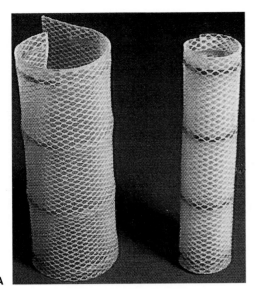
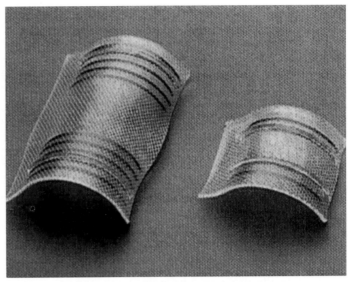

FIGURE 15–5. Nova stent coiled (**A**) and uncoiled (**B**) version. (Reprinted with permission from Bolliger CT, Mathur PN. Expandable airway stents. In: Beamis JF, Mathur PN, eds. Interventional Pulmonology. New York: McGraw-Hill, 1999:113–127.)

than with the silicone stent. This stent combines the advantage of both the silicone stent and the metallic stents in providing better anchorage to the tracheobronchial tree. Although tested in only 10 patients with both malignant and benign disease in the trachea, it has shown no migration over a 4- to 18-month follow-up.[72] In a later article by the same authors, the use of the screw-thread device was compared to the conventional Dumon stent in 46 patients (23 with benign disease, 23 with malignant) with comparable obstructive characteristics. No significant difference in efficacy was noted. Stent migration was more common with the Dumon stent but did not reach statistical significance. However, significant difference in

the incidence of migration was observed between benign and malignant stenosis and within the subgroup of benign stenosis between Dumon stent and the screw-thread device. The latter shares the same characteristics of easy insertion and removal as the Dumon silicon stent but is only one-third of the cost of the Dumon and does not require special insertion equipment.[73]

The wall thickness of the original silicon stents prompted use of other synthetic material for stent manufacture. The Polyflex stent (Willy Rusch AG, Kernen, Germany) is a synthetic self-expandable stent made of polyester wire mesh (Trevira) impregnated with a thin layer of silicone (Fig. 15–7). In a mini-pig model of

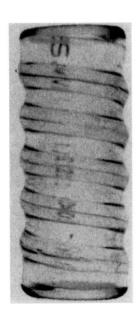

FIGURE 15–6. Reynder's stent. (Reprinted with permission from Noppen M, Maysman M, Ingeborg C, D'Haese J, Vincken W. Screw thread versus Dumon endoprosthesis in the management of tracheal stenosis. Chest 1999;115:532–535.)

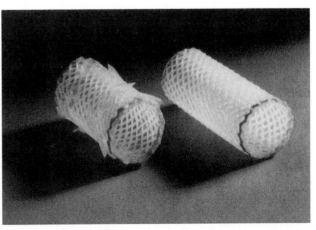

FIGURE 15–7. Polyflex stent with and without external studs. (Reprinted with permission from Bolliger CT, Wyser C, Wu X, et al. Evaluation of a new self-expandable silicone stent in an experimental tracheal stenosis. Chest 1999;115: 496–501.)

fibromalacic tracheal stenosis, both smooth-walled stents and stents with external silicone studs were deployed. Granuloma formation occurred at the ends of both stents as well as of the control Dumon stents. However, significant migration was seen only in the cases of smooth Polyflex stents and the Dumon stents, making the addition of external spikes more conducive to stent retainment.[74] Wasserman et al[17] reported initial results of the use of Polyflex stents in 19 patients (17 with malignancy) with 33 stent placements. Although major granulation tissue formation was not reported, bronchoscopic evidence of a glue-like sticky mucus was observed early in the postoperative course with frequent and repetitive isolation of *Staphylococcus aureus, Pseudomonas aeruginosa,* and *Escherichia coli.* Electron microscopy did not reveal any bio-degeneration of the synthetic material and it was assumed that the bacteria have a propensity to adhere to the preformed irregular landscape of the stent. In two patients the inner silicone of the prosthesis became detached from the filament meshwork and had to be replaced. Similar to the pig model of tracheal stenosis, both patients with benign stenosis experienced stent migration, which raised the question of whether the stent is suitable in benign diseases. Unlike the silicone-based stents, these stents readily adapt to uneven bronchial contours such as conical and step-shaped strictures and are likely to be useful in complex obstructions without an excessive decrease in luminal availability or increased risks of dislodgment.

Metal Stents

Experimentation by a number of investigators with different metals and alloys have ultimately identified certain metals that are inherently inert, noncorrosive, and eminently acceptable without significant tissue reaction. These include stainless steel, nickel titanium, and several alloys incorporating cobalt, chromium, and molybdenum (Vitallium, Nobillium). Experience with animal models and anecdotal reports on patients has paved the way for today's metallic stents.[75,76] Harkin[77] used a stent made from Nobillium and reported complications related to inspissated mucus and swelling or edema, both above and below the tube. Belsey[78] and Bucher and colleagues[79] used stainless steel wire mesh in tracheal reconstruction in two patients, each achieving good functional results. The clinical application of tube stents and the realization that metal mesh stents in the esophageal, biliary, and vascular tree, have ultimately led to the development of the metallic tracheobronchial stents.[80,81]

Metallic stents are by and large easy to insert, can be deployed endoscopically or fluoroscopically using either rigid or fiberoptic bronchoscope, and are radiopaque. They are classified as fixed diameter, requiring balloon dilatation, or as self-expandable, which spring back to

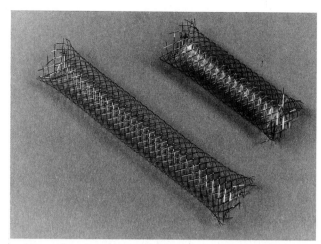

FIGURE 15–8. Uncovered (left) and silicone covered (right) Wallstent (U.S. version).

their preset diameter when released. The stents are available in their bare metallic form or coated with synthetic material such as silicone, nylon, or polyurethane. The nature and extent of these coverings varies among the manufacturers (Figs. 15–8 and 15–9). Tissue overgrowth (granulomas or tumor) may occur through the bare stents, which can be minimized by the addition of synthetic coverings, although they could and do tend to occur at the edges. We had a patient who developed granuloma through the coverings of a Wallstent (Fig. 15–10). Granulomas or tumor overgrowth can be dealt with by cryotherapy, electrocautery, or laser photoresection, but the latter could present a fire hazard with the covered stents.[82] If the covered stent is placed across a

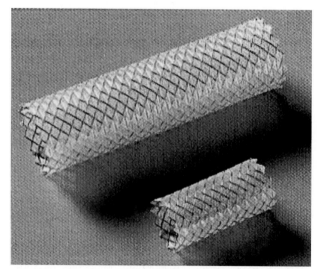

FIGURE 15–9. Covered Wallstent (European version). (Reprinted with permission from Bolliger CT, Mathur PN. Expandable airway stents. In Beamis JF, Mathur PN, eds. Interventional Pulmonology. New York: McGraw-Hill, 1999;113–127.)

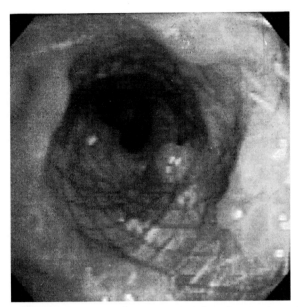

FIGURE 15–10. Covered Wallstent in left main stem bronchi. Note granulation tissue protruding through the cracks in the silicon coating.

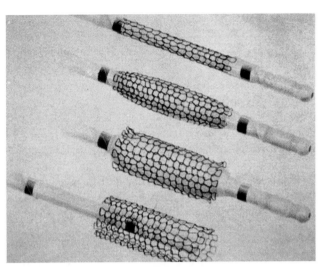

FIGURE 15–12. Strecker stent in different stages of deployment as shown from top to bottom. (Reprinted with permission from Bolliger CT, Mathur PN. Expandable airway stents. In: Beamis JF, Mathur PN, eds. Interventional Pulmonology. New York: McGraw-Hill, 1999:113–127.)

lobar orifice, unlike the bare stent it can obstruct the ventilation and cause collapse.

The balloon expandable stents are either the Palmaz stent (Johnson and Johnson Interventional Systems Co., Warren, NJ; Fig. 15–11) or the Strecker stent (Boston Scientific Vascular, Natick, MA; Fig. 15–12). The Palmaz stent exhibits plastic rather than elastic behavior and, as such, once it is deformed is unable to regain its original contours, producing significant obstruction. Thus, it is probably unsuitable for use in the tracheobronchial tree. The majority of the experience with these stents is in children, although some experience in adults has been reported.[18,19,55] The Strecker stent, in contrast, consists of a flexible, knitted tantalum wire mesh that cannot be expanded beyond its predetermined size and thus has no potential for airway perforation. It does get

occluded because of the general problems associated with the metallic stent.[20] None of these stents are available in the covered form.

The Gianturco stent (Cook, Inc., Bloomington, IN) is a self-expandable stent and has had widespread use in Europe (Fig. 15–13). There have been significant complications reported with its use including dislodgment and unraveling with the use of suction catheters, migration, tracheopharyngeal fistulas, strut fractures, mucosal ischemia at pressure points, and perforation and fatal erosion of the pulmonary artery. Although stent coverings with nylon, polyvinylchloride, and Dacron have been used, covered Gianturco stents are not available commercially.[22,23,82–89]

The maximal experience with the covered metallic stents has been seen with the use of the metallic Wallstents

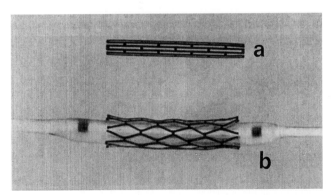

FIGURE 15–11. Palmaz stent (**a**) and its delivery system (**b**). (Reprinted with permission from Nesbitt JC, Carrasco H. Expandable stents. Chest Surg Clin North Am 1996;6:305–328.)

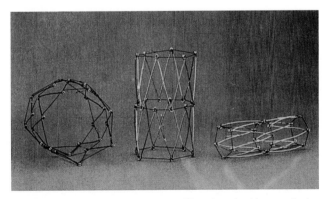

FIGURE 15–13. Gianturco stent. (Reprinted with permission from Nesbitt JC, Carrasco H. Expandable stents. Chest Surg Clin North Am 1996;6:305–328.)

(Boston Scientific Vascular, Natick, MA).[24-33] The European version (Airway stent) is covered in its entirety on the outside by polyurethane coating, whereas the U.S. counterpart has a silicone coating only in the body of the stent, leaving the uncovered metallic ends free to embed in the mucosa. We have inserted a total of 64 stents (covered as well as uncovered) in 45 patients with a mean follow-up of 11 months. Availability of these stents in a fixed length for any given diameter has created technical problems with appropriate sizing such that they may project well beyond the confines of the stenosis and cover lobar orifices. Under such circumstances controlled destruction of some of the covering filaments by laser would eliminate the problem without causing significant structural damage to the stent.[90] Apart from granuloma formation in six patients, retained secretions or migration was not encountered. In contrast, there was an increased incidence of both retained secretions and migration in both the studies by Bolliger et al,[30] and the multicenter study reported by Monnier et al[31] selectively employing the covered Airway stent (Table 15–5). It is tempting to speculate that design variation between the European (no free metallic ends) and the U.S. Wallstent may have potentiated migration in these patients. The flexibility of the Wallstent also makes it the only covered stent that can be inserted in a conical stenosis.[91]

Another exciting stent made of nitinol (Ultraflex, Boston Scientific, NatiZazzSSSSSSSSSSzxck, MA) is currently available (Fig. 15–14). It is made of nickel-tantalum alloy and exhibits shape memory characteristics such that it deforms plastically at low temperatures (martensitic effect) and regains its own shape at higher

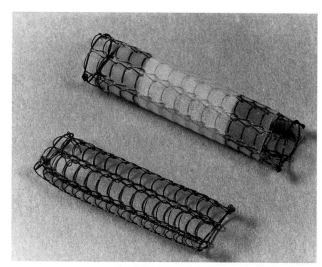

FIGURE 15–14. Covered and uncovered Ultraflex stent.

temperatures (austenitic state) in the body. Although both bare and coated version are available for the tracheobronchial tree, published expertise is still scant and longer-term data is still awaited.[34-36]

■ Conclusion

The cumulative experience with a variety of stents by numerous investigators has demonstrated significant palliation in malignant diseases and midterm to long-term subjective as well as objective benefits in benign stenosis. Whether silicone or metallic stents should be used is a

TABLE 15–5. Experience with Silicone Tracheobronchial Stents (Selected Large Series)

Author	No. of Patients	Outcome
Colt et al[64] (1993)	206	Complications usually minor (migration 15%, granulation 20%, obstruction by secretion or tumor 3%); follow-up up to 3 years
Bolliger et al[63] (1993)	31	90% had lasting improvement; complications in 26%; migration in 13%; fire hazard in one patient; median survival 2.5 months in patients with malignancy
Diaz-Jimenez et al[65] (1994)	90	Stent could not be placed in 5 patients (severe extrinsic compression); migration (13%), granuloma (9%), hypersecretion (2%); higher rate of complications in benign disease
Strausz et al[66] (1994)	38	Deployed with FB; mixed malignant (17 patients) and benign (21 patients); migration in 32%; follow-up to 5 months
Sonett et al[67] (1995)	57	Stent adjustment frequently required; all patients had symptomatic relief; median survival in cancer 3 to 10 months; migration most frequent in transplant patients
Martinez-Ballarin et al[58] (1996)	63	Migration 18%, granuloma 6%, obstruction 6%; follow-up to 18 months
Dumon et al[52] (1996)	1,058	Multicenter study, 7-year experience; migration 10%, secretion 4%, granulation 8%; mean duration (benign disease) 14 months, (malignancy) 4 months; higher rate of complications in benign disease

Adapted from ref. 9, with permission.
FB, flexible bronchoscope.

matter of some debate and is often dictated by individual preferences. Silicone stents have the clear advantage of easy removal, whereas metallic stents eventually get epithelialized and then removal is extremely difficult.[92] Thus, the selection of a specific stent is very important. In situations where there is underlying inflammation, as occurs after radiation or lung transplantation, sequential stenting initially with a silicone stent followed by a metallic stent is advocated.[93] Both stents are generally well tolerated, although migration is enhanced with the silicone stents. It is believed that in the future some form of covered stent that combines the best attributes of silicone and metal stents will be used. Increasing interest is expected in other synthetic stents (e.g., Polyflex stent, Reynder's stent) and in the covered variety of the nitinol stent. The use of stents in the relief of short-term obstruction has prompted the development of bioabsorbable stents that are now being tested in animal models.[94–96] Radiation-emitting stents as well as stents impregnated with chemotherapeutic agents on a bioabsorbable material, when developed, may offer significant advancement in the palliative management of obstructive diseases. Extensive work in animal models to develop an ideal stent as well as recent data from clinical studies from a variety of stents are being awaited. Until then the silicone stent and the covered Wallstent will probably continue to hold sway.

REFERENCES

1. Petrou M, Goldstraw P. The management of tracheobronchial obstruction: a review of endoscopic techniques. Eur J Cardiothorac Surg 1994;8:436–441.
2. Dweik RA, Mehta AC. Bronchoscopic management of malignant airway disease. Clin Pulmon Med 1996;3:43–51.
3. Cavaliere S, Venuta F, Foccoli P, et al. Endoscopic treatment of malignant airway obstruction in 2008 patients. Chest 1996;110:1536–1542.
4. Bond CJ. Note on the treatment of tracheal stenosis by a new T-shaped tracheotomy tube. Lancet 1891;1:539.
5. Colt HG, Dumon JF. Airway stents: present and future. Clin Chest Med 1995;16:465–478.
6. Nesbitt JC, Carrasco H. Expandable stents. Chest Surg Clin North Am 1996;6:305–328.
7. Becker HD. Stenting of the central airways. J Bronchol 1995;2:98–106.
8. Bolliger CT. Airway stents. Semin Respir Crit Care Med 1997;18:563–570.
9. Colt H. Silicone airway stents. In: Beamis JF, Mathur PN, eds. Interventional Bronchology. New York: McGraw-Hill, 1999:97–112.
10. Bolliger CT, Mathur PN. Expandable endobronchial stents. In: Beamis JF, Mathur PN, eds. Interventional Pulmonology. New York: McGraw-Hill, 1999:113–127.
11. Montgomery WW. T-tube tracheal stent. Arch Otolaryngol 1965; 82:320–321.
12. Neville WE, Hamouda F, Anderson J et al. Replacement of the intrathoracic trachea and both stem bronchi with a molded Silastic prosthesis. J Thorac Cardiovasc Surg 1972;63:569–576.
13. Westaby S, Jackson JW, Pearson FG. A bifurcated silicone rubber stent for relief of tracheobronchial obstruction. J Thorac Cardiovasc Surg 1982;83:414–417.
14. Dumon JF. A dedicated tracheobronchial stent. Chest 1990; 97:328–332.
15. Cooper JD, Pearson FG, Patterson GA, et al. Use of silicone stents in the management of airway problems. Ann Thorac Surg 1989;47:371–378.
16. Freitag L, Tekolf E, Stamatis G, Greschuchna D. Clinical evaluation of a new bifurcated dynamic airway stent: a 5-year experience with 135 patients. Thorac Cardiovasc Surg 1997;45:6–12.
17. Wasserman K, Koch A, Muller-Ehmsen J, et al. Clinical and laboratory evaluation of a new thin-walled self-expanding tracheobronchial silicone stent: progress and pitfalls. J Thorac Cardiovasc Surg 1997;114:527–534.
18. Filler FM, Forte V, Chait P. Tracheobronchial stenting for the treatment of airway obstruction. J Pediatr Surg 1998;33:304–311.
19. Slonim SM, Razavi M, Kee S, et al. Transbronchial Palmaz stent placement for tracheobronchial stenosis. J Vasc Intervent Radiol 1998;9:153–160.
20. Hauck RW, Lembeck RM, Emslander HP, et al. Implantation of Accuflex and Strecker stents in malignant bronchial stenosis by flexible bronchoscopy. Chest 1997;112:134–144.
21. Susanto I, Peters JI, Levine SM, et al. Use of balloon expandable metallic stents in the management of bronchial stenosis and bronchomalacia after lung transplantation. Chest 1998;114:1330–1335.
22. Kishi K, Kobayashi H, Suruda T, et al. Treatment of malignant tracheobronchial stenosis by Dacron covered Z-stents. Cardiovasc Intervent Radiol 1994;17:33–35.
23. George PJM, Irving JD, Mantell BS, Rudd RM. Covered expandable metal stent for recurrent tracheal obstruction. Lancet 1990; 335:582–584.
24. Carre P, Rousseau H, Lombart L, et al, and the Toulouse Lung Transplantation Group. Balloon dilatation and self-expanding metal Wallstent insertion for management of bronchostenosis following lung transplantation. Chest 1994;105:343–348.
25. Carre P, Rousseau H, Dahan M, et al. Therapeutic management of posttransplant bronchial stenosis by balloon dilatation and self-expandable metallic Wallstent insertion. Transplant Proc 1994;26:253.
26. Brichon PY, Blanc-Jouvan F, Rousseau H, et al. Endovascular stents for bronchial stenosis after lung transplantation. Transplant Proc 1992;24:2656–2659.
27. Dasgupta A, Dolmatch BL, Abi-Saleh WJ, et al. Self-expandable metallic airway stent insertion employing flexible bronchoscopy: preliminary results. Chest 1998;114:106–109.
28. Rousseau H, Dahan M, Lauque D, et al. Self-expandable prosthesis in the tracheobronchial tree. Radiology 1993;188:199–203.
29. Spinelli P, Meroni E, Cerrai FG. Self-expanding tracheobronchial stents using flexible bronchoscopy. Preliminary clinical experience. Surg Endosc 1994;8:411–413.
30. Bolliger CT, Heitz M, Hauser R, et al. An airway Wallstent for the treatment of tracheobronchial malignancies. Thorax 1996;51:1127–1129.
31. Monnier P, Mudry A, Stanzel F, et al. The use of the covered Wallstent for the palliative treatment of inoperable tracheobronchial cancers. Chest 1996;110:1161–1168.
32. Tan BS, Watkinson AF, Dussek JE, et al. Metallic endoprostheses for malignant tracheobronchial obstruction: initial experience. Cardiovasc Intervent Radiol 1996;19:91–96.
33. Wang KP. Preliminary experiences of self-expandable wire stent or "Wallstent" for bronchial obstruction. J Bronchol 1997;4:120–124.
34. Vinnograd I, Klin B, Brosh T, et al. A new intratracheal stent made from nitinol, an alloy with "shape memory effect." J Thorac Cardiovasc Surg 1994;107:1255–1266.
35. Yanagihara K, Mizuno H, Wada H, et al. Tracheal stenosis treated with self-expanding nitinol stent. Ann Thorac Surg 1997;63:1786–1790.
36. Yang L, Yue S, Naikang Z, Xiaomai H. Nitinol alloy endotracheal stent for treatment of tracheal stenosis. Chin Med J 1997;110:540–542.

37. Freitag L, Tekolf E, Steveling H, et al. Management of malignant esophagotracheal fistulas with airway stenting and double stenting. Chest 1996;110:1155–1160.

38. Colt HG, Meric B, Dumon JF. Double stents for carcinoma of the esophagus invading the tracheobronchial tree. Gastrointest Endosc 1992;38:485–489.

39. Nicholson DA. Tracheal and esophageal stenting for carcinoma of the upper esophagus invading the tracheo-bronchial tree. Clin Radiol 1998;53:760–763.

40. Strausz J. Management of postintubation tracheal stenosis with stent implantation. J Bronchol 1997;4:294–296.

41. Han JK, Im JG, Park JG, et al. Bronchial stenosis due to endobronchial tuberculosis: successful treatment with self-expanding metallic stent. Am J Roent 1992;159:971–972.

42. Sawada S, Fujiwara Y, Furui S, et al. Treatment of tuberculous bronchial stenosis with expandable metallic stents. Acta Radiol 1993;34:263–265.

43. Gebauer PW. Plastic reconstruction of tuberculous bronchostenosis with dermal grafts. J Thorac Surg 1950;19:604–628.

44. Colt HG, Gumpert BC, Harrell JH. Tracheobronchial obstruction caused by *Klebsiella rhinoscleromatis*: diagnosis, pathologic features, and treatment. J Bronchol 1994;1:31–36.

45. Daum TE, Specks U, Colby TV, et al. Tracheobronchial involvement in Wegener's granulomatosis. Am J Respir Crit Care Med 1995;15:522–526.

46. Novick RJ, Ahmad D, Menkis AH, et al. The importance of acquired diffuse bronchomalacia in heart-lung transplant recipients with obliterative bronchiolitis. J Thorac Cardiovasc Surg 1991;101:643–648.

47. Schafers HJ, Haydock DA, Cooper JD. The prevalence and management of bronchial anastomotic complications in lung transplantation. J Thorac Cardiovasc Surg 1991;101:1044–1052.

48. Dunne JA, Sabanathan S. Use of metallic stents in relapsing polychondritis. Chest 1994;105:864–867.

49. Sacco O, Fregonese B, Oddone M, et al. Severe endobronchial obstruction in a grid with relapsing polychondritis: treatment with Nd-YAG laser and endobronchial silicon stent. Eur Respir J 1997;10:494–496.

50. Goldstein LS, Walsh JJ, Mehta AC. Mounier-Kuhn syndrome. Bronchoscopic image. J Bronchol 1997;4:148–149.

51. Tsang V, Goldstraw P. Self-expanding metal stent for tracheobronchial strictures. Eur J Cardiothorac Surg 1992;6:555–559.

52. Dumon JF, Cavaliere S, Diaz-Jimenez JP, et al. Seven-year experience with the Dumon prosthesis. J Bronchol 1996;31:6–10.

53. Fisseler-Eckhoff A, Hofken G, Gillisen A, et al. Laryngotracheal papillomatosis due to HPV infection or stent therapy? In situ hybridization of papillomavirus DNA and immunohistochemical detection of Ki67 antigen. J Bronchol 1997;4:32–38.

54. Al-Kattan K, Simonds A, Chung KF, et al. Kyphoscoliosis and bronchial torsion. Chest 1997;111:1134–1137.

55. Cook CH, Bhattacharya N, King DR. Aortobronchial fistula after expandable metal stent insertion for pediatric bronchomalacia. J Pediatr Surg 1998;33:1306–1308.

56. Subramanian V, Anstead M, Cottrill CM, et al. Tetralogy of Fallot with absent pulmonary valve and bronchial compression: treatment with endobronchial stents. Pediatr Cardiol 1997;18:237–239.

57. Ewart R, Mutze S, Meyer R, et al. Stent implantation in severe tracheal and bronchial compression caused by aortic aneurysm (German). Pneumologie 1997;51:19–23.

58. Martinez-Ballarin JI, Diaz-Jimenez JP, Castro M, Moya JA. Silicone stents in the management of benign tracheobronchial stenosis. Chest 1996;109:626–629.

59. Berrisford RG, Oo A, Walshaw MJ, et al. Tracheal obstruction in achalasia: a role for airway stenting? Ann Thorac Surg 1998;66:939–941.

60. Dasgupta A, Jain P, Sandur S, et al. Airway complications of esophageal stent placement. Gastrointest Endosc 1998;47:532–535.

61. Colt HG, Harrel J, Neumann TR, et al. External fixation of tracheal stents. Chest 1994;105:1653–1657.

62. Temes RT, Weruly JA, Cooper JD, et al. Internal fixation of high tracheal stents. Ann Thorac Surg 1995;59:1023–1024.

63. Bolliger CT, Probst R, Tschopp K, Soler M, Perruchoud AP. Silicone stents in the management of inoperable tracheobronchial stenosis: indications and limitations. Chest 1993;104:1653–1659.

64. Colt HG, Dumon JF. Tracheobronchial stents: indications and applications. Lung Cancer 1993;9:301–306.

65. Diaz-Jimenez JP, Munoz EF, Martinez-Ballarin JI, Kovitz KL, Presas FM. Silicone stents in the management of obstructive tracheobronchial lesions: a 2 year experience. J Bronchiol 1994;1:15–18.

66. Strausz J, Kis S, Papai Z, Szima B, Juhasz J, Bolcskei P. Tracheobronchial silicone stent implantation with the flexible bronchoscope. J Bronchol 1994;1:123–125.

67. Sonett JR, Keenan RJ, Ferson PF, Griffith BP, Landreneau RJ. Endobronchial management of benign, malignant, and lung transplantation airway stenosis. Ann Thorac Surg 1995;59:1417–1422.

68. Freitag L, Eicker R, Linz B, et al. Theoretical and experimental basis for the development of a dynamic airway stent. Eur Respir J 1994;7:2038–2045.

69. Freitag L, Eicker K, Donovan TJ, Dimov D. Mechanical properties of airway stents. J Bronchol 1995;2:270–278.

70. Freitag L, Tekolf E, Bortel J, et al. Bifurcated dynamic airway stent insertion using flexible bronchoscopy. J Bronchol 1995;2:130–134.

71. Wassermann K, Eckel HE, Michel O, Muller RP. Emergency stenting of malignant obstruction of the upper airways: long term follow-up with two types of silicone prosthesis. J Thorac Cardiovasc Surg 1996;112:859–866.

72. Noppen M, Dhaese J, Meysman M, et al. A new screw-thread tracheal endoprosthesis. J Bronchol 1996;3:22–26.

73. Noppen M, Meysman M, Ingeborg C, D'Haese J, Vincken W. Screw-thread versus Dumon endoprosthesis in the management of tracheal stenosis. Chest 1999;115:532–535.

74. Bolliger CT, Wyser C, Wu X, et al. Evaluation of a new self-expandable silicone stent in an experimental tracheal stenosis. Chest 1999;115:496–501.

75. Pearse HE. Results from using Vitallium tubes in biliary surgery. Ann Surg 1946;124:1020–1029.

76. Daniel RA Jr. The regeneration of defects of the trachea and bronchi. J Thorac Surg 1948;17:335–349.

77. Harkin WB. An endotracheal metallic prosthesis in the treatment of stenosis of the upper trachea. Ann Otology Rhinol Laryngol 1952;61:932–935.

78. Belsey R. Resection and reconstruction of the intrathoracic trachea. Br J Surg 1951;51:200.

79. Bucher RM, Busenette WE, Rosemond GE. Experimental reconstruction of tracheal and bronchial defects with stainless steel wire mesh. J Thorac Surg 1951;21:572.

80. Moores DWO, Ilves R. Treatment of esophageal obstruction with covered self-expanding esophageal Wallstents. Ann Thorac Surg 1996;62:963–967.

81. Murphy TP, Webb MS, Lambiase RE, et al. Percutaneous revascularisation of complex iliac artery stenosis and occlusions with use of Wallstents: three-year experience. J Vasc Intervent Radiol 1996;7:21–27.

82. Witt C, Zietz G, Petri F, Ewert R, Baumann G. Flexible bronchoscopic stenting followed by radiation in malignant obstruction of central airways. J Bronchol 1995;2:118–122.

83. Witt C, Dinges S, Schmidt B, Ewert R, Budach V, Baumann G. Temporary tracheobronchial stenting in malignant stenosis. Eur J Cancer 1997;33:204–208.

84. Wilson GE, Walshaw MJ, Hind CRK. Treatment of large airway obstruction in lung cancer using expandable metal stents inserted under direct vision via the fiberoptic bronchoscope. Thorax 1996;51:248–252.

85. Nashef SAM, Dromer C, Velly FJ, et al. Expanding wire stents in benign tracheobronchial disease: indications and complications. Ann Thorac Surg 1992;54:937–940.

86. Carrasco CH, Nesbitt JC, Charnsangavej C, et al. Management of tracheal and bronchial stenosis with the Gianturco stent. Ann Thorac Surg 1994;58:1012–1017.

87. Coolen D, Slabbynck H, Galdermans D, et al. Insertion of a self-expandable endotracheal metal stent using topical anesthesia and a fiberoptic bronchoscope: a comfortable way to offer palliation. Thorax 1994;49:87–88.

88. Spinelli P, Cerrai FG, Spinelli A. Palliation of tracheobronchial malignant obstruction with metal stents in emergency conditions. Minerva Chir 1998;53:373–376.

89. Bolot G, Poupart M, Pignat JC, et al. Self-expanding metal stents for the management of bronchial stenosis and bronchomalacia after lung transplantation. Laryngoscope 1998;108:1230–1233.

90. Witt C, Schmidt B, Liebetruth J, et al. Nd:YAG laser and tracheobronchial metallic stents: an experimental in vitro study. Lasers Surg Med 1997;20:51–55.

91. Bolliger CT, Arnoux A, Oeggerli M, Lukic G, Perruchoud AP. Covered Wallstent insertion in a patient with conical tracheobronchial stenosis. J Bronchol 1995;2:215–218.

92. Wallace MJ, Charnsangavej C, Ogawa K, et al. Tracheobronchial tree: expandable metallic stents used in experimental and clinical applications: work in progress. Radiology 1986;158:309–312.

93. Tsang V, Williams AM, Goldstraw P. Sequential Silastic and expandable metal stenting for tracheobronchial strictures. Ann Thorac Surg 1992;53:856–860.

94. Korpela A, Aarnio P, Sariola H, et al. Bioabsorbable bronchial stents in an animal model. J Bronchol 1998;5:9–12.

95. Korpela A, Aarnio P, Sariola H, Tormala P, Harjula A. Comparison of tissue reactions in the tracheal mucosa surrounding a bioabsorbable and silicone airway stents. Ann Thorac Surg 1998;66:1772–1776.

96. Korpela A, Aarnio P, Sariola H, Tormala P, Harjula A. Bioabsorbable self-reinforced poly-L-lactide, metallic and silicone stents in the management of experimental tracheal stenosis. Chest 1999;115:490–495.

Index

Page numbers followed by "f" indicate figures; page numbers followed by "t" indicate tables.

3